Online Resources & Audiobook

Included with your purchase are multiple online resources. This includes the practice tests in an interactive format and this book in audiobook format. There is also a convenient study timer to help you manage your time.

Instructions for accessing these resources can be found on the last page of this book.

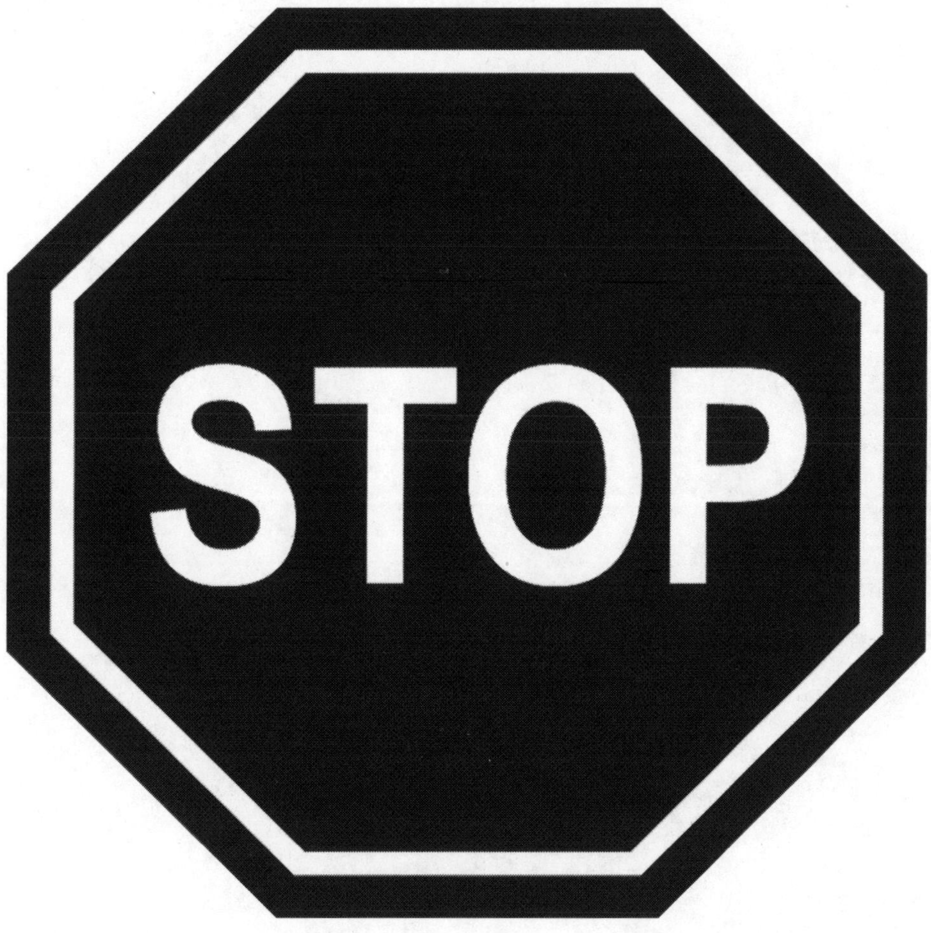

ATI TEAS® 7th Edition 2026-2027 Exam Prep

11 Practice Tests and TEAS 7 Study Guide Book [Includes Detailed Answer Explanations]

Lydia Morrison

Written and edited by TPB Publishing.

ISBN 13: 9781637756409

Table of Contents

***Welcome* ... 1**

***Quick Overview* ... 2**

***Test-Taking Strategies* ... 3**

***Introduction for the TEAS 7* ... 7**

***Study Prep Plan for the ATI TEAS 7 Exam* ... 10**

***Reading* ... 15**

Key Ideas and Details ... 15

Craft and Structure ... 22

Integration of Knowledge and Ideas ... 28

Reading Practice Quiz ... 36

Answer Explanations ... 38

***Mathematics* ... 39**

Numbers and Algebra ... 39

Measurement and Data ... 72

Mathematics Practice Quiz ... 93

Answer Explanations ... 95

***Science* ... 96**

Human Anatomy and Physiology ... 96

Biology ... 131

Chemistry ... 162

Scientific Reasoning ... 182

Science Practice Quiz ... 188

Answer Explanations ... 189

English and Language Usage ***190***

Conventions of Standard English 190

Knowledge of Language 207

Expressing Ideas in Writing 213

English & Language Usage Practice Quiz 218

Answer Explanations 219

TEAS 7 Practice Test #1 .... ***220***

Reading 220

Mathematics 237

Science 244

English and Language Usage 253

Answer Explanations #1 .... ***260***

Reading 260

Mathematics 265

Science 272

English and Language Usage 279

TEAS 7 Practice Test #2 .... ***284***

Reading 284

Mathematics 299

Science 307

English and Language Usage 315

Answer Explanations #2 .... ***323***

Reading 323

Mathematics 327

Science 332

English and Language Usage 339

Practice Tests #3–#11 .... ***344***

Index ***345***

Online Resources & Audiobook ***351***

Welcome

Dear Reader,

Welcome to your new Test Prep Books study guide! We are pleased that you chose us to help you prepare for your exam. There are many study options to choose from, and we appreciate you choosing us. Studying can be a daunting task, but we have designed a smart, effective study guide to help prepare you for what lies ahead.

Whether you're a parent helping your child learn and grow, a high school student working hard to get into your dream college, or a nursing student studying for a complex exam, we want to help give you the tools you need to succeed. We hope this study guide gives you the skills and the confidence to thrive, and we can't thank you enough for allowing us to be part of your journey.

In an effort to continue to improve our products, we welcome feedback from our customers. We look forward to hearing from you. Suggestions, success stories, and criticisms can all be communicated by emailing us at support@testprepbooks.com.

Sincerely,

Test Prep Books Team

Quick Overview

As you draw closer to taking your exam, effective preparation becomes more and more important. Thankfully, you have this study guide to help you get ready. Use this guide to help keep your studying on track and refer to it often.

This study guide contains several key sections that will help you be successful on your exam. The guide contains tips for what you should do the night before and the day of the test. Also included are test-taking tips. Knowing the right information is not always enough. Many well-prepared test takers struggle with exams. These tips will help equip you to accurately read, assess, and answer test questions.

A large part of the guide is devoted to showing you what content to expect on the exam and to helping you better understand that content. In this guide are practice test questions so that you can see how well you have grasped the content. Then, answer explanations are provided so that you can understand why you missed certain questions.

Don't try to cram the night before you take your exam. This is not a wise strategy for a few reasons. First, your retention of the information will be low. Your time would be better used by reviewing information you already know rather than trying to learn a lot of new information. Second, you will likely become stressed as you try to gain a large amount of knowledge in a short amount of time. Third, you will be depriving yourself of sleep. So be sure to go to bed at a reasonable time the night before. Being well-rested helps you focus and remain calm.

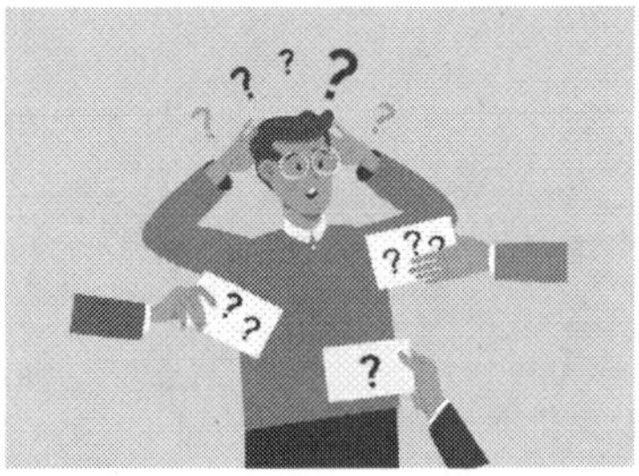

Be sure to eat a substantial breakfast the morning of the exam. If you are taking the exam in the afternoon, be sure to have a good lunch as well. Being hungry is distracting and can make it difficult to focus. You have hopefully spent lots of time preparing for the exam. Don't let an empty stomach get in the way of success!

When travelling to the testing center, leave earlier than needed. That way, you have a buffer in case you experience any delays. This will help you remain calm and will keep you from missing your appointment time at the testing center.

Be sure to pace yourself during the exam. Don't try to rush through the exam. There is no need to risk performing poorly on the exam just so you can leave the testing center early. Allow yourself to use all of the allotted time if needed.

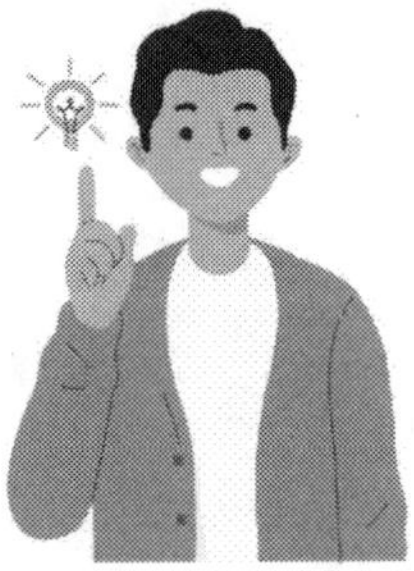

Remain positive while taking the exam even if you feel like you are performing poorly. Thinking about the content you should have mastered will not help you perform better on the exam.

Once the exam is complete, take some time to relax. Even if you feel that you need to take the exam again, you will be well served by some down time before you begin studying again. It's often easier to convince yourself to study if you know that it will come with a reward!

Test-Taking Strategies

1. Predicting the Answer

When you feel confident in your preparation for a multiple-choice test, try predicting the answer before reading the answer choices. This is especially useful on questions that test objective factual knowledge. By predicting the answer before reading the available choices, you eliminate the possibility that you will be distracted or led astray by an incorrect answer choice. You will feel more confident in your selection if you read the question, predict the answer, and then find your prediction among the answer choices. After using this strategy, be sure to still read all of the answer choices carefully and completely. If you feel unprepared, you should not attempt to predict the answers. This would be a waste of time and an opportunity for your mind to wander in the wrong direction.

2. Reading the Whole Question

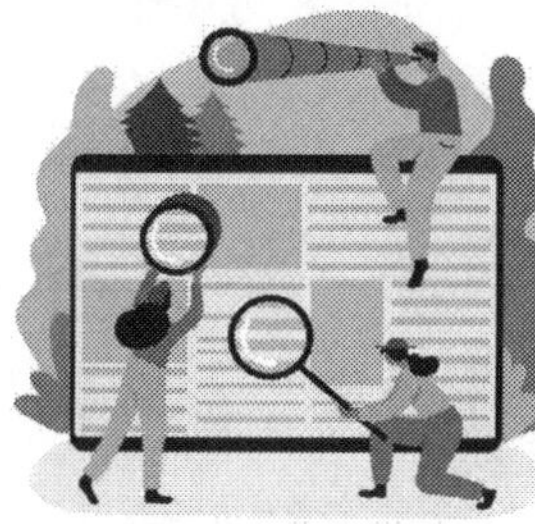

Too often, test takers scan a multiple-choice question, recognize a few familiar words, and immediately jump to the answer choices. Test authors are aware of this common impatience, and they will sometimes prey upon it. For instance, a test author might subtly turn the question into a negative, or he or she might redirect the focus of the question right at the end. The only way to avoid falling into these traps is to read the entirety of the question carefully before reading the answer choices.

3. Looking for Wrong Answers

Long and complicated multiple-choice questions can be intimidating. One way to simplify a difficult multiple-choice question is to eliminate all of the answer choices that are clearly wrong. In most sets of answers, there will be at least one selection that can be dismissed right away. If the test is administered on paper, the test taker could draw a line through it to indicate that it may be ignored; otherwise, the test taker will have to perform this operation mentally or on scratch paper. In either case, once the obviously incorrect answers have been eliminated, the remaining choices may be considered. Sometimes identifying the clearly wrong answers will give the test taker some information about the correct answer. For instance, if one of the remaining answer choices is a direct opposite of one of the eliminated answer choices, it may well be the correct answer. The opposite of obviously wrong is obviously right! Of course, this is not always the case. Some answers are obviously incorrect simply because they are irrelevant to the question being asked. Still, identifying and eliminating some incorrect answer choices is a good way to simplify a multiple-choice question.

4. Don't Overanalyze

Anxious test takers often overanalyze questions. When you are nervous, your brain will often run wild, causing you to make associations and discover clues that don't actually exist. If you feel that this may be a problem for you, do whatever you can to slow down during the test. Try taking a deep breath or counting to ten. As you read and consider the question, restrict yourself to the particular words used by the author. Avoid thought tangents about what the author *really* meant, or what he or she was *trying* to say. The only things that matter on a multiple-choice test are the words that are actually in the question. You must avoid reading too much into a multiple-choice question, or supposing that the writer meant something other than what he or she wrote.

5. No Need for Panic

It is wise to learn as many strategies as possible before taking a multiple-choice test, but it is likely that you will come across a few questions for which you simply don't know the answer. In this situation, avoid panicking. Because most multiple-choice tests include dozens of questions, the relative value of a single wrong answer is small. As much as possible, you should compartmentalize each question on a multiple-choice test. In other words, you should not allow your feelings about one question to affect your success on the others. When you find a question that you either don't understand or don't know how to answer, just take a deep breath and do your best. Read the entire question slowly and carefully. Try rephrasing the question a couple of different ways. Then, read all of the answer choices carefully. After eliminating obviously wrong answers, make a selection and move on to the next question.

6. Confusing Answer Choices

When working on a difficult multiple-choice question, there may be a tendency to focus on the answer choices that are the easiest to understand. Many people, whether consciously or not, gravitate to the answer choices that require the least concentration, knowledge, and memory. This is a mistake. When you come across an answer choice that is confusing, you should give it extra attention. A question might be confusing because you do not know the subject matter to which it refers. If this is the case, don't eliminate the answer before you have affirmatively settled on another. When you come across an answer choice of this type, set it aside as you look at the remaining choices. If you can confidently assert that one of the other choices is correct, you can leave the confusing answer aside. Otherwise, you will need to take a moment to try to better understand the confusing answer choice. Rephrasing is one way to tease out the sense of a confusing answer choice.

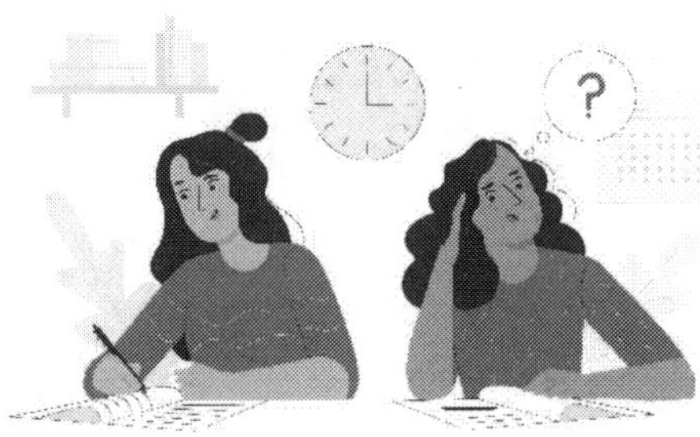

7. Your First Instinct

Many people struggle with multiple-choice tests because they overthink the questions. If you have studied sufficiently for the test, you should be prepared to trust your first instinct once you have carefully and completely read the question and all of the answer choices. There is a great deal of research suggesting that the mind can come to the correct conclusion very quickly once it has obtained all of the relevant information. At times, it may seem to you as if your intuition is working faster even than your reasoning mind. This may in fact be true. The knowledge you obtain while studying may be retrieved from your subconscious before you have a chance to work out the associations that support it. Verify your instinct by working out the reasons that it should be trusted.

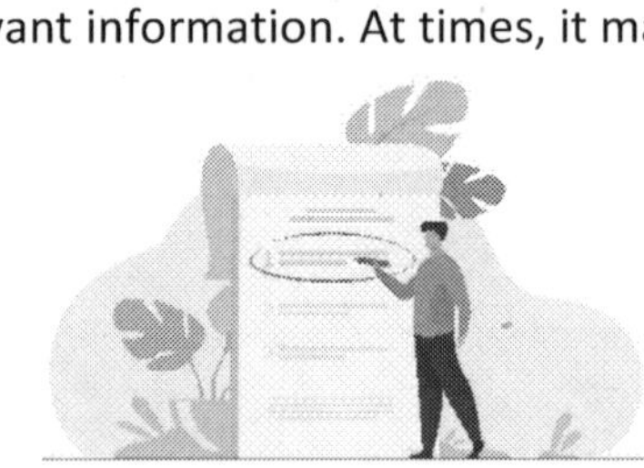

8. Key Words

Many test takers struggle with multiple-choice questions because they have poor reading comprehension skills. Quickly reading and understanding a multiple-choice question requires a mixture of skill and experience. To help with this, try jotting down a few key words and phrases on a piece of scrap paper. Doing this concentrates the process of reading and forces the mind to weigh the relative importance of the question's parts. In selecting words and phrases to write down, the test taker thinks about the question more deeply and carefully. This is especially true for multiple-choice questions that are preceded by a long prompt.

9. Subtle Negatives

One of the oldest tricks in the multiple-choice test writer's book is to subtly reverse the meaning of a question with a word like *not* or *except*. If you are not paying attention to each word in the question, you can easily be led astray by this trick. For instance, a common question format is, "Which of the following is...?" Obviously, if the question instead is, "Which of the following is not...?," then the answer will be quite different. Even worse, the test makers are aware of the potential for this mistake and will include one answer choice that would be correct if the question were not negated or reversed. A test taker who misses the reversal will find what he or she believes to be a correct answer and will be so confident that he or she will fail to reread the question and discover the original error. The only way to avoid this is to practice a wide variety of multiple-choice questions and to pay close attention to each and every word.

10. Reading Every Answer Choice

It may seem obvious, but you should always read every one of the answer choices! Too many test takers fall into the habit of scanning the question and assuming that they understand the question because they recognize a few key words. From there, they pick the first answer choice that answers the question they believe they have read. Test takers who read all of the answer choices might discover that one of the latter answer choices is actually *more* correct. Moreover, reading all of the answer choices can remind you of facts related to the question that can help you arrive at the correct answer. Sometimes, a misstatement or incorrect detail in one of the latter answer choices will trigger your memory of the subject and will enable you to find the right answer. Failing to read all of the answer choices is like not reading all of the items on a restaurant menu: you might miss out on the perfect choice.

11. Spot the Hedges

One of the keys to success on multiple-choice tests is paying close attention to every word. This is never truer than with words like *almost*, *most*, *some*, and *sometimes*. These words are called "hedges" because they indicate that a statement is not totally true or not true in every place and time. An absolute statement will contain no hedges, but in many subjects, the answers are not always straightforward or absolute. There are always exceptions to the rules in these subjects. For this reason, you should favor those multiple-choice questions that contain hedging language. The presence of qualifying words indicates that the author is taking special care with his or her words, which is certainly important when composing the right answer. After all, there are many ways to be wrong, but there is only one way to be right! For this reason, it is wise to avoid answers that are absolute when taking a multiple-choice test. An absolute answer is one that says things are either all one way or all another. They often include words like *every*, *always*, *best*, and *never*. If you are taking a multiple-choice test in a subject that doesn't lend itself to absolute answers, be on your guard if you see any of these words.

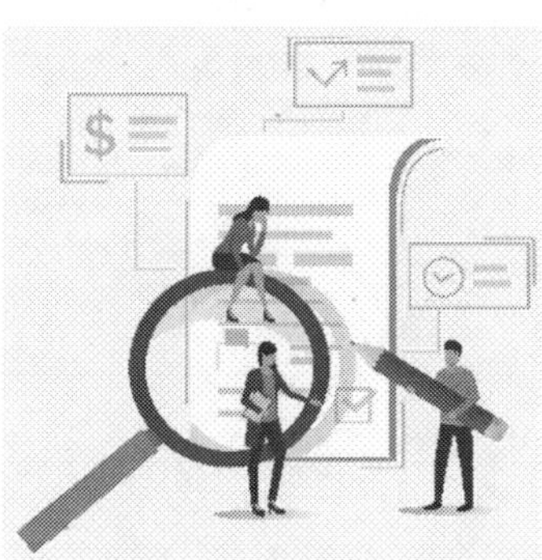

12. Long Answers

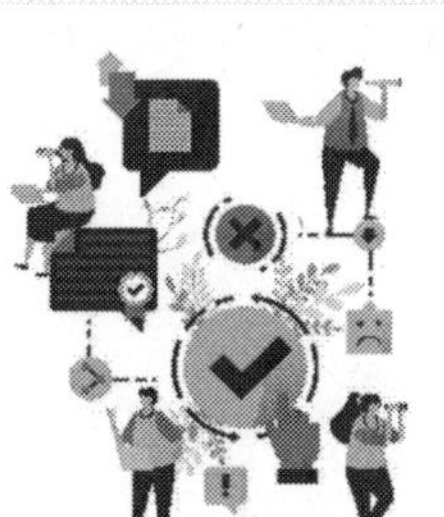

In many subject areas, the answers are not simple. As already mentioned, the right answer often requires hedges. Another common feature of the answers to a complex or subjective question are qualifying clauses, which are groups of words that subtly modify the meaning of the sentence. If the question or answer choice describes a rule to which there are exceptions or the subject matter is complicated, ambiguous, or confusing, the correct answer will require many words in order to be expressed clearly and accurately. In essence, you should not be deterred by answer choices that seem excessively long. Oftentimes, the author of the text will not be able to write the correct answer without offering some qualifications and modifications. Your job is to read the answer choices thoroughly and completely and to select the one that most accurately and precisely answers the question.

13. Restating to Understand

Sometimes, a question on a multiple-choice test is difficult not because of what it asks but because of how it is written. If this is the case, restate the question or answer choice in different words. This process serves a couple of important purposes. First, it forces you to concentrate on the core of the question. In order to rephrase the question accurately, you have to understand it well. Rephrasing the question will concentrate your mind on the key words and ideas. Second, it will present the information to your mind in a fresh way. This process may trigger your memory and render some useful scrap of information picked up while studying.

14. True Statements

Sometimes an answer choice will be true in itself, but it does not answer the question. This is one of the main reasons why it is essential to read the question carefully and completely before proceeding to the answer choices. Too often, test takers skip ahead to the answer choices and look for true statements. Having found one of these, they are content to select it without reference to the question above. The savvy test taker will always read the entire question before turning to the answer choices. Then, having settled on a correct answer choice, he or she will refer to the original question and ensure that the selected answer is relevant. The mistake of choosing a correct-but-irrelevant answer choice is especially common on questions related to specific pieces of objective knowledge.

15. No Patterns

One of the more dangerous ideas that circulates about multiple-choice tests is that the correct answers tend to fall into patterns. These erroneous ideas range from a belief that B and C are the most common right answers, to the idea that an unprepared test-taker should answer "A-B-A-C-A-D-A-B-A." It cannot be emphasized enough that pattern-seeking of this type is exactly the WRONG way to approach a multiple-choice test. To begin with, it is highly unlikely that the test maker will plot the correct answers according to some predetermined pattern. The questions are scrambled and delivered in a random order. Furthermore, even if the test maker was following a pattern in the assignation of correct answers, there is no reason why the test taker would know which pattern he or she was using. Any attempt to discern a pattern in the answer choices is a waste of time and a distraction from the real work of taking the test. A test taker would be much better served by extra preparation before the test than by reliance on a pattern in the answers.

Introduction for the TEAS 7

Background of the ATI TEAS

The Test of Essential Academic Skills (TEAS) is a standardized test created and distributed by Assessment Technologies Institute (ATI) to examine the test taker's aptitude for skillsets fundamental to a career in nursing. As such, the TEAS is used by nursing schools and allied health schools in the United States and Canada as a chief criterion for admission. The TEAS is currently in its seventh iteration.

The TEAS 7 is a nationwide test, and there is no variation in the difficulty of content among the versions given from state to state; the content of the TEAS is a standard measure for entry-level skills and abilities for nursing applicants. However, the required minimum TEAS scores can vary widely between schools and programs. Because the TEAS is used for admission to nursing and allied health programs, the majority of TEAS takers are high school diploma or GED graduates pursuing a career in nursing or are applicants to programs requiring prerequisite academic coursework. These applicants can range in background from sophomore-level collegiates to professionals looking to change careers into a healthcare field.

Test Administration

The TEAS 7 may be administered by a PSI testing center or a nursing or allied health school. The testing schedule is chosen by each individual facility, and the regularity of testing can vary from major metropolitan areas (where it may be offered multiple times per week in several locations) to sparsely populated towns (where it may be offered once per month every hundred miles). The test will also be proctored to ensure that testing protocols are enforced. Test takers can register at atitesting.com or directly through the school to which they wish to apply, as most nursing schools offer the test on-campus periodically throughout the year. The cost to take the TEAS 7 is set by the local administrator.

Students may retake the TEAS 7, but most schools have limitations regarding the number of days students must wait between attempts or the number of attempts students may make in a given period. For instance, many schools will accept the higher score of two attempts within a twelve-month period but will not consider a third attempt until twelve months has lapsed since the first attempt. Disability accommodations are generally available and can be arranged by contacting the local test administration site.

Test Format

The TEAS 7 is comprised of 150 questions. The questions are divided between four subject areas: Reading, Mathematics, Science, and English & Language Usage. There will also be 20 unscored "pretest" questions on the exam that ATI is beta testing. You will not know which questions these are, so give your best effort on every question.

Subject Area	Scored Questions	Unscored Questions	Total Questions
Reading	39	6	45
Mathematics	34	4	38
Science	44	6	50
English & Language Usage	33	4	37
Total	**150**	**20**	**170**

A certain amount of time is allotted for each section as seen below:

Subject Area	Minutes
Reading	55
Mathematics	57
Science	60
English & Language Usage	37
Total	**209 (3 hours & 39 minutes)**

Once a test taker begins a subject area, the timer will start. When the timer expires, the test taker may stretch, go to the bathroom, or otherwise relax before the timer begins for the next section. The TEAS 7 is offered in both a pencil-and-paper version and a computerized version, depending on the preference of the local test administrator. TEAS 7 test takers are not permitted to use cell phones, but four-function calculators are now permitted on the TEAS 7.

Alternate Item Types

In addition to multiple choice questions with four answer choices, the TEAS 7 includes four "alternate items types":

- Multiple-select
- Supply answer
- Ordering
- Hot spot

Multiple-Select

Multiple-select items, also referred to as *select all that apply,* are like multiple choice questions except that there may be multiple correct answers. Select every correct answer that you see. Keep in mind that there may just be one correct answer.

Supply Answer

Supply Answer items are fill-in-the blank questions. Rather than choosing from a list of choices, you must enter a number into the blank.

Ordering

For these item types, you will be given a list that needs to be put in the correct order. This may involve ranking a list from greatest to least based on some criteria or putting steps in order.

Hot Spot

For these item types, you will be given an image, and you must select a certain area of that image. For example, you may be given a diagram of the digestive system and be asked to select the stomach.

Scoring

Shortly after the examination, test takers will receive several different numbered scores with their TEAS 7 results, including scores on all the various sections and subsections. This includes the national and state-level percentile rankings that a test taker has achieved. This rank is equal to the percentage of test takers from nationwide samples that scored equal to or lower than the test taker. Higher percentiles indicate more correct answers and fewer people who scored higher than the given test taker. However, although this may be of interest to the test taker, schools do not use this score as a basis for acceptance decisions.

Instead, schools typically look at the Composite Individual Total Score. The composite score is a good determination of the test taker's performance and is calculated by averaging the test taker's performance from each section of the test. The national average composite score generally lies between 65% correct and 75% correct. Many schools have a minimum required score in this range, but each school and program chooses their own minimum standards; more prestigious schools require higher minimum scores and vice versa. Besides meeting minimum requirements, TEAS scores can display the competitiveness of the applicant just like previous GPAs and extracurricular activities, though this too varies from school to school.

Recent Developments

TEAS 7 is the successor the to the TEAS 6. In January 2022, ATI announced that the transition from the 6th edition to the 7th edition would take place in June of 2022. The TEAS 7 is similar in difficulty, but with slight differences in emphasis placed on various subjects.

Study Prep Plan for the ATI TEAS 7 Exam

1. **Schedule** - Use one of our study schedules below or come up with one of your own.
2. **Relax** - Test anxiety can hurt even the best students. There are many ways to reduce stress. Find the one that works best for you.
3. **Execute** - Once you have a good plan in place, be sure to stick to it.

One Week Study Schedule

Day	Topic
Day 1	Reading
Day 2	Mathematics
Day 3	Science
Day 4	Biology
Day 5	English and Language Usage
Day 6	TEAS 7 Practice Test #1
Day 7	Take Your Exam!

Two Week Study Schedule

Day	Topic	Day	Topic
Day 1	Reading	Day 8	Biology
Day 2	Integration of Knowledge and Ideas	Day 9	Chemistry
Day 3	Mathematics	Day 10	English and Language Usage
Day 4	Comparing and Ordering Numbers	Day 11	Knowledge of Language
Day 5	Measurement and Data	Day 12	TEAS 7 Practice Test #1
Day 6	Science	Day 13	TEAS 7 Practice Test #2
Day 7	Describe the Anatomy and Physiology...	Day 14	Take Your Exam!

One Month Study Schedule

Day	Topic	Day	Topic	Day	Topic
Day 1	Reading	Day 11	Science	Day 21	Correct Sentence Structures
Day 2	Craft and Structure	Day 12	Describe the Anatomy and Physiology of the Digestive System	Day 22	Knowledge of Language
Day 3	Integration of Knowledge and Ideas	Day 13	Describe the Anatomy and Physiolog...	Day 23	TEAS 7 Practice Test #1
Day 4	Using Data from Multiple Sources	Day 14	Describe the Anatomy and Physiology of...	Day 24	TEAS 7 Practice Test #2
Day 5	Mathematics	Day 15	Biology	Day 25	TEAS 7 Practice Test #3
Day 6	Performing Arithmetic Operations	Day 16	Apply Concepts Underlying Mendel's...	Day 26	TEAS 7 Practice Test #4
Day 7	Comparing and Ordering Numbers	Day 17	Chemistry	Day 27	TEAS 7 Practice Test #5
Day 8	Using Estimation Strategies...	Day 18	Demonstrate How Conditions Affect...	Day 28	TEAS 7 Practice Test #6
Day 9	Measurement and Data	Day 19	Scientific Reasoning	Day 29	TEAS 7 Practice Test #7
Day 10	Calculating Geometric Quantities	Day 20	English and Language Usage	Day 30	Take Your Exam!

Build your own prep plan by visiting the Online Resources page.

Instructions and a QR code can be found on the last page of this guide.

As you study for your test, we'd like to take the opportunity to remind you that you are capable of great things! With the right tools and dedication, you truly can do anything you set your mind to. The fact that you are holding this book right now shows how committed you are. In case no one has told you lately, you've got this! Our intention behind including this coloring page is to give you the chance to take some time to engage your creative side when you need a little brain-break from studying. As a company, we want to encourage people like you to achieve their dreams by providing good quality study materials for the tests and certifications that improve careers and change lives. As individuals, many of us have taken such tests in our careers, and we know how challenging this process can be. While we can't come alongside you and cheer you on personally, we can offer you the space to recall your purpose, reconnect with your passion, and refresh your brain through an artistic practice. We wish you every success, and happy studying!

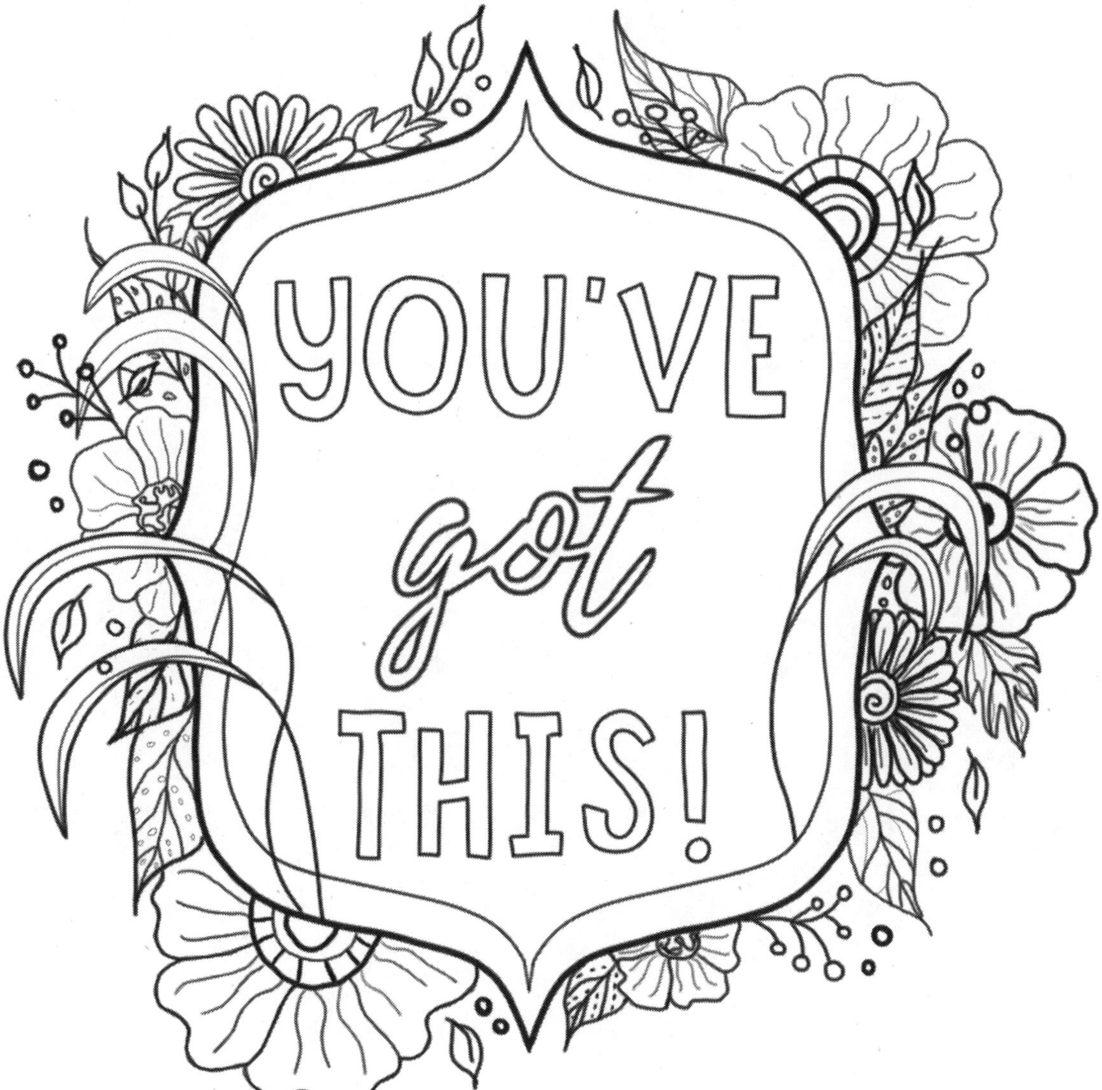

Key Ideas and Details

Summarizing a Multi-Paragraph Text

A summary is a shortened version of the original text, written by the reader in their own words. In order to effectively summarize a more complex text, it is necessary to fully understand the original source, and to highlight the major points covered. It may be helpful to outline the original text to get a big picture view of it, and to avoid getting bogged down in the minor details. For example, a summary wouldn't need to include a specific statistic from the original source unless it was the major focus of the piece. Summaries must include relevant, key points while leaving out descriptive details that are not necessary to convey the main point. Also, it's important for readers to use their own words, but to retain the original meaning of the passage. The key to a good summary is to emphasize the main idea without changing the focus of the original information.

Paraphrasing calls for the reader to take a small part of the passage and list or describe its main points. Paraphrasing is more than rewording the original passage, though. As with summary, a paraphrase should be written in the reader's own words, while still retaining the meaning of the original source. The main difference between summarizing and paraphrasing is the length of the original passage. A summary would be appropriate for a much larger piece, while paraphrase might focus on just a few lines of text. Effective paraphrasing will indicate an understanding of the original source, yet still help the reader expand on their interpretation. A paraphrase should neither add new information nor remove essential facts that will change the meaning of the source.

Topic Versus the Main Idea

It is very important to know the difference between the topic and the main idea of the text. Even though these two are similar because they both present the central point of a text, they have distinctive differences. A **topic** is the subject of the text. This can usually be described in a concise one- to two-word phrase. On the other hand, the **main idea** is more detailed and provides the author's central point of the text. It can be expressed through a complete sentence and is often found in the beginning, the middle, or the end of a paragraph. In most nonfiction books, the first sentence of the passage usually (but not always) states the main idea

Review the passage below to explore the topic versus the main idea:

Cheetahs

Cheetahs are one of the fastest mammals on the land, reaching up to 70 miles an hour over short distances. Even though cheetahs can run as fast as 70 miles an hour, they usually only have to run half that speed to catch up with their choice of prey. Cheetahs cannot maintain a fast pace over long periods of time because their bodies will overheat. After a chase, cheetahs need to rest for approximately 30 minutes prior to eating or returning to any other activity.

In the example above, the topic of the passage is "Cheetahs" simply because that is the subject of the text. The main idea of the text is "Cheetahs are one of the fastest mammals on the land but can only maintain a fast pace for shorter distances." While it covers the topic, it is more detailed and refers to the text in its entirety. The text continues to provide additional details called **supporting details**.

Supporting Details

Supporting details help readers better develop and understand the main idea. Supporting details answer questions like **who**, **what**, **where**, **when**, **why**, and **how**. Different types of supporting details include examples, facts and statistics, anecdotes, and sensory details.

Persuasive and informative texts often use supporting details. In persuasive texts, authors attempt to make readers agree with their points of view, and supporting details are often used as "selling points." If authors make a statement, they need to support the statement with evidence in order to adequately persuade readers. Informative texts use supporting details such as examples and facts to inform readers. Review the previous "Cheetahs" passage to find examples of supporting details.

Cheetahs

> *Cheetahs are one of the fastest mammals on the land, reaching up to 70 miles an hour over short distances. Even though cheetahs can run as fast as 70 miles an hour, they usually only have to run half that speed to catch up with their choice of prey. Cheetahs cannot maintain a fast pace over long periods of time because their bodies will overheat. After a chase, cheetahs need to rest for approximately 30 minutes prior to eating or returning to any other activity.*

In the example, supporting details include:

- Cheetahs reach up to 70 miles per hour over short distances.
- They usually only have to run half that speed to catch up with their prey.
- Cheetahs will overheat if they exert a high speed over longer distances.
- Cheetahs need to rest for 30 minutes after a chase.

Look at the diagram below (applying the cheetah example) to help determine the hierarchy of topic, main idea, and supporting details.

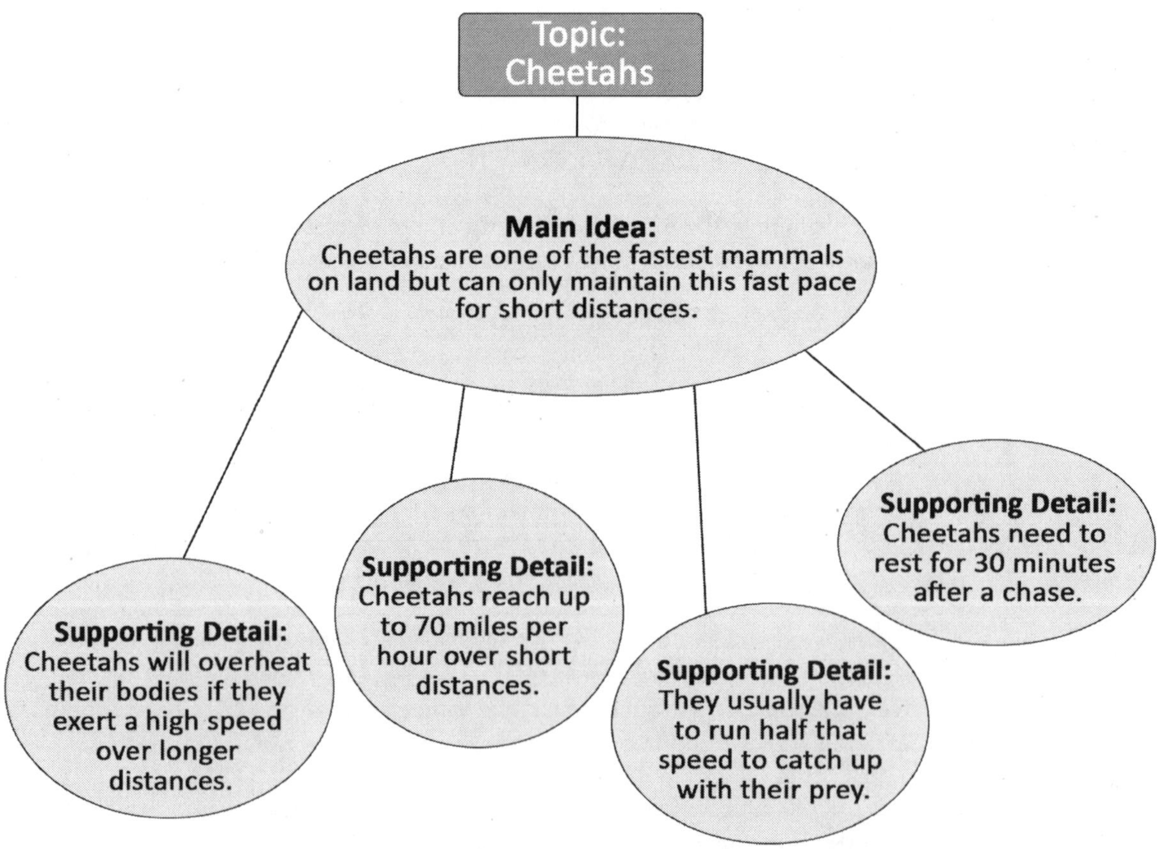

Making Inferences and Drawing Conclusions

Determining conclusions requires being an active reader, as a reader must analyze facts and supporting evidence to determine a conclusion. A reader should identify evidence, such as key words in a passage, to determine the logical conclusion or outcome that flows from the information presented. Consider the passage below:

> Lindsay, covered in flour, moved around the kitchen frantically. Her mom yelled from another room, "Lindsay, we're going to be late!"

You can conclude that Lindsay's next steps are to finish baking, clean herself up, and head off somewhere with her baked goods. Notice that the conclusion cannot be verified factually. Sometimes, authors explicitly state the conclusion that they want readers to understand. Alternatively, a conclusion may not be directly stated. In that case, readers must rely on the implications to form a logical conclusion. Here's another example:

> On the way to the bus stop, Michael realized his homework wasn't in his backpack. He ran back to the house to get it and made it back to the bus just in time.

In this example, although it's never explicitly stated, it can be inferred that Michael is a student on his way to school in the morning. When forming a conclusion from implied information, it's important to read the text carefully to find several pieces of evidence to support the conclusion.

Written Directions

When you read a comic or magazine, it's not necessary to understand everything. However, other more technical readings, such as directions for setting up a coffeemaker or a new phone app, require more attention to detail. Read each step all the way through, and don't skip ahead. While you may think that you know all or some of the steps, it's important to read directions in the manner that the writer intended. This aids in comprehension and ensures that you catch all relevant information. Take your time and reread sentences and passages if necessary. Look up unfamiliar words or concepts (outside of testing conditions), and jot comments, called annotations, in the margins.

Most often, written directions will come in the form of a numbered list, which clearly indicates the order in which to complete the steps. In the absence of such formatting, look out for words such as *first*, *second*, *then*, *next*, etc., that will make the directions easier to follow. Directions are written in chronological order, and often it is impossible to complete a later step if the previous ones are skipped. Therefore, identify task priority by the order in which they appear.

Keep in mind that there may be mistakes or confusing language in the directions. It might be helpful to read them in their entirety before beginning the task; this could help identify any contradictions or missing information. If there are contradictions or missing information, use logical reasoning to determine the correct course of action. Utilize the available information and knowledge of the final product to form a conclusion.

Locating Specific Information

Sometimes it is unnecessary to read an entire text to find relevant information. Be sure to utilize text features that will point you to information specific to your query, problem, or decision. Use critical reading skills to determine what information is relevant, and ask good questions to direct your research.

Using Text Features

Text features are used to bring clarity or to affect the meaning of it. Sometimes a publication will follow a certain style guide/manual of style, which is a set of standards for how to write and format a publication. Some examples are APA, MLA, and the Chicago Manual of Style. If the publication is following one of those standards then the text features will be in accordance with that style guide.

Writers can come up with their own uses for text features based on what they feel is best. However, text features are generally used for a specific purpose. It's important to catch on to that purpose to maximize comprehension.

A clear layout is essential for good reader comprehension. Even with the use of many text features, the text needs to be laid out in a clear, consistent manner.

Bolding, Italics, and Underlining

Bolding, italics, and underlining are all used to make words stand out. **Bolded** words are often key concepts and can usually be found in summary statements at the end of chapters and in indexes. *Italics* can be used to identify words of another language or to add extra emphasis to a word or phrase. Writers will sometime place words in italics when the word is being referred to as the word itself. Quotation marks can be used for this as well, as long as there is consistency. Italics are also used to represent a character's thoughts.

> Entering Jessica's room, Jessica's mom stepped over a pile of laundry, a stack of magazines, and a pile of dishes. *My messy daughter*, she thought, shaking her head.

Text can be <u>underlined</u> for a number of reasons, but generally it's to indicate a key term or important point.

Color can also be a text feature, as different color text can be used to make certain parts stand out or to indicate that a new section is beginning. Even if something is in black and white, the text may be in different shades of grey.

Formatting

In addition, formatting—such as indentation or bullet points—helps to clearly present content. Content may also be left justified, centered, or right justified:

Left Justified

Centered

Right Justified

Text is often centered to stand out and catch the reader's eye.

Analyzing Headings and Subheadings

Headings and subheadings are used in writing to organize discussions and allow the reader to find information quickly. Headings show a complete change in thought. Subheadings, which fall below headings, show different aspects of the same topic. For instance, if you saw the title *Government* and the heading *Forms of Government*, you might see the subheadings *Monarchy*, *Oligarchy*, *Democracy*, *Socialism*, and *Totalitarianism*.

Note the headings that got you to this point:

> # Reading
>
> Key Ideas and Details
>
> **Using Text Features**
>
> <u>Analyzing Headings and Subheadings</u>

As well as providing organization and structure, headings and subheadings also put more white space on a page, which places less strain on the reader's eyes. It's a good idea to skim a document and get familiar with headings and subheadings. Write down the title, headings, and subheadings before you begin reading to provide structure to your notes and thoughts.

Locating Information

Many longer pieces of writing, such as booklets or books, have additional textual features that help the reader locate specific information within the larger text. A table of contents, placed at the beginning, displays the sections into which the text is divided and provides the starting page numbers. A glossary is usually found at the end of a text or a section of text. It provides a list of key terms and their descriptions or definitions. An index also lists key terms, but instead of defining them, it shows the page numbers where information on that term can be found.

Additionally, technology can be used to look up information easily. Internet search engines provide an abundance of information on any given topic at the click of a button. Many specific websites have their own internal search engines as well.

Charts, Graphs, and Other Visuals

Texts may have graphic representations to help illustrate and visually support assertions made. For example, graphics can be used to express samples or segments of a population or demonstrate growth or decay. Three of the most popular graphic formats include line graphs, bar graphs, and pie charts.

Line graphs rely on a horizontal *X*-axis and a vertical *Y*-axis to establish baseline values. A point is plotted for each data value where the *x*-value and *y*-value of the data point intersect the axes, and those points are connected with lines. Compared to bar graphs or pie charts, line graphs are more useful for looking at the past and present and predicting future outcomes. For instance, a potential investor would look for stocks that demonstrated steady growth over many decades when examining the stock market. Note that severe spikes up and down indicate instability, while line graphs that display a slow but steady increase may indicate good returns.

Here's an example of a bar graph:

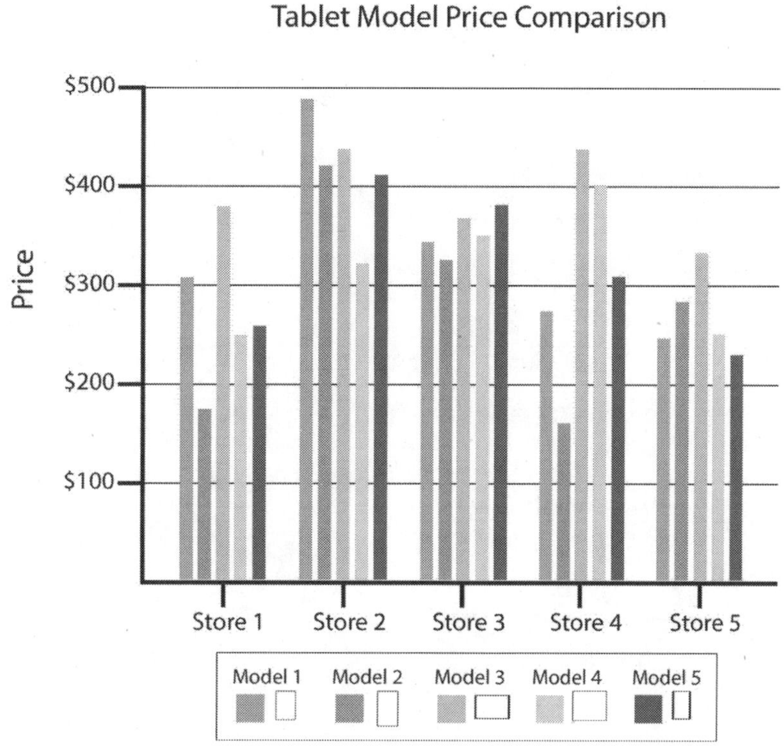

Bar graphs are usually displayed on a vertical *Y*-axis. The bars themselves can be two- or three-dimensional, depending on the designer's tastes. Unlike a line graph, which shows the fluctuation of only one variable, the *X*-axis on a bar graph is excellent for making comparisons because it shows differences between several variables. For instance, if an electronics store wanted to visually represent the number tablet sales for the year, a bar graph could have a bar for each type of tablet offered. To provide additional information, the store could show quarterly sales by constructing a bar for each type of tablet for each quarter in the fiscal year. The height of the bar would indicate the number of sales. The tablet types would be displayed along the *x*-axis with groups of four bars per tablet—one for each quarter.

A pie chart is divided into wedges that represent a numerical piece of the whole. Pie charts are useful for demonstrating how different categories add up to 100 percent. However, pie charts are not useful in comparing dissimilar items. High schools tend to use pie charts to track where students end up after graduation. Each wedge, for instance, might be labeled *vocational school, two-year college, four-year college, workforce,* or *unemployed.* By calculating the size of each wedge, schools can offer classes in the same ratios as where students will end up after high school. Pie charts are also useful for tracking finances. Items such as car payments, insurance, rent, credit cards, and entertainment would each get their own wedge proportional to the amount spent in a given time period. If one wedge is inordinately bigger than the rest, or if a wedge is expendable, it might be time to create a new financial strategy.

Using Legends and Map Keys

Legends and map keys are placed on maps to identify what the symbols on the map represent. Generally, map symbols stand for things like railroads, national or state highways, and public parks. Legends and maps keys can generally be found in the bottom right corner of a map. They are necessary to avoid the needless repetition of the same information because of the large amounts of information condensed onto a map. In addition, there may be a compass rose that shows the directions of north, south, east, and west. Most maps are oriented such that the top of the map is north.

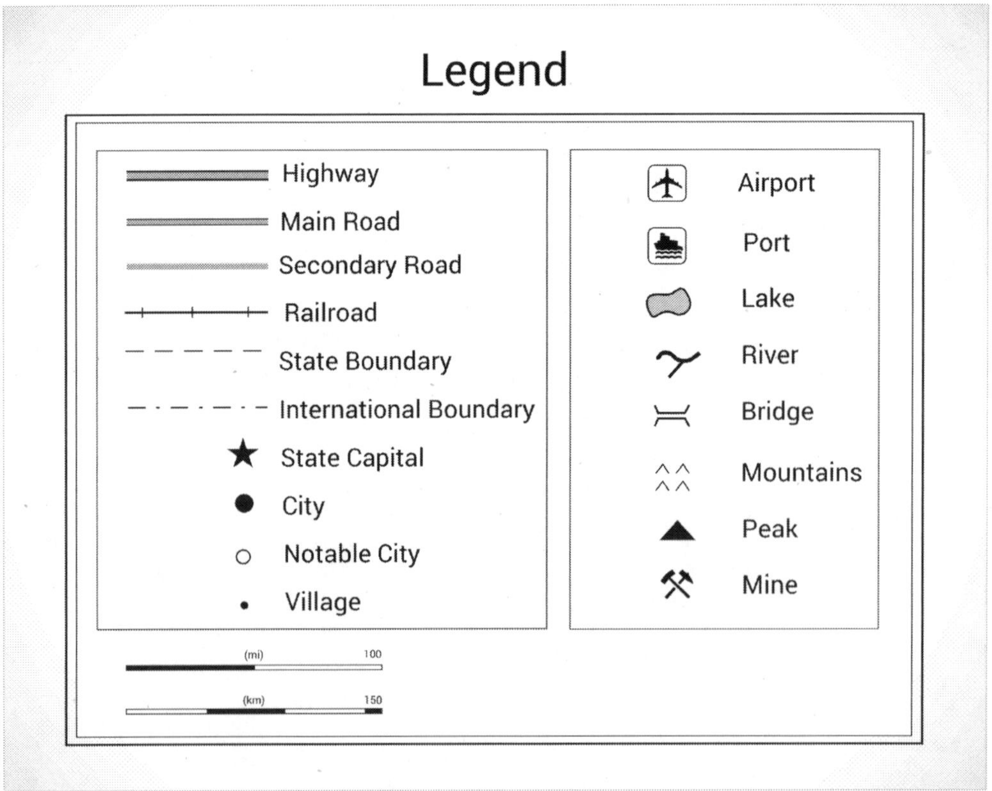

Interpreting Graphical Representations

As with written text, information presented in graphic form should be carefully evaluated. Authors can use images or graphs with biased or skewed information to help prove their point. Approach such information with a critical eye, and if any of it seems misleading or tainted by bias, it would be a good idea to cross-check it with other sources.

Authors might include visuals that seem relevant but are actually red herrings (distractions from the main point that look or sound good but do not contribute to the argument). They might also leave out pertinent information that harms their position. Do your best to determine what additional information might be necessary to evaluate an argument thoroughly.

Events in a Sequence

Ideas within texts should be organized, connected, or related in some way. In sequential relationships, ideas or events have a temporal relationship; they occur in some sort of order. Every passage has a plot, whether it is from a short story, a manual, a newspaper article or editorial, or a history text. And each plot has a logical order, which is also known as a sequence. Some of the most straightforward sequences can be found in technology directions, science experiments, instructional materials, and recipes. These forms of writing list actions that must occur in a proper sequence in order to get sufficient results. Other forms of writing, however, use style and ideas in ways that completely change the sequence of events. Poetry, for instance, may introduce repetitions that make the events seem cyclical. Postmodern writers are famous for experimenting with different concepts of place and time, creating "cut scenes" that distort straightforward sequences and abruptly transport the audience to different contexts or times. Even everyday newspaper articles, editorials, and historical sources may experiment with different sequential forms for stylistic effect.

In some cases, sequence can be found through comprehension techniques. For example, more literal passages might number the sequences or use key words such as *firstly*, *secondly*, *finally*, *next*, or *then*. The sequences of these stories can be found by rereading the passage and charting these numbers or key words. In most cases, however, readers must correctly order events through inferential and evaluative reading techniques; they have to place events in a logical order without explicit cues. They may also have to use inferences to fill in gaps that are not explicitly stated in the text.

Ideas in a text can also have a **comparative** relationship wherein certain qualities are shown to overlap or be the same between two different things. In comparative relationships, similarities are drawn out. Words like *as, like, also, similarly, in the same way,* and *too* are often used.

Passages that have a **cause-and-effect** relationship demonstrate a specific type of connection between ideas or events wherein one (or multiple) caused another. Words such as *if, since, because, then*, or *consequently* indicate a relationship.

Understanding the Meaning and Purpose of Transition Words

The writer should act as a guide, showing the reader how all the sentences fit together. Consider this example:

> Seat belts save more lives than any other automobile safety feature. Many studies show that airbags save lives as well. Not all cars have airbags. Many older cars don't. Air bags aren't entirely reliable. Studies show that in 15% of accidents, airbags don't deploy as designed. Seat belt malfunctions are extremely rare.

There's nothing wrong with any of these sentences individually, but together they're disjointed and difficult to follow. The best way for the writer to communicate information is through the use of transition words. Here are examples of transition words and phrases that tie sentences together, enabling a more natural flow:

- To show causality: as a result, therefore, and consequently
- To compare and contrast: however, but, and on the other hand
- To introduce examples: for instance, namely, and including
- To show order of importance: foremost, primarily, secondly, and lastly

Note: This is not a complete list of transitions. There are many more that can be used; however, most fit into these or similar categories. The point is that the words should clearly show the relationship between sentences, supporting information, and the main idea.

Here is an update to the previous example using transition words. These changes make it easier to read and bring clarity to the writer's points:

> Seat belts save more lives than any other automobile safety feature. Many studies show that airbags save lives as well; however, not all cars have airbags. For instance, some older cars don't. Furthermore, air bags aren't entirely reliable. For example, studies show that in 15% of accidents, airbags don't deploy as designed; but, on the other hand, seat belt malfunctions are extremely rare.

Also, be prepared to analyze whether the writer is using the best transition word or phrase for the situation. Take this sentence for example: "As a result, seat belt malfunctions are extremely rare." This sentence doesn't make sense in the context above because the writer is trying to show the contrast between seat belts and airbags, not the causality.

Craft and Structure

Distinguishing Between Fact and Opinion

A **fact** is information that is true. If information can be disproved, it is not a fact. For example, water freezes at or below thirty-two degrees Fahrenheit. An argument stating that water freezes at seventy degrees Fahrenheit cannot be supported by data and is therefore not a fact. Facts tend to be associated with science, mathematics, and statistics.

Opinions are information open to debate. Opinions are often tied to subjective concepts like feelings, desires, or manners. They can also be controversial.

Biases and stereotypes are viewpoints based in opinion and held despite evidence that they are incorrect. A **bias** is an individual prejudice. Biased people ignore evidence that contradicts their position while offering as proof any evidence that supports it. A **stereotype** is a widely held belief projected onto a group. Those who stereotype tend to make assumptions based on what others have told them and usually have little firsthand experience with the group or item in question.

Readers must read critically to discern between fact and opinion and to notice bias and stereotypes.

Tone

Tone refers to the writer's attitude toward the subject matter. Tone conveys how the writer feels about characters, situations, events, ideas, etc.

A lot of nonfiction writing has a neutral tone, which is an important one for the writer to use. A neutral tone demonstrates that the writer is presenting a topic impartially and letting the information speak for itself. On the other hand, nonfiction writing can be just as effective and appropriate if the tone isn't neutral. The following short passage provides an example of tone in nonfiction writing:

> Seat belts save more lives than any other automobile safety feature. Many studies show that airbags save lives as well; however, not all cars have airbags. For instance, some older cars don't. Furthermore, air bags aren't entirely reliable. For example, studies show that in 15% of accidents airbags don't deploy as designed, but, on the other hand, seat belt malfunctions are extremely rare. The number of highway fatalities has plummeted since laws requiring seat belt usage were enacted.

In this passage, the writer mostly chooses to retain a neutral tone when presenting information. If instead, the author chose to include their own personal experience of losing a friend or family member in a car accident, the tone would change dramatically. Or, if the author used words and phrases such as, "Ever since the government required individuals to wear seat belts, the amount of hard working American lives that have been saved is extraordinary!" The tone would no longer be neutral and would show the reader the seriousness, joy, sadness, etc. of the situation.

Using Context to Determine Meaning

Most experts agree that learning new words is worth your time. It helps you understand what you're reading, and it expands your vocabulary. An extensive vocabulary improves your ability to think. When you add words to your vocabulary, you are better able to make sense of the world around you.

One of the fastest ways to decode a word is through context. Context, or surrounding words, gives clues as to what unknown words mean. Take the following example: *When the students in the classroom teased Johnny, he was so discombobulated that he couldn't finish a simple math problem.* Even though you might be unfamiliar with the word *discombobulated*, you can use context clues in the sentence to make sense of the word. In this case, you can deduce that *discombobulated* means confused or distracted.

Context clues help readers understand unfamiliar words.
Synonyms are words or phrases that have nearly, if not exactly, the same meaning as other words or phrases

> *Large* boxes are needed to pack *big* items.

Antonyms are words or phrases that have opposite definitions. Antonyms, like synonyms, can serve as context clues, although more cryptically.

> *Large* boxes are not needed to pack *small* items.

Definitions are sometimes included within a sentence to define uncommon words.

> They practiced the *rumba*, a *type of dance*, for hours on end.

Explanations provide context through elaboration.

> Large boxes holding items weighing over 60 pounds were stacked in the corner.

Contrast provides ways in which things are different.

> These *miniscule* creatures were much different than the *huge* mammals that the zoologist was accustomed to dealing with.

Connotation refers to the emotion evoked by a word.

Marta was feeling *blue* today.

Blue is a color, though its connotation refers to emotions like *sad, down, depressed, etc.*

Denotation refers to the exact definition of a word.

Marta was feeling *sad* today.

There is no open interpretation for the meaning of sad in this sentence.

Determining the Denotative Meaning of Words

Connotation refers to the implied meaning of a word or phrase. Connotations are the ideas or feelings that words or phrases invoke other than their literal meaning. An example of the use of connotation is in people's use of the word *cheap*. While the literal meaning is something of low cost, people use the word to suggest something is poor in value or to negatively describe a person as reluctant to spend money. When something or someone is described this way, the reader is more inclined to have a particular image or feeling about it or them. Thus, connotation can be a very effective language tool in creating emotion and swaying opinion. However, connotations are sometimes hard to pin down because varying emotions can be associated with a word. Generally, though, connotative meanings tend to be fairly consistent within a specific cultural group.

Denotation is the literal definition of a word or phrase. The denotative meaning of a word is the one you would find in a dictionary. To present hard facts or vocabulary terms, it is helpful for a writer to use words which are mainly known for their denotative meanings rather than their connotative ones. In those instances, the words *inexpensive* and *frugal* are better because they do not carry the negative connotations that cheap does. *Inexpensive* refers to the cost of something, not its value, and *frugal* indicates that a person is conscientiously watching their spending. These terms do not elicit the same emotions that cheap does.

Authors sometimes choose to use both, but what they choose and when they use it is what critical readers need to differentiate. One method isn't inherently better than the other; however, one may create a better effect, depending upon an author's intent. If, for example, an author's purpose is to inform, to instruct, and to familiarize readers with a difficult subject, their use of connotation may be helpful. However, it may also undermine credibility and confuse readers. An author who wants to create a credible, scholarly effect in their text would most likely use denotation, which emphasizes literal, factual meaning and examples.

Use a dictionary to find the denotative meaning of words. Though context clues provide a rudimentary understanding of a word, using a dictionary can provide the reader with a more comprehensive meaning. Printed dictionaries list words in alphabetical order, and all versions, including those online, include a word's multiples meanings. Typically, the first definition is the most widely used or known. The second, third, and subsequent entries move toward the more unusual or archaic. Dictionaries also indicate the part of speech of each word, such as noun, verb, adjective, etc.

Keep in mind that dictionaries are not fixed in time. The English language today looks nothing like it did in Shakespeare's time, and Shakespeare's English is vastly different from Chaucer's. The English language is constantly evolving, as evidenced by the deletion of old words and the addition of new. *Ginormous* and *bling-bling*, for example, can both be found in Merriam-Webster's latest edition.

Figurative Language

Similes and **metaphors** are types of figurative language that are used as rhetorical devices. Both are comparisons between two things, but their formats differ slightly. A simile says that two things are similar and makes a comparison using "like" or "as"—*A* is like *B,* or *A* is as [some characteristic] as *B*—whereas a metaphor states that two things are exactly the same—*A* is *B*. In both cases, similes and metaphors invite the reader to think more deeply about the characteristics of the two subjects and consider where they overlap. Sometimes the poet develops a complex metaphor throughout the entire poem; this is known as an extended metaphor. An example of metaphor can be found in the sentence: "His pillow was a fluffy cloud". An example of simile can be found in the first line of Robert Burns' famous poem:

> My love is like a red, red rose

This is comparison using "like," and the two things being compared are love and a rose. Some characteristics of a rose are that it is fragrant, beautiful, blossoming, colorful, vibrant—by comparing his love to a red, red rose, Burns asks the reader to apply these qualities of a rose to his love. In this way, he implies that his love is also fresh, blossoming, and brilliant.

In addition to rhetorical devices that play on the *meanings* of words, there are also rhetorical devices that use the sounds of words. These devices are most often found in poetry, but may also be found in other types of literature and in nonfiction writing like texts for speeches.

Alliteration and **assonance** are both varieties of sound repetition. Other types of sound repetition include: **anaphora**—repetition that occurs at the beginning of the sentences; **epiphora**—repetition occurring at the end of phrases; antimetabole—repetition of words in a succession; and antiphrasis—a form of denial of an assertion in a text.

Alliteration refers to the repetition of the first sound of each word. Recall Robert Burns' opening line:

> My love is like a red, red rose

This line includes two instances of alliteration: "love" and "like" (repeated *L* sound), as well as "red" and "rose" (repeated *R* sound). Next, assonance refers to the repetition of vowel sounds and can occur anywhere within a word (not just the opening sound). Here is the opening of a poem by John Keats:

> When I have fears that I may cease to be
>
> Before my pen has glean'd my teeming brain

Assonance can be found in the words "fears," "cease," "be," "glean'd," and "teeming," all of which stress the long *E* sound. Both alliteration and assonance create a harmony that unifies the writer's language.

Another sound device is **onomatopoeia**—words whose spelling mimics the sound they describe. Words such as "crash," "bang," and "sizzle" are all examples of onomatopoeia. Use of onomatopoetic language adds auditory imagery to the text.

Readers are probably most familiar with the technique of using a **pun**. A pun is a play on words, taking advantage of two words that have the same or similar pronunciation. Puns can be found throughout Shakespeare's plays, for instance:

> Now is the winter of our discontent
>
> Made glorious summer by this son of York

These lines from *Richard III* contain a play on words. Richard III refers to his brother—the newly crowned King Edward IV—as the "son of York," referencing their family heritage from the house of York. However, while drawing a comparison between the political climate and the weather (times of political trouble were the "winter," but now the new king brings "glorious summer"), Richard's use of the word "son" also implies another word with the same pronunciation, "sun"—so Edward IV is also like the sun, bringing light, warmth, and hope to England. Puns are a clever way for writers to suggest two meanings at once.

Evaluating the Author's Purpose

All authors write with a purpose, whether that be to entertain, persuade, inform, or describe (or, a combination of these). Often, the purpose is clear from the beginning, but readers may need to utilize critical thinking and logical reasoning to infer what it is. Once the purpose is identified, engaged readers should take note of the key points and evidence that support or promote the message of the text. Readers should also take note of the author's tone and incorporate that into their analysis of the text. For example, a news article may be written in a factual style but actually be satirical, or sarcastic. The tone can alter the text's meaning completely, so it is important to identify it as soon as possible.

Types of Writing

Writing can be classified under four passage types: narrative, expository, descriptive (sometimes called technical), and persuasive. Though these types are not mutually exclusive, one form tends to dominate the rest. By recognizing the type of passage you're reading, you gain insight into how you should read. If you're reading a narrative, you can assume the author intends to entertain, which means you may skim the text without losing meaning. A technical document might require a close read because skimming the passage might cause the reader to miss salient details.

1. **Narrative writing**, at its core, is the art of storytelling. For a narrative to exist, certain elements must be present. First, it must have characters. While many characters are human, **characters** could be defined as anything that thinks, acts, and talks like a human. For example, many recent movies, such as *Lord of the Rings* and *The Chronicles of Narnia*, include animals, fantastical creatures, and even trees that behave like humans. Second, it must have a plot or sequence of events. Typically, those events follow a standard plot diagram, but recent trends start **in medias res** or in the middle (near the climax). In this instance, foreshadowing and flashbacks often fill in plot details. Finally, along with characters and a plot, there must also be conflict. Conflict is usually divided into two types: internal and external. **Internal conflict** indicates the character is in turmoil and is presented through the character's thoughts. **External conflicts** are visible. Types of external conflict include a person versus nature, another person, or society.

2. **Expository writing** is detached and to the point. Since expository writing is designed to instruct or inform, it usually involves directions and steps written in second person ("you" voice) and lacks any persuasive or narrative elements. Sequence words such as *first, second*, and *third*, or *in the first place*, *secondly,* and *lastly* are often given to add fluency and cohesion. Common examples of expository writing include instructor's lessons, cookbook recipes, and repair manuals.

3. Due to its empirical nature, **technical writing** is filled with steps, charts, graphs, data, and statistics. The goal of technical writing is to advance understanding in a field through the scientific method. Experts such as teachers, doctors, or mechanics use words unique to the profession in which they operate. These words, which often incorporate acronyms, are called **jargon**. Technical writing is a type of expository writing but is not meant to be understood by the general public. Instead, technical writers assume readers have received a formal education in a particular field of study and need no explanation as to what the jargon means. Imagine a doctor trying to understand a diagnostic reading for a car or a mechanic trying to interpret lab results. Only professionals with proper training will fully comprehend the text.

4. **Persuasive writing** is designed to change opinions and attitudes. The topic, stance, and arguments are found in the thesis, positioned near the end of the introduction. Later supporting paragraphs offer relevant quotations, paraphrases, and summaries from primary or secondary sources, which are then interpreted, analyzed, and evaluated. The goal of persuasive writers is not to stack quotes but to develop original ideas by using sources as a starting point. Good persuasive writing makes powerful arguments with valid sources and thoughtful analysis. Poor persuasive writing is riddled with bias and logical fallacies. Sometimes logical and illogical arguments are

sandwiched together in the same piece. Therefore, readers should display skepticism when reading persuasive arguments.

Fact and Opinion, Biases, and Stereotypes

It is important to distinguish between facts and opinions when reading a piece of writing. When an author presents **facts**, such as statistics or data, readers should be able to check those facts to verify that they are accurate. When authors share their own thoughts and feelings about a subject, they are expressing their **opinions**.

Authors often use words like *think, feel, believe,* or *in my opinion* when expressing an opinion, but these words won't always appear in an opinion piece, especially if it is formally written. An author's opinion may be backed up by facts, which gives it more credibility, but that opinion should not be taken as fact. A critical reader should be wary of an author's opinion, especially if it is only supported by other opinions.

Fact	**Opinion**
There are nine innings in a game of baseball.	Baseball games run too long.
James Garfield was assassinated on July 2, 1881.	James Garfield was a good president.
McDonald's® has stores in 118 countries.	McDonald's® has the best hamburgers.

Critical readers examine the facts used to support an author's argument. They check the facts against other sources to be sure those facts are correct. They also check the validity of the sources used to be sure those sources are credible, academic, and/or peer reviewed. When an author uses another person's opinion to support their argument, even if it is an expert's opinion, it is still only an opinion and should not be taken as fact. A strong argument uses valid, measurable facts to support ideas. Even then, the reader may disagree with the argument.

An authoritative argument may use the facts to sway the reader. In the example of global warming, many experts differ in their opinions of which alternative fuels can be used to aid in offsetting it. Because of this, a writer may choose to only use the information and experts' opinions that supports their viewpoint. For example, if the argument is that wind energy is the best solution, the author will use facts that support this idea. That same author may leave out relevant facts on solar energy. The way the author uses facts can influence the reader, so it's important to consider the facts being used, how those facts are being presented, and what information might be left out.

Evaluating the Author's Point of View or Perspective

Readers should always identify the author's point of view or perspective in a text. The author may write with a sole perspective, or they may present more than one. No matter how objective a piece may seem, assume the author has preconceived beliefs. Reduce the likelihood of accepting an invalid argument by looking for multiple articles on the topic, including those with varying opinions. If several opinions point in the same direction, and are backed by reputable peer-reviewed sources, it's more likely the author has a valid argument. Positions that run contrary to widely held beliefs and existing data should invite scrutiny. There are exceptions to the rule, so be a careful consumer of information.

Evaluating the Credibility of a Print or Digital Source

There are several additional criteria that need to be examined before using a source for a research topic. The following questions will help determine whether a source is credible:

Author

1. Who is he or she?
2. Does he or she have the appropriate credentials—e.g., M.D, PhD?
3. Is this person authorized to write on the matter through their job or personal experiences?

4. Is he or she affiliated with any known credible individuals or organizations?
5. Has he or she written anything else?

Publisher

1. Who published/produced the work? Is it a well-known journal, like *National Geographic*, or a tabloid, like *The National Enquirer*?
2. Is the publisher from a scholarly, commercial, or government association?
3. Do they publish works related to specific fields?
4. Have they published other works?
5. If a digital source, what kind of website hosts the text? Does it end in .edu, .org, or .com?

Bias

1. Is the writing objective? Does it contain any loaded or emotional language?
2. Does the publisher/producer have a known bias, such as Fox News or CNN?
3. Does the work include diverse opinions or perspectives?
4. Does the author have any known bias—e.g., Michael Moore, Bill O'Reilly, or the Pope? Is he or she affiliated with any organizations or individuals that may have a known bias—e.g., Citizens United or the 5. National Rifle Association?
6. Does the magazine, book, journal, or website contain any advertising?

References

1. Are there any references?
2. Are the references credible? Do they follow the same criteria as stated above?
3. Are the references from a related field?

Accuracy/reliability

1. Has the article, book, or digital source been peer reviewed?
2. Are all of the conclusions, supporting details, or ideas backed with published evidence?
3. If a digital source, is it free of grammatical errors, poor spelling, and improper English?
4. Do other published individuals have similar findings?

Coverage

1. Is the topic successfully addressed and appropriate for the intended audience?
2. Does the work add new information or theories to those of their sources?

Integration of Knowledge and Ideas

Using Evidence from the Text

Predictions

Some texts use suspense and foreshadowing to captivate readers. For example, an intriguing aspect of murder mysteries is that the reader is never sure of the culprit until the author reveals the individual's identity. Authors often build suspense and add depth and meaning to a work by leaving clues to provide hints or predict future events in the story; this is called foreshadowing. While some instances of foreshadowing are subtle, others are quite obvious.

Inferences

Making an **inference** requires the reader to read between the lines and look for what is implied rather than what is directly stated. That means, using information that is known from the text, the reader is able to make a logical assumption about information that is not explicitly stated but is probably true.

Authors employ literary devices such as tone, characterization, and theme to engage the audience by showing details of the story instead of merely telling them. For example, if an author said *Bob is selfish*, there's little left to infer. If the author said, *Bob cheated on his test, ignored his mom's calls, and parked illegally*, the reader can infer Bob is selfish. Authors also make implications through character dialogue, thoughts, effects on others, actions, and looks. Like in life, readers must assemble all the clues to form a complete picture.

Read the following passage:

> "Hey, do you want to meet my new puppy?" Jonathan asked.
> "Oh, I'm sorry but please don't—" Jacinta began to protest, but before she could finish, Jonathan had already opened the passenger side door of his car and a perfect white ball of fur came bouncing towards Jacinta.
> "Isn't he the cutest?" beamed Jonathan.
> "Yes—achoo!—he's pretty—aaaachooo!!—adora—aaa—aaaachoo!" Jacinta managed to say in between sneezes. "But if you don't mind, I—I—achoo!—need to go inside."

Which of the following can be inferred from Jacinta's reaction to the puppy?

a. She hates animals.
b. She is allergic to dogs.
c. She prefers cats to dogs.
d. She is angry at Jonathan.

An inference requires the reader to consider the information presented and then form their own idea about what is probably true. Based on the details in the passage, what is the best answer to the question? Important details to pay attention to in the passage include the tone of Jacinta's dialogue, as well as her reaction itself, which is a long string of sneezes. Answer choices (a) and (d) both express strong emotions ("hates" and "angry") that are not evident in Jacinta's speech or actions. Answer choice (c) mentions cats, but there is nothing in the passage to indicate Jacinta's feelings about cats. Answer choice (b), "she is allergic to dogs," is the most logical choice. Based on the fact that she began sneezing as soon as a fluffy dog approached her, it makes sense to infer that Jacinta is allergic to dogs even though she never directly states it in the passage.

Making inferences is crucial because literary texts often avoid presenting complete and direct information to readers about characters' thoughts or feelings, or they present the information in an unclear way, leaving it up to the reader to interpret clues given in the text. In order to make inferences while reading, readers should ask themselves:

- What details are being presented in the text?
- Is there any important information that seems to be missing?
- Based on the information that the author does include, what else is probably true?
- Is this inference reasonable based on what is already known?

Conclusions

Active readers should also draw conclusions. When doing so, the reader should ask the following questions: What is this piece about? What does the author believe? Does this piece have merit? Do I believe the author? Would this piece support my argument? The reader should first determine the author's intent. Identify the author's viewpoint and connect relevant evidence to support it. Readers may then move to the most important step: deciding whether to agree and determining whether they are correct. Always read cautiously and critically. Interact with text, and record reactions in the margins. These active reading skills help determine not only what the author thinks, but what you think as the reader.

Comparing and Contrasting Themes

Identifying Theme or Central Message

The **theme** is the central message of a fictional work, whether that work is structured as prose, drama, or poetry. It is the heart of what an author is trying to say to readers through the writing, and theme is largely conveyed through literary elements and techniques.

In literature, a theme can often be determined by considering the overarching narrative conflict within the work. Though there are several types of conflicts and several potential themes within them, the following are the most common:

- *Individual against the self*—relevant to themes of self-awareness, internal struggles, pride, coming of age, facing reality, fate, free will, vanity, loss of innocence, loneliness, isolation, fulfillment, failure, and disillusionment
- *Individual against nature*— relevant to themes of knowledge vs. ignorance, nature as beauty, quest for discovery, self-preservation, chaos and order, circle of life, death, and destruction of beauty
- *Individual against society*— relevant to themes of power, beauty, good, evil, war, class struggle, totalitarianism, role of men/women, wealth, corruption, change vs. tradition, capitalism, destruction, heroism, injustice, and racism
- *Individual against another individual*— relevant to themes of hope, loss of love or hope, sacrifice, power, revenge, betrayal, and honor

For example, in Hawthorne's *The Scarlet Letter*, one possible narrative conflict could be the individual against the self, with a relevant theme of internal struggles. This theme is alluded to through characterization—Dimmesdale's moral struggle with his love for Hester and Hester's internal struggles with the truth and her daughter, Pearl. It's also alluded to through plot—Dimmesdale's suicide and Hester helping the very townspeople who initially condemned her.

Sometimes, a text can convey a *message* or *universal lesson*—a truth or insight that the reader infers from the text, based on analysis of the literary and/or poetic elements. This message is often presented as a statement. For example, a potential message in Shakespeare's *Hamlet* could be "Revenge is what ultimately drives the human soul." This message can be immediately determined through plot and characterization in numerous ways, but it can also be determined through the setting of Norway, which is bordering on war.

How Authors Develop Theme

Authors employ a variety of techniques to present a theme. They may compare or contrast characters, events, places, ideas, or historical or invented settings to speak thematically. They may use analogies, metaphors, similes, allusions, or other literary devices to convey the theme. An author's use of diction, syntax, and tone can also help convey the theme. Authors will often develop themes through the development of characters, use of the setting, repetition of ideas, use of symbols, and through contrasting value systems. Authors of both fiction and nonfiction genres will use a variety of these techniques to develop one or more themes.

Regardless of the literary genre, there are commonalities in how authors, playwrights, and poets develop themes or central ideas.

Authors often do research, the results of which contribute to theme. In prose fiction and drama, this research may include real historical information about the setting the author has chosen or include elements that make fictional characters, settings, and plots seem realistic to the reader. In nonfiction, research is critical since information contained within this literature must be accurate and, moreover, accurately represented.

In fiction, authors present a narrative conflict that will contribute to the overall theme. This conflict may involve the storyline itself and some trouble within characters that needs resolution. In nonfiction, this conflict may be an explanation or commentary on factual people and events.

Authors will sometimes use character motivation to convey theme, such as in the example from *Hamlet* regarding revenge. In fiction, the characters an author creates will think, speak, and act in ways that effectively convey the theme to readers. In nonfiction, the characters are factual, as in a biography, but authors pay particular attention to presenting those motivations to make them clear to readers.

Authors also use literary devices as a means of conveying theme. For example, the use of moon symbolism in Mary Shelley's *Frankenstein* is significant as its phases can be compared to the phases that the Creature undergoes as he struggles with his identity.

The selected point of view can also contribute to a work's theme. The use of first-person point of view in a fiction or nonfiction work engages the reader's response differently than third person point of view. The central idea or theme from a first-person narrative may differ from a third-person limited text.

In literary nonfiction, authors usually identify the purpose of their writing, which differs from fiction, where the general purpose is to entertain. The purpose of nonfiction is usually to inform, persuade, or entertain the audience. The stated purpose of a nonfiction text will drive how the central message or theme, if applicable, is presented.

Authors identify an audience for their writing, which is critical in shaping the theme of the work. For example, the audience for J.K. Rowling's *Harry Potter* series would be different than the audience for a biography of George Washington. The audience an author chooses to address is closely tied to the purpose of the work. The choice of an audience also drives the choice of language and level of diction an author uses. Ultimately, the intended audience determines the level to which that subject matter is presented and the complexity of the theme.

Cultural Influence on Themes

Regardless of culture, place, or time, certain themes are universal to the human condition. Because all humans experience certain feelings and engage in similar experiences—birth, death, marriage, friendship, finding meaning, etc.—certain themes span cultures. However, different cultures have different norms and general beliefs concerning these themes. For example, the theme of maturing and crossing from childhood to adulthood is a global theme; however, the literature from one culture might imply that this happens in someone's twenties, while another culture's literature might imply that it happens in the early teenage years.

It's important for the reader to be aware of these differences. Readers must avoid being **ethnocentric**, which means believing the aspects of one's own culture to be superior to that of other cultures.

Evaluating an Argument

It's important to evaluate the author's supporting details to be sure that the details are credible, provide evidence of the author's point, and directly support the main idea. Though shocking statistics grab readers' attention, their use could be ineffective information in the piece. Details like this are crucial to understanding the passage and evaluating how well the author presents their argument and evidence.

Readers draw **conclusions** about what an author has presented. This helps them better understand what the writer has intended to communicate and whether or not they agree with what the author has offered. There are a few ways to determine a logical conclusion, but careful reading is the most important. It's helpful to read a passage a few times, noting details that seem important to the piece. Sometimes, readers arrive at a conclusion that is different than what the writer intended or come up with more than one conclusion.

Evidence

It is important to distinguish between fact and opinion when reading a piece of writing. When an author presents **facts**, such as statistics or data, readers should be able to check those facts and make sure they are accurate. When authors use **opinion**, they are sharing their own thoughts and feelings about a subject.

Textual evidence within the details helps readers draw a conclusion about a passage. **Textual evidence** refers to information—facts and examples that support the main point. Textual evidence will likely come from outside sources and can be in the form of quoted or paraphrased material. In order to draw a conclusion from evidence, it's important to examine the credibility and validity of that evidence as well as how (and if) it relates to the main idea.

Credibility

Critical readers examine the facts used to support an author's argument. They check the facts against other sources to be sure those facts are correct. They also check the validity of the sources used to be sure those sources are credible, academic, and/or peer reviewed. Consider that when an author uses another person's opinion to support their argument, even if it is an expert's opinion, it is still only an opinion and should not be taken as fact. A strong argument uses valid, measurable facts to support ideas. Even then, the reader may disagree with the argument as it may be rooted in their personal beliefs.

An authoritative argument may use the facts to sway the reader. Because of this, a writer may choose to only use the information and expert opinion that supports their viewpoint.

Counter-Arguments

If an author presents a differing opinion or a **counter argument** in order to refute it, the reader should consider how and why the information is being presented. It is meant to strengthen the original argument and shouldn't be confused with the author's intended conclusion, but it should also be considered in the reader's final evaluation. On the contrary, sometimes authors will concede to an opposing argument by recognizing the validity the other side has to offer. A concession will allow readers to see both sides of the argument in an unbiased light, thereby increasing the credibility of the author.

Authors can also reflect **bias** if they ignore an opposing viewpoint or present their side in an unbalanced way. A strong argument considers the opposition and finds a way to refute it. Critical readers should look for an unfair or one-sided presentation of the argument and be skeptical, as a bias may be present. Even if this bias is unintentional, if it exists in the writing, the reader should be wary of the validity of the argument.

Rhetorical Devices

Authors utilize a wide range of techniques to tell a story or communicate information. Readers should be familiar with the most common of these techniques. Writing techniques are also known as **rhetorical devices**.

In nonfiction writing, authors employ argumentative techniques to present their opinions to readers in the most convincing way. Persuasive writing usually includes at least one type of **appeal**: an appeal to logic (**logos**), emotion (**pathos**), or credibility and trustworthiness (**ethos**). When writers appeal to logic, they are asking readers to agree with them based on research, evidence, and an established line of reasoning. An author's argument might also appeal to readers' emotions, perhaps by including personal stories and **anecdotes** (a short narrative of a specific event). A final type of appeal—appeal to authority—asks the reader to agree with the author's argument on the basis of their expertise or credentials. Three different approaches to arguing the same opinion are exemplified below:

Logic (Logos)

> Our school should abolish its current ban on campus cell phone use. The ban was adopted last year as an attempt to reduce class disruptions and help students focus more on their lessons. However, since the rule was enacted, there has been no change in the number of disciplinary problems in class. Therefore, the rule is ineffective and should be done away with.

The above is an example of an appeal to logic. The author uses evidence to disprove the logic of the school's rule (the rule was supposed to reduce discipline problems, but the number of problems has not been reduced; therefore, the rule is not working) and to call for its repeal.

Emotion (Pathos)

An author's argument might also appeal to readers' emotions, perhaps by including personal stories and anecdotes.

The next example presents an appeal to emotion. By sharing the personal anecdote of one student and speaking about emotional topics like family relationships, the author invokes the reader's empathy in asking them to reconsider the school rule.

> Our school should abolish its current ban on campus cell phone use. If students aren't able to use their phones during the school day, many of them feel isolated from their loved ones. For example, last semester, one student's grandmother had a heart attack in the morning. However, because he couldn't use his cell phone, the student didn't know about his grandmother's accident until the end of the day—when she had already passed away, and it was too late to say goodbye. By preventing students from contacting their friends and family, our school is placing undue stress and anxiety on students.

Credibility (Ethos)

Finally, an appeal to authority includes a statement from a relevant expert. In this case, the author uses a doctor in the field of education to support the argument. All three examples begin from the same opinion—the school's phone ban needs to change—but rely on different argumentative styles to persuade the reader.

> Our school should abolish its current ban on campus cell phone use. According to Dr. Bartholomew Everett, a leading educational expert, "Research studies show that cell phone usage has no real impact on student attentiveness. Rather, phones provide a valuable technological resource for learning. Schools need to learn how to integrate this new technology into their curriculum." Rather than banning phones altogether, our school should follow the advice of experts and allow students to use phones as part of their learning.

Using Data from Multiple Sources

Finding Relevant Information

With a wealth of information at your fingertips in this digital age, it's important to not only know the type of information you're looking for, but also in what medium you're most likely to find it. Information needs to be specific and reliable. For example, if you're repairing a car, an encyclopedia would be mostly useless. While an encyclopedia might include information about cars, an owner's manual will contain the specific information needed for repairs. Information must also be credible, or trustworthy. A well-known newspaper may have reliable information, but a peer-reviewed journal article will have likely gone through a more rigorous check for validity. Determining bias can be helpful in determining credibility. If the information source (person, organization, or company) has something to gain from the reader forming a certain view on a topic, it's likely the information is skewed. For example, if you are trying to find the unemployment rate, the Bureau of Labor Statistics is a more credible source than a politician's speech.

Identifying Primary Sources in Various Media

Primary sources are best defined as records or items that serve as historical evidence. To be considered primary, the source documents or objects must have been created during the time period in which they reference. Examples include diaries, newspaper articles, speeches, government documents, photographs, and historical artifacts. In today's digital age, primary sources, which were once in print, often are embedded in secondary sources. **Secondary sources**, such as websites, history books, databases, or reviews, contain analysis or commentary on primary sources. Secondary sources borrow information from primary sources through the process of quoting, summarizing, or paraphrasing.

Today's students often complete research online through electronic sources. Electronic sources offer advantages over print and can be accessed on virtually any computer, while libraries or other research centers are limited to fixed locations and specific catalogs. Electronic sources are also efficient and yield massive amounts of data in seconds. The user can tailor a search based on key words, publication years, and article length. Lastly, many databases provide the user with instant citations, saving the user the trouble of manually assembling sources.

Though electronic sources yield powerful results, researchers must use caution. While there are many reputable and reliable sources on the internet, just as many are unreliable or biased sources. It's up to the researcher to examine and verify the reliability of sources. Wikipedia, for example, may or may not be accurate, depending on the contributor. Many databases, such as EBSCO or SIRS, offer peer reviewed articles, meaning the publications have been reviewed for the quality of their content.

Constructing Arguments Through Evidence

Using only one form of supporting evidence is not nearly as effective as using a variety to support a claim. Presenting only a list of statistics can be boring to the reader, but providing a true story that's both interesting and humanizing helps. In addition, one example isn't always enough to prove the writer's larger point, so combining it with other examples in the writing is extremely effective. Thus, when reading a passage, readers should not just look for a single form of supporting evidence.

For example, although most people can't argue with the statement, "Seat belts save lives", its impact on the reader is much greater when supported by additional content. The writer can support this idea by:

- Providing statistics on the rate of highway fatalities alongside statistics of estimated seat belt usage.
- Explaining the science behind car accidents and what happens to a passenger who doesn't use a seat belt.
- Offering anecdotal evidence or true stories from reliable sources on how seat belts prevent fatal injuries in car crashes.

Another key aspect of supporting evidence is a **reliable source**. Does the writer include the source of the information? If so, is the source well-known and trustworthy? Is there a potential for bias? For example, a seat belt study done by a seat belt manufacturer may have its own agenda to promote.

Logical Sequence

Even if the writer includes plenty of information to support their point, the writing is only effective when the information is in a logical order. **Logical sequencing** is really just common sense, but it's also an important writing technique. First, the writer should introduce the main idea, whether for a paragraph, a section, or the entire text.

Then, they should present evidence to support the main idea by using transitional language. This shows the reader how the information relates to the main idea and to the sentences around it. The writer should then take time to interpret the information, making sure necessary connections are obvious to the reader. Finally, the writer can summarize the information in the closing section.

NOTE: Although most writing follows this pattern, it isn't a set rule. Sometimes writers change the order for effect. For example, the writer can begin with a surprising piece of supporting information to grab the reader's attention, and then transition to the main idea. Thus, if a passage doesn't follow the logical order, readers should not immediately assume it's wrong. However, most writing that has a nontraditional beginning usually settles into a logical sequence.

Integrate Data

It's important to find multiple relevant and credible sources for data. Rather than just reading one article from a credible newspaper regarding a current event, read several articles from different newspapers. Journalists will differ in how they report a story and in which details they choose to include. Utilize visual data in conjunction with written information. Charts, graphs, and other visuals can enhance writing and provide additional evidence that supports the conclusion.

The same principle holds true for scientific or academic research. Multiple sources help give one a more thorough and balanced perspective. Be sure to find data from multiple types of sources as well. For instance, if you were to research the results of U.S. presidential elections it would be helpful to combine books with graphs and articles to get a comprehensive understanding.

Always consider the data from one source or type of source in light of data from other sources. A chart may convince you to think one way until you read a book that goes more into depth about the factors affecting the date.

Reading Practice Quiz

Questions 1-2 refer to the passage below:

> I believe that this was the first moving line ever installed. The idea came in a general way from the overhead trolley that the Chicago packers use in dressing beef. We had previously assembled the fly-wheel magneto in the usual method. With one workman doing a complete job he could turn out from thirty-five to forty pieces in a nine-hour day, or about twenty minutes to an assembly. What he did alone was then spread into twenty-nine operations; that cut down the assembly time to thirteen minutes, ten seconds. Then we raised the height of the line eight inches—this was in 1914—and cut the time to seven minutes. Further experimenting with the speed that the work should move at cut the time down to five minutes. In short, the result is this: by the aid of scientific study one man is now able to do somewhat more than four did only a comparatively few years ago. That line established the efficiency of the method and we now use it everywhere. The assembling of the motor, formerly done by one man, is now divided into eighty-four operations—those men do the work that three times their number formerly did. In a short time we tried out the plan on the chassis.

Excerpt from *My Life and My Work* by Henry Ford, 1922

1. According to the passage, which one of the following best describes the primary economic benefit of this innovation?
    a. The innovation increased workers' ability to multitask.
    b. The innovation decreased labor costs per worker.
    c. The innovation increased productivity in terms of both speed and quantity.
    d. The innovation decreased the size of the industrial workforce.

2. According to the passage, how did this new method of production improve over time?
    a. The method improved by adopting the exact practices of other industries.
    b. The method improved after it was applied to the chassis.
    c. The method improved by continually increasing the number of operations per product.
    d. The method improved progressively through experimentation.

3. Which of the following most accurately describes the meaning of the underlined word in the following passage?

> As long as the reason of man continues to be fallible, and he is at liberty to exercise it, different opinions will be formed. As long as the connection subsists between his reason and his self-love, his opinions and his passions will have a reciprocal influence on each other; and the former will be objects to which the latter will attach themselves. The diversity in the faculties of men, from which the rights of property originate, is not less an insuperable obstacle to a uniformity of interests.

    a. Achievable
    b. Unconquerable
    c. Difficult
    d. Unexpected

4. Which rhetorical device is being used in the following passage?

> ... we here highly resolve that these dead shall not have died in vain—that this nation, under God, shall have a new birth of freedom—and that government of the people, by the people, for the people, shall not perish from the earth.

a. Antimetabole
b. Antiphrasis
c. Anaphora
d. Epiphora

5. What is the effect of Lincoln's statement in the following passage?

> But, in a larger sense, we cannot dedicate—we cannot consecrate—we cannot hallow—this ground. The brave men, living and dead, who struggled here, have consecrated it, far above our poor power to add or detract.

a. His comparison emphasizes the great sacrifice of the soldiers who fought in the war.
b. His comparison serves as a reminder of the inadequacies of his audience.
c. His comparison serves as a catalyst for guilt and shame among audience members.
d. His comparison suggests that the dedication ceremony was inappropriate.

See answers on the next page.

Answer Explanations

1. C: The innovation's primary economic benefit was to increase productivity in terms of both speed and quantity. The passage contains several examples of how the assembly increased the production of fly-wheel magnetos and motors. For example, at the end of the passage, Ford claims that the assembly line tripled the productivity for motors. Thus, Choice *C* is the correct answer. The innovation is that each worker is assigned one single operation to be completed on every product, which is the opposite of multitasking. So, Choice *A* is incorrect. Although the innovation might have decreased labor costs by standardizing tasks, the passage doesn't reference labor costs. Therefore, Choice *B* is incorrect. Choice *D* is the second-best answer choice. Ford mentions that men can perform three times the amount of work, but it's unclear whether this means the workforce decreased. In other words, the workforce could've remained the same or even increased to support mass production. As such, Choice *D* is incorrect.

2. D: The method improved progressively through experimentation. Ford describes how he first got the idea from the overhead trolley used by Chicago beef packers and then they later elevated the height of the assembly line. In addition, the passage explicitly references "experimenting with the speed" of the line and making use of "scientific study." Thus, Choice *D* is the correct answer. Choice *A* is the second best answer choice because the Chicago beef packing industry influenced Ford. However, Ford claims it was only loosely based on the beef industry's overhead trolley, and he repeatedly describes experimenting with the height and speed. So, Choice *A* is incorrect. The passage ends with Ford stating his intention to test the new method on a chassis, which is the automobile's frame. As such, the chassis didn't improve the method as described in the passage, so Choice *B* is incorrect. Choice *C* is incorrect because the increased number of operations was a consequence of Ford's experimentation; the method didn't improve simply because the number of operations increased. So, Choice *C* is incorrect.

3. D: Choice *B* is the correct answer because *unconquerable* is the word that best fits the meaning of *insuperable*. In this context, *insuperable* means that the obstacle is insurmountable as it talks about the uniformity of interests in men. The word *unconquerable* aligns with this meaning. Choice *A* is incorrect because *achievable* has the opposite meaning to the author's intention. Choice *C* is incorrect because although the obstacle may be considered difficult, that is not the purpose of the word *insuperable*. Choice *D* is incorrect because there is no element of surprise in this context.

4. D: Choice *D* is the correct answer because of the repetition of the word *people* at the end of the passage. Choice A, antimetabole, is the repetition of words in a phrase or clause but in reverse order, such as: "I do what I like, and like what I do." Choice *B*, *antiphrasis*, is a form of denial of an assertion in a text. Choice *C*, *anaphora*, is the repetition that occurs at the beginning of sentences.

5. A: Choice *A* is correct because Lincoln's intention was to memorialize the soldiers who had fallen as a result of war as well as celebrate those who had put their lives in danger for the sake of their country. Choices *B* and *C* are incorrect because Lincoln's speech was supposed to foster a sense of pride among the members of the audience while connecting them to the soldiers' experiences. Choice *D* is incorrect because Lincoln does not make a distinction between soldiers and civilians but rather points his audience toward the sacrifices made by the soldiers on the battlefield at Gettysburg.

Mathematics

Numbers and Algebra

Numbers usually serve as an adjective representing a quantity of objects. They function as placeholders for a value. Numbers can be better understood by their type and related characteristics.

Definitions

A few definitions:

Whole numbers – describes a set of numbers that does not contain any fractions or decimals. The set of whole numbers includes zero.

Example: 0, 1, 2, 3, 4, 189, 293 are all whole numbers.

Integers – describes whole numbers and their negative counterparts. (Zero does not have a negative counterpart here. Instead, zero is its own negative.)

Example: -1, -2, -3, -4, -5, 0, 1, 2, 3, 4, 5 are all integers.

-1, -2, -3, -4, -5 are considered negative integers, and 1, 2, 3, 4, 5 are considered positive integers.

Absolute value – describes the value of a number regardless of its sign. The symbol for absolute value is | |.

Example: The absolute value of 24 is 24 or |24| = 24.

The absolute value of -693 is 693 or |-693| = 693.

Even numbers – describes any number that can be divided by 2 evenly, meaning the answer has no decimal or remainder portion.

Example: 2, 4, 9082, -2, -16, -504 are all considered even numbers, because they can be divided by 2, without leaving a remainder or forming a decimal. It does not matter whether the number is positive or negative.

Odd numbers – describes any number that does not divide evenly by 2.

Example: 1, 21, 541, 3003, -9, -63, -1257 are all considered odd numbers, because they cannot be divided by 2 without a remainder or a decimal.

Prime numbers – describes a number that is only evenly divisible, resulting in no remainder or decimal, by 1 and itself.

Example: 2, 3, 7, 13, 113 are all considered prime numbers because each can only be evenly divided by 1 and itself.

Composite numbers – describes a positive integer that is formed by multiplying two smaller integers together. Composite numbers can be divided evenly by numbers other than 1 or itself.

Example: 9, 24, 45, 66, 2348, 1,0002 are all considered composite numbers because they are the result of multiplying two smaller integers together.

Decimals – designated by a decimal point which indicates that what follows the point is a value that is less than 1 and is added to the integer number preceding the decimal point. The digit immediately following the decimal point is in the tenths place, the digit following the tenths place is in the hundredths place, and so on.

For example, the decimal number 1.735 has a value greater than 1 but less than 2. The 7 represents seven tenths of the unit 1 (0.7 or $\frac{7}{10}$); the 3 represents three hundredths of 1 (0.03 or $\frac{3}{100}$); and the 5 represents five thousandths of 1 (0.005 or $\frac{5}{1,000}$).

Real numbers – describes rational numbers and irrational numbers.

Rational numbers – describes any number that can be expressed as a fraction, with a non-zero denominator. Since any integer can be written with 1 in the denominator without changing its value, all integers are considered rational numbers. Every rational number has a decimal expression that terminates or repeats. That is, any rational number either will have a countable number of nonzero digits or will end with an ellipsis or a bar (3.6666... or $3.\overline{6}$) to depict repeating decimal digits. Some examples of rational numbers include 12, -3.54, $110.\overline{256}$, $\frac{-35}{10}$, and $4.\overline{7}$.

Irrational numbers – describes numbers that cannot be written as a finite decimal. Pi (π) is considered to be an irrational number because its decimal portion is unending or a non-repeating decimal. Pi (π) is the most common irrational number, but there are other well-known irrational numbers like *e* and $\sqrt{2}$.

Factorization

Factors are the numbers multiplied to achieve a product. Thus, every product in a multiplication equation has, at minimum, two factors. Of course, some products will have more than two factors. For the sake of most discussions, assume that factors are positive integers.

To find a number's factors, start with 1 and the number itself. Then divide the number by 2, 3, 4, and so on, seeing if any divisors can divide the number without a remainder, keeping a list of those that do. Stop upon reaching either the number itself or another factor.

Let's find the factors of 45. Start with 1 and 45. Then try to divide 45 by 2, which fails. Now divide 45 by 3. The answer is 15, so 3 and 15 are now factors. Dividing by 4 doesn't work, and dividing by 5 leaves 9. Lastly, dividing 45 by 6, 7, and 8 all don't work. The next integer to try is 9, but this is already known to be a factor, so the factorization is complete. The factors of 45 are 1, 3, 5, 9, 15 and 45.

Prime Factorization

Prime factorization involves an additional step after breaking a number down to its factors: breaking down the factors until they are all prime numbers. A prime number is any number that can only be divided by 1 and itself. The prime numbers between 1 and 20 are 2, 3, 5, 7, 11, 13, 17, and 19. As a simple test, numbers that are even or end in 5 are not prime.

Let's break 129 down into its prime factors. First, the factors are 3 and 43. Both 3 and 43 are prime numbers, so we're done. But if 43 was not a prime number, then it would also need to be factorized until all of the factors are expressed as prime numbers.

Common Factor

A common factor is a factor shared by two numbers. Let's take 45 and 30 and find the common factors:

The factors of 45 are: 1, 3, 5, 9, 15, and 45.

The factors of 30 are: 1, 2, 3, 5, 6, 10, 15, and 30.
The common factors are 1, 3, 5, and 15.

Greatest Common Factor

The greatest common factor is the largest number among the shared, common factors. From the factors of 45 and 30, the common factors are 3, 5, and 15. Thus, 15 is the greatest common factor, as it's the largest number.

Least Common Multiple

The least common multiple is the smallest number that's a multiple of two numbers. Let's try to find the least common multiple of 4 and 9. The multiples of 4 are 4, 8, 12, 16, 20, 24, 28, 32, 36, and so on. For 9, the multiples are 9, 18, 27, 36, 45, 54, etc. Thus, the least common multiple of 4 and 9 is 36, the lowest number where 4 and 9 share multiples.

If two numbers share no factors besides 1 in common, then their least common multiple will be simply their product. If two numbers have common factors, then their least common multiple will be their product divided by their greatest common factor. This can be visualized by the formula $LCM = \frac{x \times y}{GCF}$, where x and y are some integers and **LCM** and **GCF** are their least common multiple and greatest common factor, respectively.

Converting Fractions, Decimals, and Percentages

Fractions

A fraction is an expression that represents a part of a whole but can also be used to present ratios or division problems. An example of a fraction is $\frac{x}{y}$. In this example, x is called the numerator, while y is the denominator. The numerator represents the number of parts, and the denominator is the total number of parts. They are separated by a line or slash, known as a fraction bar. In simple fractions, the numerator and denominator can be nearly any integer. However, the denominator of a fraction can never be zero because dividing by zero is a function that is undefined.

Imagine that an apple pie has been baked for a holiday party, and the full pie has eight slices. After the party, there are five slices left. How could the amount of the pie that remains be expressed as a fraction? The numerator is 5 since there are 5 pieces left, and the denominator is 8 since there were eight total slices in the whole pie. Thus, expressed as a fraction, the leftover pie totals $\frac{5}{8}$ of the original amount.

Fractions come in three different varieties: proper fractions, improper fractions, and mixed numbers. Proper fractions have a numerator less than the denominator, such as $\frac{3}{8}$, but improper fractions have a numerator greater than the denominator, such as $\frac{7}{2}$. Mixed numbers combine a whole number with a proper fraction, such as $3\frac{1}{2}$. Any mixed number can be written as an improper fraction by multiplying the integer by the denominator, adding the product to the value of the numerator, and dividing the sum by the original denominator. For example:

$$3\frac{1}{2} = \frac{3 \times 2 + 1}{2} = \frac{7}{2}$$

Whole numbers can also be converted into fractions by placing the whole number as the numerator and making the denominator 1. For example, $3 = \frac{3}{1}$.

One of the most fundamental concepts of fractions is their ability to be manipulated by multiplication or division. This is possible since $\frac{n}{n} = 1$ for any non-zero integer. As a result, multiplying or dividing by $\frac{n}{n}$ will not alter the original fraction since any number multiplied or divided by 1 doesn't change the value of that number. Fractions of the same value are known as equivalent fractions.

For example, $\frac{2}{4}, \frac{4}{8}, \frac{50}{100}$, and $\frac{75}{150}$ are equivalent, as they all equal $\frac{1}{2}$.

Although many equivalent fractions exist, they are easier to compare and interpret when reduced or simplified. The numerator and denominator of a simple fraction will have no factors in common other than 1. When reducing or simplifying fractions, divide the numerator and denominator by the greatest common factor. A simple strategy is to divide the numerator and denominator by low numbers, like 2, 3, or 5 until arriving at a simple fraction, but the same thing could be achieved by determining the greatest common factor for both the numerator and denominator and dividing each by it. Using the first method is preferable when both the numerator and denominator are even, end in 5, or are obviously a multiple of another number. However, if no numbers seem to work, it will be necessary to factor the numerator and denominator to find the GCF. Here are some examples:

1) Simplify the fraction $\frac{6}{8}$:

Dividing the numerator and denominator by 2 results in $\frac{3}{4}$, which is a simple fraction.

2) Simplify the fraction $\frac{12}{36}$:

Dividing the numerator and denominator by 2 leaves $\frac{6}{18}$. This isn't a simple fraction, as both the numerator and denominator have factors in common. Dividing each by 3 results in $\frac{2}{6}$, but this can be further simplified by dividing by 2 to get $\frac{1}{3}$. This is the simplest fraction, as the numerator is 1. In cases like this, multiple division operations can be avoided by determining the greatest common factor between the numerator and denominator. The greatest common factor of $\frac{12}{36}$ is 12 because it divides evenly into both numbers, equaling $\frac{1}{3}$.

3) Simplify the fraction $\frac{18}{54}$ by dividing by the greatest common factor:

First, determine the factors for the numerator and denominator. The factors of 18 are 1, 2, 3, 6, 9, and 18. The factors of 54 are 1, 2, 3, 6, 9, 18, 27, and 54. Thus, the greatest common factor is 18. Dividing $\frac{18}{54}$ by 18 leaves $\frac{1}{3}$, which is the simplest fraction. This method takes slightly more work, but it definitively arrives at the simplest fraction.

A ratio is a comparison between the relative sizes of two parts of a whole, separated by a colon. It's different from a fraction because, in a ratio, the second number represents the number of parts that aren't currently being referenced, while in a fraction, the second or bottom number represents the total number of parts in the whole. For example, if 3 pieces of an 8-piece pie were eaten, the number of uneaten parts expressed as a ratio to the number of eaten parts would be 5:3.

Equivalent ratios work just like equivalent fractions. For example, let's find two ratios equivalent to 1:3. Both 3:9 and 20:60 are equivalent ratios because both can be simplified to 1:3.

Recognizing Equivalent Fractions and Mixed Numbers

The value of a fraction does not change if multiplying or dividing both the numerator and the denominator by the same number (other than 0). In other words, $\frac{x}{y} = \frac{a \times x}{a \times y} = \frac{x \div a}{y \div a}$, as long as *a* is not 0. This means that $\frac{2}{5} = \frac{4}{10}$, for example. If *x* and *y* are integers that have no common factors, then the fraction is said to be **simplified**. This means $\frac{2}{5}$ is simplified, but $\frac{4}{10}$ is not.

Often when working with fractions, the fractions need to be rewritten so that they all share a single denominator—this is called finding a **common denominator** for the fractions. Using two fractions, $\frac{a}{b}$ and $\frac{c}{d}$, the numerator and denominator of the left fraction can be multiplied by *d*, while the numerator and denominator of the right fraction can be multiplied by *b*. This provides the fractions $\frac{a \times d}{b \times d}$ and $\frac{c \times b}{d \times b}$ with the common denominator $b \times d$.

A fraction whose numerator is smaller than its denominator is called a **proper fraction**. A fraction whose numerator is bigger than its denominator is called an **improper fraction**. These numbers can be rewritten as a combination of integers and fractions, called a **mixed number**. For example:

$$\frac{6}{5} = \frac{5}{5} + \frac{1}{5} = 1 + \frac{1}{5}$$

It can be written as $1\frac{1}{5}$.

Percentages

Think of percentages as fractions with a denominator of 100. In fact, percentage means "per hundred." Problems often require converting numbers from percentages, fractions, and decimals. The following explains how to work through those conversions.

Converting Fractions to Percentages: Convert the fraction by using an equivalent fraction with a denominator of 100. For example:

$$\frac{3}{4} = \frac{3}{4} \times \frac{25}{25} = \frac{75}{100} = 75\%$$

Converting Percentages to Fractions: Percentages can be converted to fractions by turning the percentage into a fraction with a denominator of 100. Be wary of questions asking the converted fraction to be written in the simplest form. For example, $35\% = \frac{35}{100}$ which, although correctly written, has a numerator and denominator with a greatest common factor of 5 and can be simplified to $\frac{7}{20}$.

Percent Problems

The basic percent equation is the following:

$$\frac{is}{of} = \frac{\%}{100}$$

The placement of numbers in the equation depends on what the question asks.

Example 1

Find 40% of 80.

Basically, the problem is asking, "What is 40% of 80?" The 40 is the percent, and 80 is the number to find the percent "of." The equation is:

$$\frac{x}{80} = \frac{40}{100}$$

After cross-multiplying, the problem becomes $100x = 80(40)$. Solving for x produces the answer: $x = 32$.

Example 2

What percent of 100 is 20?

20 fills in the "is" portion, while 100 fills in the "of." The question asks for the percent, so that will be x, the unknown. The following equation is set up:

$$\frac{20}{100} = \frac{x}{100}$$

Cross-multiplying yields the equation $100x = 20(100)$. Solving for x gives the answer: 20%.

Example 3

30% of what number is 30?

The following equation uses the clues and numbers in the problem:

$$\frac{30}{x} = \frac{30}{100}$$

Cross-multiplying results in the equation $30(100) = 30x$. Solving for x gives the answer: $x = 100$.

Decimals

Recognition of Decimals

The **decimal system** is a way of writing out numbers that uses ten different numerals: 0, 1, 2, 3, 4, 5, 6, 7, 8, and 9. This is also called a "base ten" or "base 10" system. Other bases are also used. For example, computers work with a base of 2. This means they only use the numerals 0 and 1.

The **decimal place** denotes how far to the right of the decimal point a numeral is. The first digit to the right of the decimal point is in the **tenths** place. The next is the **hundredths**. The third is the **thousandths**.

So, 3.142 has a 1 in the tenths place, a 4 in the hundredths place, and a 2 in the thousandths place.

The **decimal point** is a period used to separate the **ones** place from the **tenths** place when writing out a number as a decimal.

A **decimal number** is a number written out with a decimal point instead of as a fraction, for example, 1.25 instead of $\frac{5}{4}$. Depending on the situation, it can sometimes be easier to work with fractions and sometimes easier to work with decimal numbers.

A decimal number is terminating if it stops at some point. It is called repeating if it never stops but repeats over and over. It is important to note that every rational number can be written as a terminating decimal or as a repeating decimal.

Conversions

Decimals and Percentages: Since a percentage is based on "per hundred," decimals and percentages can be converted by multiplying or dividing by 100. Practically speaking, this always amounts to moving the decimal point two places to the right or left, depending on the conversion. To convert a percentage to a decimal, move the decimal point two places to the left and remove the % sign. To convert a decimal to a percentage, move the decimal point two places to the right and add a % sign. Here are some examples:

65% = 0.65
0.33 = 33%
0.215 = 21.5%
99.99% = 0.9999
500% = 5.00
7.55 = 755%

Fractions and Percentages: Remember that a percentage is a number per one hundred. So, a percentage can be converted to a fraction by making the number in the percentage the numerator and putting 100 as the denominator:

$$43\% = \frac{43}{100}$$

$$97\% = \frac{97}{100}$$

Note that the percent symbol (%) kind of looks like a 0, a 1, and another 0. So, think of a percentage like 54% as 54 over 100.

To convert a fraction to a percent, follow the same logic. If the fraction happens to have 100 in the denominator, you're in luck. Just take the numerator and add a percent symbol:

$$\frac{28}{100} = 28\%$$

Otherwise, divide the numerator by the denominator to get a decimal:

$$\frac{9}{12} = 0.75$$

Then convert the decimal to a percentage:

$$0.75 = 75\%$$

Another option is to make the denominator equal to 100. Be sure to multiply the numerator and the denominator by the same number. For example:

$$\frac{3}{20} \times \frac{5}{5} = \frac{15}{100}$$

$$\frac{15}{100} = 15\%$$

Fractions and Decimals: To convert a fraction to a decimal, divide the numerator by the denominator:

$$\frac{5}{20} = 0.25$$

The other option is to multiply the numerator and denominator by whatever is needed to make the denominator equal to 100:

$$\frac{5}{20} \times \frac{5}{5} = \frac{25}{100}$$

When the denominator is equal to 100, the numerator can be turned into a decimal directly:

$$\frac{25}{100} = 0.25$$

To convert a fraction to a decimal, follow the same logic:

$$0.65 = \frac{65}{100}$$

Then you can simplify, if possible:

$$\frac{65}{100} = \frac{13}{20}$$

Performing Arithmetic Operations

Addition

Addition is the combination of two numbers; their quantities are added together cumulatively. The sign for an addition operation is the $+$ symbol. For example, $9 + 6 = 15$. The 9 and 6 combine to achieve a cumulative value, called a sum. Addition follows the Commutative Property, which means that the order of the numbers in an addition equation can be switched without altering the result. The formula for the commutative property is:

$$a + b = b + a$$

Let's look at a few examples to see how the commutative property works:

$$7 = 3 + 4 = 4 + 3 = 7$$

$$20 = 12 + 8 = 8 + 12 = 20$$

Addition also follows the Associative Property, which means that the grouping of numbers doesn't matter in an addition problem. In other words, the presence or absence of parentheses is irrelevant. The formula for the associative property is $(a + b) + c = a + (b + c)$. Here are some examples of the associative property at work:

$$30 = (6 + 14) + 10 = 6 + (14 + 10) = 30$$

$$35 = 8 + (2 + 25) = (8 + 2) + 25 = 35$$

There are set columns for addition: ones, tens, hundreds, thousands, ten-thousands, hundred-thousands, millions, and so on. To add how many units there are total, each column needs to be combined, starting from the right, or the ones column.

THOUSANDS	HUNDREDS	TENS	ONES

Every 10 units in the ones column equals one in the tens column, and every 10 units in the tens column equals one in the hundreds column, and so on.

Example: The number 5,432 has 2 ones, 3 tens, 4 hundreds, and 5 thousands. The number 371 has 3 hundreds, 7 tens and 1 one. To combine, or add, these two numbers, simply add up how many units of each column exist. The best way to do this is by lining up the columns:

$$\begin{array}{r} 5\,4\,3\,2 \\ +\quad 3\,7\,1 \\ \hline \end{array}$$

The ones column adds $2 + 1$ for a total (sum) of 3.

The tens column adds $3 + 7$ for a total of 10; since 10 of that unit was collected, add 1 to the hundreds column to denote the total in the next column:

$$\begin{array}{r} 1 \\ 5\,4\,3\,2 \\ +\quad 3\,7\,1 \\ \hline 0\,3 \end{array}$$

When adding the hundreds column, this extra 1 needs to be combined, so it would be the sum of 4, 3, and 1.

$$4 + 3 + 1 = 8$$

The last, or thousands, column listed would be the sum of 5. Since there are no other numbers in this column, that is the final total.

The answer would look as follows:

$$\begin{array}{r} 5\,4\,3\,2 \\ +\quad 3\,7\,1 \\ \hline 5\,8\,0\,3 \end{array}$$

Example

Find the sum of 9,734 and 895.

Set up the problem:

$$\begin{array}{r} 9\,7\,3\,4 \\ +\quad 8\,9\,5 \\ \hline \end{array}$$

Total the columns:

$$\begin{array}{r} 9\,7\,3\,4 \\ +\quad 8\,9\,5 \\ \hline 1\,0\,6\,2\,9 \end{array}$$

In this example, another column (ten-thousands) is added to the left of the thousands column, to denote a carryover of 10 units in the thousands column. The final sum is 10,629.

When adding using all negative integers, the total is negative. The integers are simply added together and the negative symbol is tacked on.

$$(-12) + (-435) = -447$$

To add decimal numbers, each number needs to be lined up by the decimal point in vertical columns. For each number being added, the zeros to the right of the last number need to be filled in so that each of the numbers has the same number of places to the right of the decimal. Then, the columns can be added together.

Here is an example of $2.45 + 1.3 + 8.891$ written in column form:

$$\begin{array}{r} 2.450 \\ 1.300 \\ +\,8.891 \\ \hline \end{array}$$

Zeros have been added in the columns so that each number has the same number of places to the right of the decimal.

Added together, the correct answer is 12.641:

$$\begin{array}{r} 2.450 \\ 1.300 \\ +\,8.891 \\ \hline 12.641 \end{array}$$

Subtraction

Subtraction is taking away one number from another, so their quantities are reduced. The sign designating a subtraction operation is the – symbol, and the result is called the difference. For example, $9 - 6 = 3$. The number *6* detracts from the number *9* to reach the difference *3*.

Unlike addition, subtraction follows neither the commutative nor associative properties. The order and grouping in subtraction impact the result.

$$15 = 22 - 7 \neq 7 - 22 = -15$$

$$3 = (10 - 5) - 2 \neq 10 - (5 - 2) = 7$$

When working through subtraction problems involving larger numbers, it's necessary to regroup the numbers. Let's work through a practice problem using regrouping:

$$\begin{array}{r} 3\,2\,5 \\ -\;7\,7 \\ \hline \end{array}$$

Here, it is clear that the ones and tens columns for 77 are greater than the ones and tens columns for 325. To subtract this number, borrow from the tens and hundreds columns. When borrowing from a column, subtracting 1 from the lender column will add 10 to the borrower column:

$$\begin{array}{rrr} 3-1 & 10+2-1 & 10+5 \\ - & 7 & 7 \\ \hline \end{array} = \begin{array}{rrr} 2 & 11 & 15 \\ - & 7 & 7 \\ \hline 2 & 4 & 8 \end{array}$$

After ensuring that each digit in the top row is greater than the digit in the corresponding bottom row, subtraction can proceed as normal, and the answer is found to be 248.

When subtracting decimal numbers, the decimals are lined up in vertical columns just as they are when adding decimals. Here is $7.89 - 4.235$ written in column form:

$$\begin{array}{r} 7.890 \\ -\underline{4.235} \\ 3.655 \end{array}$$

A zero has been added in the column so that each number has the same number of places to the right of the decimal.

Multiplication

Multiplication involves adding together multiple copies of a number. It is indicated by an × symbol or a number immediately outside of a parenthesis. For example:

$$5(8-2)$$

The two numbers being multiplied together are called factors, and their result is called a product. For example, $9 \times 6 = 54$. This can be shown alternatively by expansion of either the 9 or the 6:

$$9 \times 6 = 9 + 9 + 9 + 9 + 9 + 9 = 54$$

$$9 \times 6 = 6 + 6 + 6 + 6 + 6 + 6 + 6 + 6 + 6 = 54$$

Like addition, multiplication holds the commutative and associative properties:

$$115 = 23 \times 5 = 5 \times 23 = 115$$

$$84 = 3 \times (7 \times 4) = (3 \times 7) \times 4 = 84$$

Multiplication also follows the distributive property, which allows the multiplication to be distributed through parentheses. The formula for distribution is $a \times (b + c) = ab + ac$. This is clear after the examples:

$$45 = 5 \times 9 = 5(3 + 6) = (5 \times 3) + (5 \times 6) = 15 + 30 = 45$$

$$20 = 4 \times 5 = 4(10 - 5) = (4 \times 10) - (4 \times 5) = 40 - 20 = 20$$

For larger-number multiplication, the way the numbers are lined up can make it easier to obtain the product. It is simplest to put the number with the most digits on top and the number with fewer digits on the bottom. If they have the same number of digits, select one for the top and one for the bottom. Line up the problem, and begin by multiplying the far-right column on the top and the far-right column on the bottom. If the answer to a column is more than 9, the ones place digit will be written below that column and the tens place digit will carry to the top of the next column to be added after those digits are multiplied. Write the answer below that column. Move to the next column to the left on the top, and multiply it by the same far-right column on the bottom. Keep moving to the left one column at a time on the top number until the end.

Example
Multiply 37×8

Line up the numbers, placing the one with the most digits on top.

$$\begin{array}{r} 3\;7 \\ \times\quad 8 \\ \hline \end{array}$$

Multiply the far-right column on the top with the far-right column on the bottom (7 x 8). Write the answer, 56, as below: The ones value, 6, gets recorded, the tens value, 5, is carried.

$$\begin{array}{r} {\scriptstyle +5}\;\; \\ 3\;7 \\ \text{X}\quad 8 \\ \hline 6 \end{array}$$

Move to the next column left on the top number and multiply with the far-right bottom (3 x 8). Remember to add any carry over after multiplying: 3 x 8 = 24, 24 + 5 = 29. Since there are no more digits on top, write the entire number below.

$$\begin{array}{r} {\scriptstyle +5}\;\; \\ 3\;7 \\ \text{X}\quad 8 \\ \hline 2\;9\;6 \end{array}$$

The solution is 296

If there is more than one column to the bottom number, move to the row below the first strand of answers, mark a zero in the far-right column, and then begin the multiplication process again with the far-right column on top and the second column from the right on the bottom. For each digit in the bottom number, there will be a row of answers, each padded with the respective number of zeros on the right. Finally, add up all of the answer rows for one total number.

Example: Multiply 512×36.

Line up the numbers (the one with the most digits on top) to multiply. Begin with the right column on top and the right column on bottom (2×6).

$$\begin{array}{r} 5\;1\;2 \\ \text{X}\quad 3\;6 \\ \hline \end{array}$$

Move one column left on top and multiply by the far-right column on the bottom (1×6). Add the carry over after multiplying: $1 \times 6 = 6, 6 + 1 = 7$.

$$\begin{array}{r} {\scriptstyle +1}\;\;\; \\ 5\;1\;2 \\ \times\quad 3\;6 \\ \hline 7\;2 \end{array}$$

Move one column left on top and multiply by the far-right column on the bottom (5×6). Since this is the last digit on top, write the whole answer below.

$$\begin{array}{r} 512 \\ \times\ \ 36 \\ \hline 3072 \end{array}$$

Now move on to the second column on the bottom number. Starting on the far-right column on the top, repeat this pattern for the next number left on the bottom (2×3). Write the answers below the first line of answers; remember to begin with a zero placeholder on the far-right.

$$\begin{array}{r} 512 \\ \times\ \ 36 \\ \hline 3072 \\ 60 \end{array}$$

Continue the pattern (1×3).

$$\begin{array}{r} 512 \\ \times\ \ 36 \\ \hline 3072 \\ 360 \end{array}$$

Since this is the last digit on top, write the whole answer below.

$$\begin{array}{r} 512 \\ \times\ \ 36 \\ \hline 3072 \\ 15360 \end{array}$$

Now add the answer rows together. Pay attention to ensure they are aligned correctly.

$$\begin{array}{r} 512 \\ \times\ \ 36 \\ \hline 3072 \\ 15360 \\ \hline 18432 \end{array}$$

The solution is 18,432.

Multiplication becomes slightly more complicated when multiplying numbers with decimals. The easiest way to answer these problems is to ignore the decimals and multiply as if they were whole numbers. After multiplying the factors, place a decimal in the product. The placement of the decimal is determined by taking the cumulative number of decimal places in the factors.

For example:

$$\begin{array}{r} 0.7 \\ \times 3\ \ \\ \hline 2.1 \end{array} \qquad \begin{array}{r} 2.6 \\ \times\ \ 4.2 \\ \hline 10.92 \end{array} \qquad \begin{array}{r} 1.5 \\ \times 6.4 \\ \hline 9.60 \end{array}$$

Let's tackle the first example. First, ignore the decimal and multiply the numbers as though they were whole numbers to arrive at a product: 21. Second, count the number of digits that follow a decimal (one). Finally, move the decimal place that many positions to the left, as the factors have only one decimal place. The second example works the same way, except that there are two total decimal places in the factors, so the product's decimal is moved two places over. In the third example, the decimal should be moved over two digits, but the digit zero is no longer needed, so it is erased, and the final answer is 9.6.

The simplest way to multiply decimals is to calculate the product as if the decimals are not there, then count the number of decimal places in the original problem. Use that total to place the decimal the same number of places over in your answer, counting from right to left. For example, 0.5×1.25 can be rewritten and multiplied as 5×125, which equals 625. Then the decimal is added three places from the right for 0.625.

The final answer will have the same number of decimal **places** as the total number of decimal **places** in the problem. The first number has one decimal place, and the second number has two decimal places. Therefore, the final answer will contain three decimal places:

$$0.5 \times 1.25 = 0.625$$

Division

Division and multiplication are inverses of each other in the same way that addition and subtraction are opposites. The signs designating a division operation are the ÷ and / symbols. In division, the second number divides into the first.

The number before the division sign is called the dividend or, if expressed as a fraction, the numerator. For example, in a ÷ b, a is the dividend, while in $\frac{a}{b}$, a is the numerator.

The number after the division sign is called the divisor or, if expressed as a fraction, the denominator. For example, in a ÷ b, b is the divisor, while in $\frac{a}{b}$, b is the denominator.

Like subtraction, division doesn't follow the commutative property, as it matters which number comes before the division sign, and division doesn't follow the associative or distributive properties for the same reason. For example:

$$\frac{3}{2} = 9 \div 6 \neq 6 \div 9 = \frac{2}{3}$$

$$2 = 10 \div 5 = (30 \div 3) \div 5 \neq 30 \div (3 \div 5) = 30 \div \frac{3}{5} = 50$$

$$25 = 20 + 5 = (40 \div 2) + (40 \div 8) \neq 40 \div (2 + 8) = 40 \div 10 = 4$$

If a divisor doesn't divide into a dividend evenly, whatever is left over is termed the remainder. The remainder can be further divided out into decimal form by using long division; however, this doesn't always give a quotient with a finite number of decimal places, so the remainder can also be expressed as a fraction over the original divisor.

Example

Divide 1050 by 42, or $1050 \div 42$.

Set up the problem with the denominator being divided into the numerator:

$$42\overline{)1050}$$

Check for divisibility into the first unit of the numerator, 1.
42 cannot go into 1, so add on the next unit in the denominator, 0.
42 cannot go into 10, so add on the next unit in the denominator, 5.
42 can be divided into 105 two times. Write the 2 over the 5 in 105 and multiply 42×2. Write the 84 under 105 for subtraction and note the remainder, 21 is less than 42.

$$\begin{array}{r} 2 \\ 42\overline{)1050} \\ -84 \\ \hline 21 \end{array}$$

Drop the next digit in the numerator down to the remainder (making 21 into 210) to create a number 42 can divide into. 42 divides into 210 five times. Write the 5 over the 0 and multiply 42×5.

$$\begin{array}{r} 25 \\ 42\overline{)1050} \\ -84 \\ \hline 210 \end{array}$$

Write the 210 under 210 for subtraction. The remainder is 0.

$$\begin{array}{r} 25 \\ 42\overline{)1050} \\ -84 \\ \hline 210 \\ -210 \\ \hline 0 \end{array}$$

The solution is 25.

Example

Divide $\frac{375}{4}$ or $375 \div 4$.

Set up the problem.

$$4\overline{)375}$$

4 cannot divide into 3, so add the next unit from the numerator, 7. 4 divides into 37 nine times, so write the 9 above the 7. Multiply $4 \times 9 = 36$. Write the 36 under the 37 for subtraction. The remainder is 1 (1 is less than 4).

$$\begin{array}{r} 9 \\ 4\overline{)375} \\ -36 \\ \hline 1 \end{array}$$

Drop the next digit in the numerator, 5, making the remainder 15. 4 divides into 15, three times, so write the 3 above the 5. Multiply 4×3. Write the 12 under the 15 for subtraction, remainder is 3 (3 is less than 4).

```
     9 3
  4|3 7 5
  - 3 6
  ------
     1 5
   - 1 2
  ------
       3
```

The solution is 93 remainder 3 or 93 ¾ (the remainder can be written over the original denominator).

Division with decimals is similar to multiplication with decimals in that when dividing a decimal by a whole number, ignore the decimal and divide as if it were a whole number.

Upon finding the answer, or quotient, place the decimal at the decimal place equal to that in the dividend.

$$15.75 \div 3 = 5.25$$

When the divisor is a decimal number, multiply both the divisor and dividend by 10. Repeat this until the divisor is a whole number, then complete the division operation as described above.

$$17.5 \div 2.5 = 175 \div 25 = 7$$

Dividing a decimal by a whole number entails using long division first by ignoring the decimal point. Then, the decimal point is moved the number of places given in the problem.

For example, $6.8 \div 4$ can be rewritten as $68 \div 4$, which is 17. There is one non-zero integer to the right of the decimal point, so the final solution would have one decimal place to the right of the solution. In this case, the solution is 1.7.

Dividing a decimal by another decimal requires changing the divisor to a whole number by moving its decimal point. The decimal place of the dividend should be moved by the same number of places as the divisor. Then, the problem is the same as dividing a decimal by a whole number.

For example, $5.72 \div 1.1$ has a divisor with one decimal place. The expression can be rewritten as $57.2 \div 11$ by moving each decimal to the right to eliminate the decimal. The long division can be completed as $572 \div 11$ with a result of 52. Since there is one non-zero integer to the right of the decimal point in the problem, the final solution is 5.2.

In another example, $8 \div 0.16$ has a divisor with two decimal places. The expression can be rewritten as $800 \div 16$ by moving each decimal point two places to the right to eliminate the decimal in the divisor. The long division can be completed with a result of 50.

Exponents

An exponent is an operation used as shorthand for a number multiplied or divided by itself for a defined number of times:

$$3^7 = 3 \times 3 \times 3 \times 3 \times 3 \times 3 \times 3$$

In this example, the 3 is called the base, and the 7 is called the exponent. The exponent is typically expressed as a superscript number near the upper-right side of the base but can also be identified as the number following a caret symbol (^). This operation would be verbally expressed as "3 to the 7th power" or "3 raised to the power of 7."

Common exponents are 2 and 3. A base raised to the power of 2 is referred to as having been "squared," while a base raised to the power of 3 is referred to as having been "cubed."

Several special rules apply to exponents. First, the Zero Power Rule finds that any number raised to the zero power equals 1. For example, 100^0, 2^0, $(-3)^0$and 0^0 all equal 1 because the bases are raised to the zero power.

Second, exponents can be negative. With negative exponents, the equation is expressed as a fraction, as in the following example:

$$3^{-7} = \frac{1}{3^7} = \frac{1}{3 \times 3 \times 3 \times 3 \times 3 \times 3 \times 3}$$

Third, the Power Rule concerns exponents being raised by another exponent. When this occurs, the exponents are multiplied by each other:

$$(x^2)^3 = x^6 = (x^3)^2$$

Fourth, when multiplying two exponents with the same base, the Product Rule requires that the base remains the same, and the exponents are added. For example, $a^x \times a^y = a^{x+y}$. Since addition and multiplication are commutative, the two terms being multiplied can be in any order.

$$x^3x^5 = x^{3+5} = x^8 = x^{5+3} = x^5x^3$$

Fifth, when dividing two exponents with the same base, the Quotient Rule requires that the base remains the same, but the exponents are subtracted. So,

$$a^x \div a^y = a^{x-y}$$

Since subtraction and division are not commutative, the two terms must remain in order.

$$x^5x^{-3} = x^{5-3} = x^2 = x^5 \div x^3 = \frac{x^5}{x^3}$$

Additionally, 1 raised to any power is still equal to 1, and any number raised to the power of 1 is equal to itself. In other words, $a^1 = a$ and $14^1 = 14$.

Exponents play an important role in scientific notation to present extremely large or small numbers as follows: $a \times 10^b$. To write the number in scientific notation, the decimal is moved until there is only one digit on the left side of the decimal point, indicating that the number a has a value between 1 and 10. The number of times the decimal moves indicates the exponent to which 10 is raised, here represented by b. If the decimal moves to the left, then b is positive, but if the decimal moves to the right, then b is negative.

See the following examples:

$$3{,}050 = 3.05 \times 10^3$$

$$-777 = -7.77 \times 10^2$$

$$0.000123 = 1.23 \times 10^{-4}$$

$$-0.0525 = -5.25 \times 10^{-2}$$

Roots

The **square root symbol** is expressed as $\sqrt{\ }$ and is commonly known as the radical. Taking the root of a number is the inverse operation of multiplying that number by itself some amount of times. For example, squaring the number 7 is equal to 7×7, or 49. Finding the square root is the opposite of finding an exponent, as the operation seeks a number that when multiplied by itself equals the number in the square root symbol.

For example, $\sqrt{36} = 6$ because 6 multiplied by 6 equals 36. Note, the square root of 36 is also -6 since -6 $x - 6 =$ 36. This can be indicated using a plus/minus symbol like this: ±6. However, square roots are often just expressed as a positive number for simplicity with it being understood that the true value can be either positive or negative.

Perfect squares are squares of whole numbers. The list of perfect squares begins with 0, 1, 4, 9, 16, 25, 36, 49, 64, 81, and 100.

Determining the square root of imperfect squares requires a calculator to reach an exact figure. It's possible, however, to approximate the answer by finding the two perfect squares that the number fits between. For example, the square root of 40 is between 6 and 7 since the squares of those numbers are 36 and 49, respectively.

Square roots are the most common root operation. If the radical doesn't have a number to the upper left of the symbol $\sqrt{\ }$, then it's a square root. Sometimes a radical includes a number in the upper left, like $\sqrt[3]{27}$, as in the other common root type—the cube root. Complicated roots like the cube root often require a calculator.

Operations with Fractions

Of the four basic operations that can be performed on fractions, the one that involves the least amount of work is multiplication. To multiply two fractions, simply multiply the numerators together, multiply the denominators together, and place the products of each as a fraction. Whole numbers and mixed numbers can also be expressed as a fraction, as described above, to multiply with a fraction. Work through these examples:

1) $\frac{2}{5} \times \frac{3}{4} = \frac{6}{20} = \frac{3}{10}$

2) $\frac{4}{9} \times \frac{7}{11} = \frac{28}{99}$

Dividing fractions is similar to multiplication with one key difference. To divide fractions, flip the numerator and denominator of the second fraction, and then proceed as if it were a multiplication problem:

1) $\frac{7}{8} \div \frac{4}{5} = \frac{7}{8} \times \frac{5}{4} = \frac{35}{32}$

2) $\frac{5}{9} \div \frac{1}{3} = \frac{5}{9} \times \frac{3}{1} = \frac{15}{9} = \frac{5}{3}$

Addition and subtraction require more steps than multiplication and division, as these operations require the fractions to have the same denominator, also called a common denominator. It is always possible to find a common denominator by multiplying the denominators. However, when the denominators are large numbers, this method is unwieldy, especially if the answer must be provided in its simplest form. Thus, it's beneficial to find the least common denominator of the fractions—the least common denominator is incidentally also the least common multiple.

Once equivalent fractions have been found with common denominators, simply add or subtract the numerators to arrive at the answer:

1) $\frac{1}{2} + \frac{3}{4} = \frac{2}{4} + \frac{3}{4} = \frac{5}{4}$

2) $\frac{3}{12} + \frac{11}{20} = \frac{15}{60} + \frac{33}{60} = \frac{48}{60} = \frac{4}{5}$

3) $\frac{7}{9} - \frac{4}{15} = \frac{35}{45} - \frac{12}{45} = \frac{23}{45}$

4) $\frac{5}{6} - \frac{7}{18} = \frac{15}{18} - \frac{7}{18} = \frac{8}{18} = \frac{4}{9}$

Parentheses

Parentheses separate different parts of an equation, and operations within them should be thought of as taking place before the outside operations take place. Practically, this means that the distinction between what is inside and outside of the parentheses decides the order of operations that the equation follows. Failing to solve operations inside the parentheses before addressing the part of the equation outside of the parentheses will lead to incorrect results.

For example, let's analyze $5 - (3 + 25)$. The addition operation within the parentheses must be solved first. So $3 + 25 = 28$, leaving $5 - (28) = -23$. If this was solved in the incorrect order of operations, the solution might be found to be $5 - 3 + 25 = 2 + 25 = 27$, which would be wrong.

Equations often feature multiple layers of parentheses. To differentiate them, square brackets [ ] and braces { } are used in addition to parentheses. The innermost parentheses must be solved before working outward to larger brackets. For example, in $\{2 \div [5 - (3 + 1)]\}$, solving the innermost parentheses $(3 + 1)$ leaves $\{2 \div [5 - (4)]\}$. $[5 - (4)]$ is now the next smallest, which leaves $\{2 \div [1]\}$ in the final step, and 2 as the answer.

Order of Operations

When solving equations with multiple operations, special rules apply. These rules are known as the Order of Operations. The order is as follows: Parentheses, Exponents, Multiplication and Division from left to right, and Addition and Subtraction from left to right. A popular pneumonic device to help remember the order is Please Excuse My Dear Aunt Sally (PEMDAS).

Evaluate the following two problems to understand the Order of Operations:

1) $4 + (3 \times 2)^2 \div 4$

First, solve the operation within the parentheses: $4 + 6^2 \div 4$.
Second, solve the exponent: $4 + 36 \div 4$.
Third, solve the division operation: $4 + 9$.
Fourth, finish the operation with addition for the answer, 13.

2) $2 \times (6 + 3) \div (2 + 1)^2$

$2 \times 9 \div (3)^2$
$2 \times 9 \div 9$
$18 \div 9$
2

Positive and Negative Numbers

Signs

Aside from 0, numbers can be either positive or negative. The sign for a positive number is the plus sign or the + symbol, while the sign for a negative number is the minus sign or the – symbol. If a number has no designation, then it's assumed to be positive.

Absolute Values

Both positive and negative numbers are valued according to their distance from 0. Look at this number line for +3 and -3:

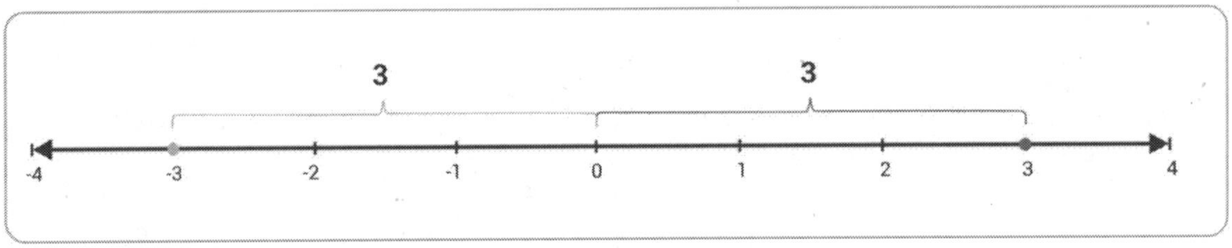

Both 3 and -3 are three spaces from 0. The distance from 0 is called its absolute value. Thus, both -3 and 3 have an absolute value of 3 since they're both three spaces away from 0.

An absolute number is written by placing | | around the number. So, $|3|$ and $|-3|$ both equal 3, as that's their common absolute value.

Implications for Addition and Subtraction

For addition, if all numbers are either positive or negative, simply add them together. For example,

$$4 + 4 = 8$$

and

$$-4 + -4 = -8$$

However, things get tricky when some of the numbers are negative, and some are positive.

Take 6 + (-4) as an example. First, take the absolute values of the numbers, which are 6 and 4. Second, subtract the smaller value from the larger. The equation becomes $6 - 4 = 2$. Third, place the sign of the original larger number on the sum. Here, 6 is the larger number, and it's positive, so the sum is 2.

Here's an example where the negative number has a larger absolute value: (-6) + 4. The first two steps are the same as the example above. However, on the third step, the negative sign must be placed on the sum, as the absolute value of (-6) is greater than 4. Thus, $-6 + 4 = -2$.

The absolute value of numbers implies that subtraction can be thought of as flipping the sign of the number following the subtraction sign and simply adding the two numbers. This means that subtracting a negative number will in fact be adding the positive absolute value of the negative number. Here are some examples:

$$-6 - 4 = -6 + -4 = -10$$

$$3 - -6 = 3 + 6 = 9$$

$$-3 - 2 = -3 + -2 = -5$$

Implications for Multiplication and Division

For multiplication and division, if both numbers are positive, then the product or quotient is always positive. If both numbers are negative, then the product or quotient is also positive. However, if the numbers have opposite signs, the product or quotient is always negative.

Simply put, the product in multiplication and quotient in division is always positive, unless the numbers have opposing signs, in which case it's negative. Here are some examples:

$$(-6) \times (-5) = 30$$

$$(-50) \div 10 = -5$$

$$8 \times |-7| = 56$$

$$(-48) \div (-6) = 8$$

If there are more than two numbers in a multiplication problem, then whether the product is positive or negative depends on the number of negative numbers in the problem. If there is an odd number of negatives, then the product is negative. If there is an even number of negative numbers, then the result is positive.

Here are some examples:

$$(-6) \times 5 \times (-2) \times (-4) = -240$$

$$(-6) \times 5 \times 2 \times (-4) = 240$$

Comparing and Ordering Numbers

A common question type asks test takers to order rational numbers from least to greatest or greatest to least. The numbers will come in a variety of formats, including decimals, percentages, roots, fractions, and whole numbers. These questions test for knowledge of different types of numbers and the ability to determine their respective values.

Comparing numbers often uses symbols to represent “greater than” and “less than.” Much like how "equals" is represented by a = sign, "greater than" is expressed by > and "less than" is represented by <. You should also be able to identify that "less than or equal to" is expressed by the inequality symbol ≤, and "greater than or equal” to is expressed as ≥.

Whether the question asks to order the numbers from greatest to least or least to greatest, the crux of the question is the same—convert the numbers into a common format. Generally, it’s easiest to write the numbers as whole numbers and decimals so they can be placed on a number line.

Follow these examples to understand this strategy.

1) Order the following rational numbers from greatest to least:

$$\sqrt{36}, 0.65, 78\%, \frac{3}{4}, 7, 90\%, \frac{5}{2}$$

Of the seven numbers, the whole number (7) and decimal (0.65) are already in an accessible form, so concentrate on the other five.

First, the square root of 36 equals 6. (If the test asks for the root of a non-perfect root, determine which two whole numbers the root lies between.) Next, convert the percentages to decimals. A percentage means "per hundred," so this conversion requires moving the decimal point two places to the left, leaving 0.78 and 0.9. Lastly, evaluate the fractions:

$$\frac{3}{4} = \frac{75}{100} = 0.75 \,; \frac{5}{2} = 2\frac{1}{2} = 2.5$$

Now, the only step left is to list the numbers in the requested order:

$$7, \sqrt{36}, \frac{5}{2}, 90\%, 78\%, \frac{3}{4}, 0.65$$

2) Order the following rational numbers from least to greatest:

$$2.5, \sqrt{9}, -10.5, 0.853, 175\%, \sqrt{4}, \frac{4}{5}$$

$$\sqrt{9} = 3$$

$$175\% = 1.75$$

$$\sqrt{4} = 2$$

$$\frac{4}{5} = 0.8$$

$$-10.5 < 0.8 < 0.853 < 1.75 < 2 < 3$$

From least to greatest, the answer is:

$$-10.5, \frac{4}{5}, 0.853, 175\%, \sqrt{4}, 2.5, \sqrt{9}$$

Solving Equations with One Variable

Solving equations with one variable is the process of isolating a variable on one side of the equation. The letters in an equation are **variables** as they stand for unknown quantities that you are trying to solve for. The numbers attached to the variables by multiplication are called **coefficients**. *X* is commonly used as a variable, though any letter can be used. For example, in $3x - 7 = 20$, the variable is $3x$, and it needs to be isolated. The numbers (also called **constants**) are -7 and 20. That means $3x$ needs to be on one side of the equals sign (either side is fine), and all the numbers need to be on the other side of the equals sign.

To accomplish this, the equation must be manipulated by performing opposite operations (or inverse operations) of what already exists. Remember that addition and subtraction are opposites and that multiplication and division are opposites. Any action taken to one side of the equation must be taken on the other side to maintain equality.

Since the 7 is being subtracted, it can be moved to the right side of the equation by adding seven to both sides:

$$3x - 7 = 20$$

$$3x - 7 + 7 = 20 + 7$$

$$3x = 27$$

Now that the variable $3x$ is on one side and the constants (now combined into one constant) are on the other side, the 3 needs to be moved to the right side. 3 and x are being multiplied together, so 3 then needs to be divided from each side.

$$\frac{3x}{3} = \frac{27}{3}$$

$$x = 9$$

Now that x has been completely isolated, we know its value.

The solution is found to be $x = 9$. This solution can be checked for accuracy by plugging $x = 9$ in the original equation. After simplifying the equation, $20 = 20$ is found, which is a true statement:

$$3 \times 9 - 7 = 20$$

$$27 - 7 = 20$$

$$20 = 20$$

Equations that require solving for a variable (**algebraic equations**) come in many forms. Here are some more examples:

No coefficient attached to the variable:

$$x + 8 = 20$$

$$x + 8 - 8 = 20 - 8$$

$$x = 12$$

A fractional coefficient:

$$\frac{1}{2}z + 24 = 36$$

$$\frac{1}{2}z + 24 - 24 = 36 - 24$$

$$\frac{1}{2}z = 12$$

Now we multiply the fraction by its inverse:

$$\frac{2}{1} \times \frac{1}{2}z = 12 \times \frac{2}{1}$$

$$z = 24$$

Multiple instances of x:

$$14x + x - 4 = 3x + 2$$

All instances of x can be combined.

$$15x - 4 = 3x + 2$$

$$15x - 4 + 4 = 3x + 2 + 4$$

$$15x = 3x + 6$$

$$15x - 3x = 3x + 6 - 3x$$

$$12x = 6$$

$$\frac{12x}{12} = \frac{6}{12}$$

$$x = \frac{1}{2}$$

Much like a scale factor can be written using an equation like $2A = B$, a **relationship** is represented by the equation $Y = kX$. X and Y are proportional because as values of X increase, the values of Y also increase. A relationship that is inversely proportional can be represented by the equation $Y = \frac{k}{X}$, where the value of Y decreases as the value of X increases and vice versa.

As an example, let's say the variable y is directly proportional to x. If $y = 3$ when $x = 5$, then what is y when $x = 20$?

The variable y is directly proportional to x, which means that whenever x is multiplied by a number, y is multiplied by that same number. When x changes from 5 to 20, it is multiplied by 4, so the original y value must also be multiplied by 4. That means $y = 3 \times 4 = 12$.

Solving Real-World Problems

Word problems can appear daunting, but don't let the verbiage psych you out. No matter the scenario or specifics, the key to answering them is to translate the words into a math problem. Always keep in mind what the question is asking and what operations could lead to that answer. The following word problem resembles one of the question types most frequently encountered on the exam.

Working with Money

Walter's Coffee Shop sells a variety of drinks and breakfast treats.

Price List	
Hot Coffee	\$2.00
Slow-Drip Iced Coffee	\$3.00
Latte	\$4.00
Muffin	\$2.00
Crepe	\$4.00
Egg Sandwich	\$5.00

Costs	
Hot Coffee	\$0.25
Slow-Drip Iced Coffee	\$0.75
Latte	\$1.00
Muffin	\$1.00
Crepe	\$2.00
Egg Sandwich	\$3.00

Walter's utilities, rent, and labor costs him \$500 per day. Today, Walter sold 200 hot coffees, 100 slow-drip iced coffees, 50 lattes, 75 muffins, 45 crepes, and 60 egg sandwiches. What was Walter's total profit today?

To accurately answer this type of question, determine the total cost of making his drinks and treats, then determine how much revenue he earned from selling those products. After arriving at these two totals, the profit is measured by deducting the total cost from the total revenue.

Walter's costs for today:

Item	Quantity	Cost Per Unit	Total Cost
Hot Coffee	200	$0.25	$50
Slow-Drip Iced Coffee	100	$0.75	$75
Latte	50	$1.00	$50
Muffin	75	$1.00	$75
Crepe	45	$2.00	$90
Egg Sandwich	60	$3.00	$180
Utilities, rent, and labor			$500
Total Costs			$1,020

Walter's revenue for today:

Item	Quantity	Revenue Per Unit	Total Revenue
Hot Coffee	200	$2.00	$400
Slow-Drip Iced Coffee	100	$3.00	$300
Latte	50	$4.00	$200
Muffin	75	$2.00	$150
Crepe	45	$4.00	$180
Egg Sandwich	60	$5.00	$300
Total Revenue			$1,530

Walter's Profit = **Revenue** – **Costs** = $1,530 – $1,020 = $510

Walter's total profit today was $510. Always make sure to label the answer to a word problem with the correct unit of measure, such as dollars in this case.

When you've completed the question, assess the reasonableness of your answer. Does your answer make sense in the context of the question? If your solution to the problem seems unreasonable, check your work to ensure that there aren't any obvious mistakes.

This strategy is applicable to other question types. For example, calculating salary after deductions, balancing a checkbook, and calculating a dinner bill are common word problems similar to business planning. Just remember to use the correct operations. When a balance is increased, use addition. When a balance is decreased, use subtraction. Common sense and organization are your greatest assets when answering word problems.

Using Percentages

Questions dealing with percentages can be difficult when they are phrased as word problems. These word problems almost always come in three varieties. The first type will ask to find what percentage of some number will equal another number. The second asks to determine what number is some percentage of another given number. The third will ask what number another number is a given percentage of.

One of the most important parts of correctly answering percentage word problems is to identify the numerator and the denominator. This fraction can then be converted into a percentage, as described above.

The following word problem shows how to make this conversion:

A department store carries several different types of footwear. The store is currently selling 8 athletic shoes, 7 dress shoes, and 5 sandals. What percentage of the store's footwear are sandals?

First, calculate what serves as the 'whole', as this will be the denominator. How many total pieces of footwear does the store sell? The store sells 20 different types (8 athletic + 7 dress + 5 sandals).

Second, what footwear type is the question specifically asking about? Sandals. Thus, 5 is the numerator.

Third, the resultant fraction must be expressed as a percentage. The first two steps indicate that $\frac{5}{20}$ of the footwear pieces are sandals. This fraction must now be converted into a percentage:

$$\frac{5}{20} \times \frac{5}{5} = \frac{25}{100} = 25\%$$

Percent Increase/Decrease

Problems dealing with percentages may involve an original value, a change in that value, and a percentage change. A problem will provide two pieces of information and ask to find the third. To do so, this formula is used: $\frac{change}{original\ value} \times 100 = \text{percent change}$.

The following word problem shows how to deal with percent increase/decrease:

Attendance at a baseball stadium has dropped 16% from last year. Last year's average attendance was 40,000. What is this year's average attendance?

Using the formula and information, the change is unknown (x), the original value is 40,000, and the percent change is 16%. The formula can be written as: $\frac{x}{40{,}000} \times 100 = 16$. When solving for x, it is determined the change was 6,400. The problem asked for this year's average attendance, so to calculate, the change (6,400) is subtracted from last year's attendance (40,000) to determine this year's average attendance is 33,600.

Using Estimation Strategies and Rounding Rules

Estimation

Estimation is finding a value that is close to a solution but is not the exact answer. For example, if there are values in the thousands to be multiplied, then each value can be estimated to the nearest thousand and the calculation performed. This value provides an approximate solution that can be determined very quickly. The derived result after completing the problem can then be evaluated by its nearness to the expected answer.

When estimating measurements (for area, length, weight, or volume), apply real-world knowledge to better understand what a problem is asking. Try to make a reasonable assumption by comparing the information that the question gives you to something that you can mentally picture. This gives you a starting point from which you can quickly understand the problem. When you complete the question, you can compare your solution to your estimated guess to see if it makes sense.

Rounding Numbers

It's often convenient to round a number, which means giving an approximate figure to make it easier to compare amounts or perform mental math. Round up when the digit is 5 or more. The digit used to determine the rounding, and all subsequent digits, become 0, and the selected place value is increased by 1. Here are some examples:

> 75 rounded to the nearest ten is 80
> 380 rounded to the nearest hundred is 400
> 22.697 rounded to the nearest hundredth is 22.70

Round down when rounding on any digit that is below 5. The rounded digit, and all subsequent digits, becomes 0, and the preceding digit stays the same. Here are some examples:

> 92 rounded to the nearest ten is 90
> 839 rounded to the nearest hundred is 800
> 22.643 rounded to the nearest hundredth is 22.64

Determining the Reasonableness of Results

When solving math word problems, the solution obtained should make sense within the given scenario. The step of checking the solution will reduce the possibility of a calculation error or a solution that may be **mathematically** correct but not applicable in the real world. Consider the following scenarios:

A problem states that Lisa got 24 out of 32 questions correct on a test and asks to find the percentage of correct answers. To solve the problem, a student divided 32 by 24 to get 1.33, and then multiplied by 100 to get 133 percent. By examining the solution within the context of the problem, the student should recognize that getting all 32 questions correct will produce a perfect score of 100 percent. Therefore, a score of 133 percent with 8 incorrect answers does not make sense, and the calculations should be checked.

A problem states that the maximum weight on a bridge cannot exceed 22,000 pounds. The problem asks to find the maximum number of cars that can be on the bridge at one time if each car weighs 4,000 pounds. To solve this problem, a student divided 22,000 by 4,000 to get an answer of 5.5. By examining the solution within the context of the problem, the student should recognize that although the calculations are mathematically correct, the solution does not make sense. Half of a car on a bridge is not possible, so the student should determine that a maximum of 5 cars can be on the bridge at the same time.

Mental Math Estimation

Once a result is determined to be logical within the context of a given problem, the result should be evaluated by its nearness to the expected answer. This is performed by approximating given values to perform mental math. Numbers should be rounded to the nearest value possible to check the initial results.

Consider the following example: A problem states that a customer is buying a new sound system for their home. The customer purchases a stereo for $435, 2 speakers for $67 each, and the necessary cables for $12. The customer chooses an option that allows him to spread the costs over equal payments for 4 months. How much will the monthly payments be?

After making calculations for the problem, a student determines that the monthly payment will be $145.25. To check the accuracy of the results, the student rounds each cost to the nearest ten ($440 + 70 + 70 + 10$) and determines that the total is approximately \$590. Dividing by 4 months gives an approximate monthly payment of \$147.50. Therefore, the student can conclude that the solution of \$145.25 is very close to what should be expected.

When rounding, the place-value that is used in rounding can make a difference. Suppose the student had rounded to the nearest hundred for the estimation. The result ($400 + 100 + 100 + 0 = 600;\ 600 \div 4 = 150$) will show that the answer is reasonable but not as close to the actual value as rounding to the nearest ten. Similarly, ensure when rounding fractions and mixed numbers that you are rounding to an appropriate place-value to find a close approximation of the answer.

Using Proportions

Much like a scale factor can be written using an equation like $2A = B$, a **relationship** is represented by the equation $Y = kX$. X and Y are proportional because as values of X increase, the values of Y also increase. A relationship that is inversely proportional can be represented by the equation $Y = \frac{k}{X}$, where the value of *Y* decreases as the value of *X* increases and vice versa.

Proportional reasoning can be used to solve problems involving ratios, percentages, and averages. Ratios can be used in setting up proportions and solving them to find unknowns. For example, if a student completes an average of 10 pages of math homework in 3 nights, how long would it take the student to complete 22 pages? Both ratios can be written as fractions. The second ratio would contain the unknown.

The following proportion represents this problem, where x is the unknown number of nights:

$$\frac{10 \text{ pages}}{3 \text{ nights}} = \frac{22 \text{ pages}}{x \text{ nights}}$$

Solving this proportion entails cross-multiplying and results in the following equation: $10x = 22 \times 3$. Simplifying and solving for x results in the exact solution: $x = 6.6$ nights. The result would be rounded up to 7 because the homework would actually be completed on the 7th night.

The following problem uses ratios involving percentages:

> If 20% of the class is girls and 30 students are in the class, how many girls are in the class?

To set up this problem, it is helpful to use the common proportion:

$$\frac{\%}{100} = \frac{is}{of}$$

Within the proportion, % is the percentage of girls, 100 is the total percentage of the class, *is* is the number of girls, and *of* is the total number of students in the class. Most percentage problems can be written using this language. To solve this problem, the proportion should be set up as $\frac{20}{100} = \frac{x}{30}$ and then solved for x. Cross-multiplying results in the equation $20 \times 30 = 100x$, which results in the solution $x = 6$. There are 6 girls in the class.

Ratios can be used to solve problems that concern length, volume, and other units. For example, A problem may ask for the volume of a cone that has a radius, $r = 7$ m and a height, $h = 16$ m. Referring to the formulas provided on the test, the volume of a cone is given as: $V = \pi r^2 \frac{h}{3}$, where r is the radius, and h is the height. Plugging $r = 7$ and $h = 16$ into the formula, the following is obtained:

$$V = \pi(7^2)\frac{16}{3}$$

Therefore, the volume of the cone is found to be approximately 821 m^3. Sometimes, answers in different units are sought. If this problem wanted the answer in liters, 821 m^3 would need to be converted. Using the equivalence statement $1\text{ m}^3 = 1{,}000\text{ L}$, the following ratio would be used to solve for liters:

$$821\text{ m}^3 \times \frac{1{,}000\text{ L}}{1\text{ m}^3}$$

Cubic meters in the numerator and denominator cancel each other out, and the answer is converted to 821,000 liters, or 8.21×10^5 L.

Other conversions can also be made between different given and final units. If the temperature in a pool is 30°C, what is the temperature of the pool in degrees Fahrenheit? To convert these units, an equation is used relating Celsius to Fahrenheit. The following equation is used:

$$T_{°F} = 1.8T_{°C} + 32$$

Plugging in the given temperature and solving the equation for T yields the result:

$$T_{°F} = 1.8(30) + 32 = 86°F$$

Units in both the metric system and U.S. customary system are widely used.

Here are some more examples of how to solve for proportions:

1) $\frac{75\%}{90\%} = \frac{25\%}{x}$

To solve for x, the fractions must be cross multiplied:

$$(75\%x = 90\% \times 25\%)$$

To make things easier, let's convert the percentages to decimals:

$$(0.9 \times 0.25 = 0.225 = 0.75x)$$

To get rid of x's coefficient, each side must be divided by that same coefficient to get the answer $x = 0.3$. The question could ask for the answer as a percentage or fraction in lowest terms, which are 30% and $\frac{3}{10}$, respectively.

2) $\frac{x}{12} = \frac{30}{96}$

Cross-multiply: $96x = 30 \times 12$
Multiply: $96x = 360$
Divide: $x = 360 \div 96$
Answer: $x = 3.75$

3) $\frac{0.5}{3} = \frac{x}{6}$

Cross-multiply: $3x = 0.5 \times 6$

Multiply: $3x = 3$
Divide: $x = 3 \div 3$
Answer: $x = 1$

You may have noticed there's a faster way to arrive at the answer. If there is an obvious operation being performed on the proportion, the same operation can be used on the other side of the proportion to solve for x. For example, in the first practice problem, 75% became 25% when divided by 3, and upon doing the same to 90%, the correct answer of 30% would have been found with much less legwork. However, these questions aren't always so intuitive, so it's a good idea to work through the steps, even if the answer seems apparent from the outset.

Using Ratios and Rates of Change

Ratios are used to show the relationship between two quantities. The ratio of oranges to apples in the grocery store may be 3 to 2. That means that for every 3 oranges, there are 2 apples. This comparison can be expanded to represent the actual number of oranges and apples, such as 36 oranges to 24 apples. Another example may be the number of boys to girls in a math class. If the ratio of boys to girls is given as 2 to 5, that means there are 2 boys to every 5 girls in the class. Ratios can also be compared if the units in each ratio are the same. The ratio of boys to girls in the math class can be compared to the ratio of boys to girls in a science class by stating which ratio is higher and which is lower.

Rates are used to compare two quantities with different units. **Unit rates** are the simplest form of rate. With unit rates, the denominator in the comparison of two units is one. For example, if someone can type at a rate of 1,000 words in 5 minutes, then their unit rate for typing is $\frac{1,000}{5} = 200$ words in one minute or 200 words per minute. Any rate can be converted into a unit rate by dividing to make the denominator one. 1,000 words in 5 minutes has been converted into the unit rate of 200 words per minute.

Ratios and rates can be used together to convert rates into different units. For example, if someone is driving 50 kilometers per hour, that rate can be converted into miles per hour by using a ratio known as the **conversion factor**. Since the given value contains kilometers and the final answer needs to be in miles, the ratio relating miles to kilometers needs to be used. There are 0.62 miles in 1 kilometer. This, written as a ratio and in fraction form, is $\frac{0.62 \text{ miles}}{1 \text{ km}}$. To convert 50km/hour into miles per hour, the following conversion needs to be set up:

$$\frac{50 \text{ km}}{\text{hour}} \times \frac{0.62 \text{ miles}}{1 \text{ km}} = 31 \text{ miles per hour}$$

The ratio between two similar geometric figures is called the **scale factor**. For example, a problem may depict two similar triangles, A and B. The scale factor from the smaller triangle A to the larger triangle B is given as 2 because the length of the corresponding side of the larger triangle, 16, is twice the corresponding side on the smaller triangle, 8. This scale factor can also be used to find the value of a missing side, x, in triangle A. Since the scale factor from the smaller triangle (A) to larger one (B) is 2, the larger corresponding side in triangle B (given as 25) can be divided by 2 to find the missing side in A (x = 12.5). The scale factor can also be represented in the equation $2A = B$ because two times the lengths of A gives the corresponding lengths of B. This is the idea behind similar triangles.

Unit Rate

Unit rate word problems will ask to calculate the rate or quantity of something in a different value. For example, a problem might say that a car drove a certain number of miles in a certain number of minutes and then ask how many miles per hour the car was traveling. These questions involve solving proportions. Consider the following examples:

1) Alexandra made $96 during the first 3 hours of her shift as a temporary worker at a law office. She will continue to earn money at this rate until she finishes in 5 more hours. How much does Alexandra make per hour? How much will Alexandra have made at the end of the day?

This problem can be solved in two ways. The first is to set up a proportion, as the rate of pay is constant. The second is to determine her hourly rate, multiply the 5 hours by that rate, and then add the $96.

To set up a proportion, put the money already earned over the hours already worked on one side of an equation. The other side has x over 8 hours (the total hours worked in the day). It looks like this:

$$\frac{96}{3} = \frac{x}{8}$$

Now, cross-multiply to get $768 = 3x$. To get x, divide by 3, which leaves $x = 256$. Alternatively, as x is the numerator of one of the proportions, multiplying by its denominator will reduce the solution by one step. Thus, Alexandra will make \$256 at the end of the day. To calculate her hourly rate, divide the total by 8, giving \$32 per hour.

Alternatively, it is possible to figure out the hourly rate by dividing \$96 by 3 hours to get \$32 per hour. Now her total pay can be figured by multiplying \$32 per hour by 8 hours, which comes out to \$256.

2) Jonathan is reading a novel. So far, he has read 215 of the 335 total pages. It takes Jonathan 25 minutes to read 10 pages, and the rate is constant. How long does it take Jonathan to read one page? How much longer will it take him to finish the novel? Express the answer in time.

To calculate how long it takes Jonathan to read one page, divide the 25 minutes by 10 pages to determine the page per minute rate. Thus, it takes 2.5 minutes to read one page.

Jonathan must read 120 more pages to complete the novel. (This is calculated by subtracting the pages already read from the total.) Now, multiply his rate per page by the number of pages. Thus,

$$120 \times 2.5 = 300$$

Expressed in time, 300 minutes is equal to 5 hours.

3) At a hotel, $\frac{4}{5}$ of the 120 rooms are booked for Saturday. On Sunday, $\frac{3}{4}$ of the rooms are booked. On which day are more of the rooms booked, and by how many more?

The first step is to calculate the number of rooms booked for each day. Do this by multiplying the fraction of the rooms booked by the total number of rooms.

Saturday: $\frac{4}{5} \times 120 = \frac{4}{5} \times \frac{120}{1} = \frac{480}{5} = 96 \text{ rooms}$

Sunday: $\frac{3}{4} \times 120 = \frac{3}{4} \times \frac{120}{1} = \frac{360}{4} = 90 \text{ rooms}$

Thus, more rooms were booked on Saturday by 6 rooms.

4) In a veterinary hospital, the veterinarian-to-pet ratio is 1:9. The ratio is always constant. If there are 45 pets in the hospital, how many veterinarians are currently in the veterinary hospital?

Set up a proportion to solve for the number of veterinarians:

$$\frac{1}{9} = \frac{x}{45}$$

Cross-multiplying results in $9x = 45$, which works out to 5 veterinarians.

Alternatively, as there are always 9 times as many pets as veterinarians, it is possible to divide the number of pets (45) by 9. This also arrives at the correct answer of 5 veterinarians.

5) At a general practice law firm, 30% of the lawyers work solely on tort cases. If 9 lawyers work solely on tort cases, how many lawyers work at the firm?

First, solve for the total number of lawyers working at the firm, which will be represented here with x. The problem states that 9 lawyers work solely on torts cases, and they make up 30% of the total lawyers at the firm. Thus, 30% multiplied by the total, x, will equal 9. Written as equation, this is:

$$30\% \times x = 9$$

It's easier to deal with the equation after converting the percentage to a decimal, leaving $0.3x = 9$. Thus, $x = \frac{9}{0.3} =$ 30 lawyers working at the firm.

6) Xavier was hospitalized with pneumonia. He was originally given 35 mg of antibiotics. Later, after his condition continued to worsen, Xavier's dosage was increased to 60 mg. What was the percent increase of the antibiotics? Round the percentage to the nearest tenth.

An increase or decrease in percentage can be calculated by dividing the difference in amounts by the original amount and multiplying by 100. Written as an equation, the formula is:

$$\frac{new\ quantity\ - old\ quantity}{old\ quantity} \times 100$$

Here, the question states that the dosage was increased from 35 mg to 60 mg, so these are plugged into the formula to find the percentage increase.

$$\frac{60 - 35}{35} \times 100 = \frac{25}{35} \times 100$$

$$0\,.7142 \times 100 = 71.4\%$$

Rate of Change

Rate of change for any line calculates the steepness of the line over a given interval. Rate of change is also known as the slope or rise/run. The TEAS will focus on the rate of change for linear functions which are straight lines. The slope is given by the change in y divided by the change in x, so the formula looks like this:

$$slope = \frac{y_2 - y_1}{x_2 - x_1}$$

In the graph below, two points are plotted. The first has the coordinates of $(0, 1)$ and the second point is $(2, 3)$. Remember that the x coordinate is always placed first in coordinate pairs. Work from left to right when identifying coordinates. Thus, the point on the left is point 1 $(0, 1)$,and the point on the right is point 2 $(2, 3)$.

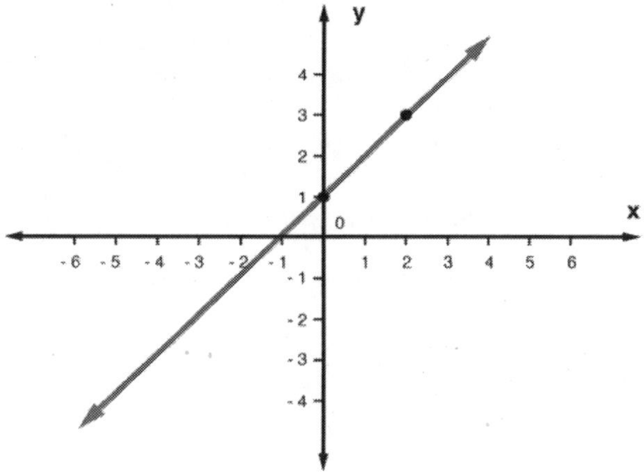

Now, we can plug those numbers into the equation:

$$slope = \frac{3-1}{2-0}$$

$$slope = \frac{2}{2}$$

$$slope = 1$$

This means that for every increase of 1 for x, y also increased by 1. You can see this in the line. When x equalled 0, y equalled 1, and when x was increased to 1, y equalled 2.

Slope can be thought of as determining the rise over run:

$$slope = \frac{rise}{run}$$

The rise being the change vertically on the y axis and the run being the change horizontally on the x axis.

Given the Slope and -Intercept

Linear equations are commonly written in slope-intercept form, $y = mx + b$, where m represents the slope of the line and b represents the y-intercept. The slope is the rate of change between the variables, usually expressed as a whole number or fraction. The y-intercept is the value of y when $x = 0$ (the point where the line intercepts the y-axis on a graph). Given the slope and y-intercept of a line, the values are substituted for m and b into the equation. A line with a slope of $\frac{1}{2}$ and y-intercept of -2 would have an equation:

$$y = \frac{1}{2}x - 2$$

Using Expressions, Equations, And Inequalities

To translate a word problem into an expression, look for a series of key words indicating addition, subtraction, multiplication, or division:

Addition: add, altogether, together, plus, increased by, more than, in all, sum, and total
Subtraction: minus, less than, difference, decreased by, fewer than, remain, and take away
Multiplication: *times*, *twice*, *of*, *double*, and *triple*
Division: divided by, cut up, half, quotient of, split, and shared equally

By identifying the variables (unknown quantities) in the word problem, you can use the identified operations to create a mathematical expression, equation, or inequality. Solve the real-world problem defined in the question, making sure that your answer uses the correct units of measure.

If a question asks to give words to a mathematical expression and says "equals," then an = sign must be included in the answer. Similarly, "less than or equal to" is expressed by the inequality symbol ≤, and "greater than or equal to" is expressed as ≥. Furthermore, "less than" is represented by <, and "greater than" is expressed by >.

Measurement and Data

Table, Charts, and Graphs

Interpretation of Tables, Charts, and Graphs

Data can be represented in many ways. It is important to be able to organize the data into categories that could be represented using one of these methods. Equally important is the ability to read these types of diagrams and interpret their meaning.

Data in Tables

One of the most common ways to express data is in a table. The primary reason for plugging data into a table is to make interpretation more convenient. It's much easier to look at the table than to analyze results in a narrative paragraph. When analyzing a table, pay close attention to the title, variables, and data.

Let's analyze a theoretical antibiotic study. The study has 6 groups, named A through F, and each group receives a different dose of medicine. The results of the study are listed in the table below.

Results of Antibiotic Studies

Group	Dosage of Antibiotics in milligrams (mg)	Efficacy (% of participants cured)
A	0 mg	20%
B	20 mg	40%
C	40 mg	75%
D	60 mg	95%
E	80 mg	100%
F	100 mg	100%

Tables generally list the title immediately above the data. The title should succinctly explain what is listed below. Here, "Results of Antibiotic Studies" informs the audience that the data pertains to the results of a scientific study on antibiotics.

Identifying the variables at play is one of the most important parts of interpreting data. Remember, the independent variable is intentionally altered, and its change is independent of the other variables. Here, the dosage of antibiotics administered to the different groups is the independent variable. The study is intentionally manipulating the strength of the medicine to study the related results. Efficacy is the dependent variable since its results **depend** on a different variable, the dose of antibiotics. Generally, the independent variable will be listed before the dependent variable in tables.

Also, pay close attention to the variables' labels. Here, the dose is expressed in milligrams (mg) and efficacy in percentages (%). Keep an eye out for questions referencing data in a different unit of measurement, or questions asking for a raw number when only the percentage is listed.

Now that the nature of the study and variables at play have been identified, the data itself needs be interpreted. Group A did not receive any of the medicine. As discussed earlier, Group A is the control, as it reflects the amount of people cured in the same timeframe without medicine. It's important to see that efficacy positively correlates with the dosage of medicine. A question using this study might ask for the lowest dose of antibiotics to achieve 100% efficacy. Although Group E and Group F both achieve 100% efficacy, it's important to note that Group E reaches 100% with a lower dose.

Data in Graphs

Graphs provide a visual representation of data. The variables are placed on the two axes. The bottom of the graph is referred to as the horizontal axis or x-axis. The left-hand side of the graph is known as the vertical axis or y-axis. Typically, the independent variable is placed on the x-axis, and the dependent variable is located on the y-axis. Sometimes the x-axis is a timeline, and the dependent variables for different trials or groups have been measured throughout points in time; time is still an independent variable but is not always immediately thought of as the independent variable being studied.

The most common types of graphs are the bar graph and the line graph.

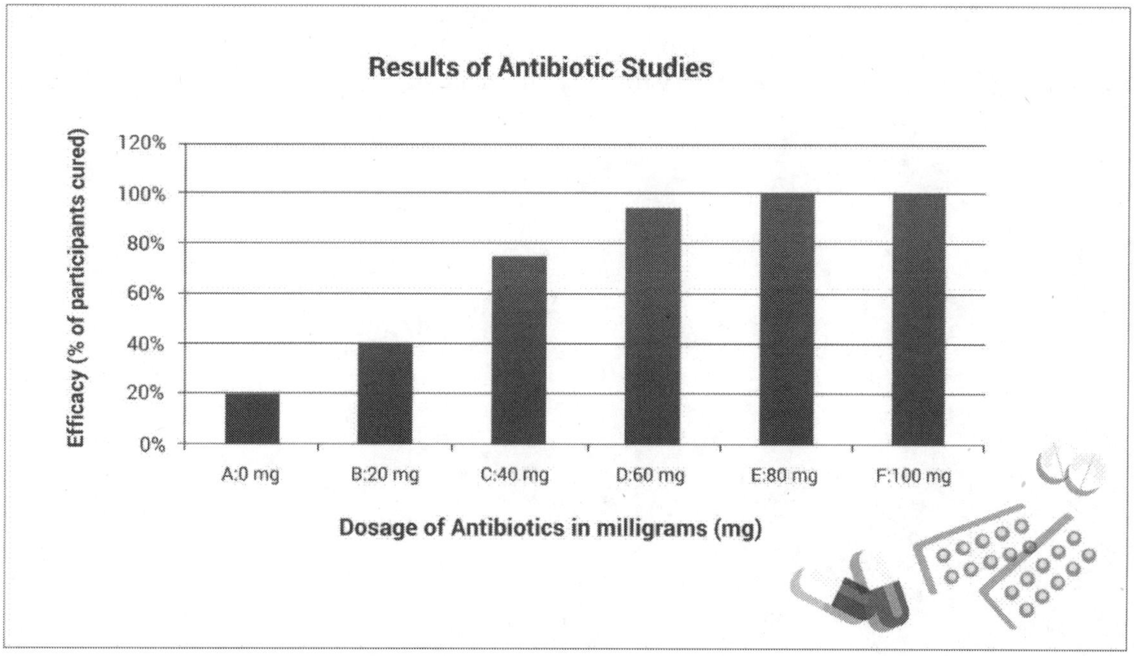

The **bar graph** above expresses the data from the table entitled "Results of Antibiotic Studies." To interpret the data for each group in the study, look at the top of their bars and read the corresponding efficacy on the y-axis.

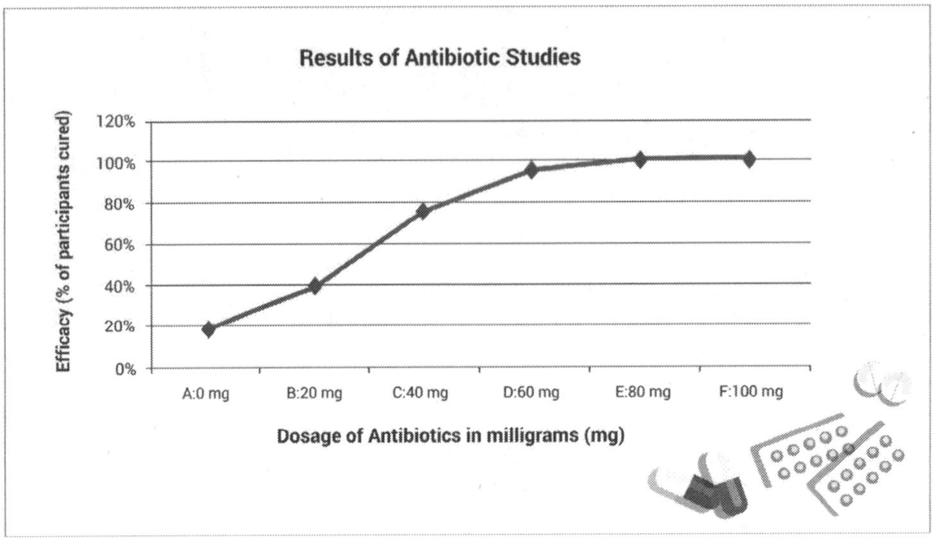

Here, the same data is expressed on a **line graph**. The points on the line correspond with each data entry. Reading the data on the line graph works like the bar graph. The data trend is measured by the slope of the line.

Data in Other Charts

Chart is a broad term that refers to a variety of ways to represent data.

To graph relations, the **Cartesian plane** is used. This means to think of the plane as being given a grid of squares, with one direction being the x-axis and the other direction the y-axis. Generally, the independent variable is placed along the horizontal axis, and the dependent variable is placed along the vertical axis. Any point on the plane can be specified by saying how far to go along the x-axis and how far along the y-axis with a pair of numbers (x, y). Specific values for these pairs can be given names such as $C = (-1, 3)$.

Negative values mean to move left or down; positive values mean to move right or up. The point where the axes cross one another is called the **origin**. The origin has coordinates $(0, 0)$ and is usually called O when given a specific label. An illustration of the Cartesian plane, along with the plotted points $(2, 1)$ and $(-1, -1)$, is below.

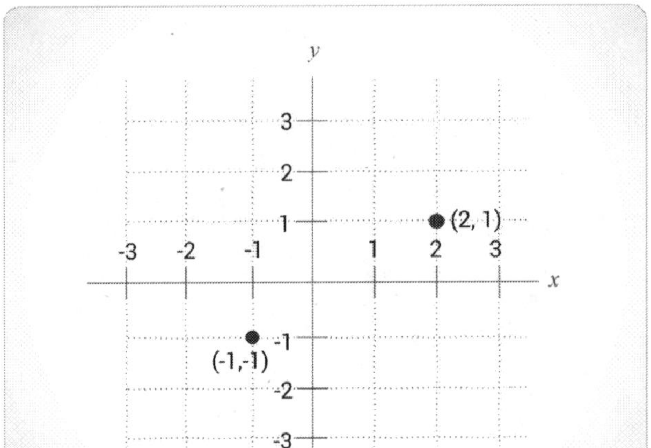

A **line plot** is a diagram that shows quantity of data along a number line. It is a quick way to record data in a structure similar to a bar graph without needing to do the required shading of a bar graph. Here is an example of a line plot:

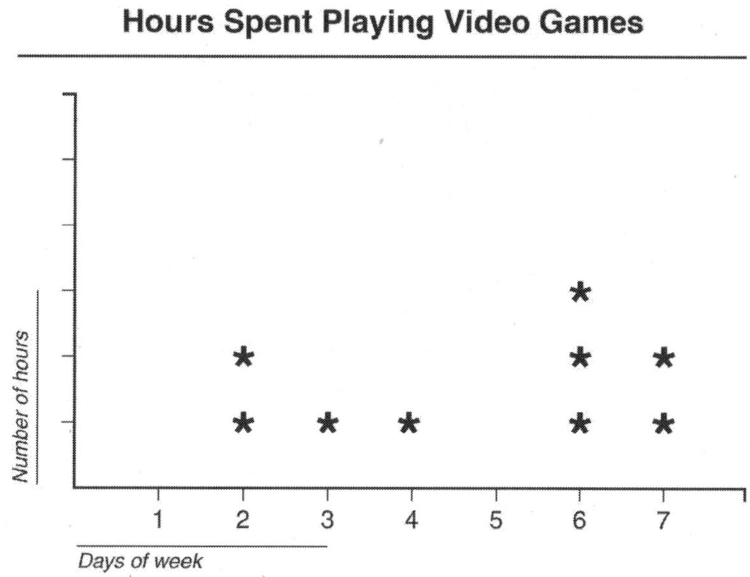

A **tally chart** is a diagram in which tally marks are utilized to represent data. Tally marks are a means of showing a quantity of objects within a specific classification. Here is an example of a tally chart:

Number of days with rain	Number of weeks
0	||
1	𝍸 |
2	𝍸 ||||
3	𝍸 𝍸 𝍸
4	𝍸
5	𝍸 |
6	𝍸
7	|

Data is often recorded using fractions, such as half a mile, and understanding fractions is critical because of their popular use in real-world applications. Also, it is extremely important to label values with their units when using data. For example, regarding length, the number 2 is meaningless unless it is attached to a unit. A measurement of 2 cm is much different than 2 miles.

A **picture graph** is a diagram that shows pictorial representations of data being discussed. The symbols used can represent a certain number of objects. Notice how each fruit symbol in the following graph represents a count of two fruits. One drawback of picture graphs is that they can be less accurate if each symbol represents a large number. For example, if each banana symbol represented ten bananas, and students consumed 22 bananas, it may be challenging to draw and interpret two and one-fifth bananas as a frequency count of 22.

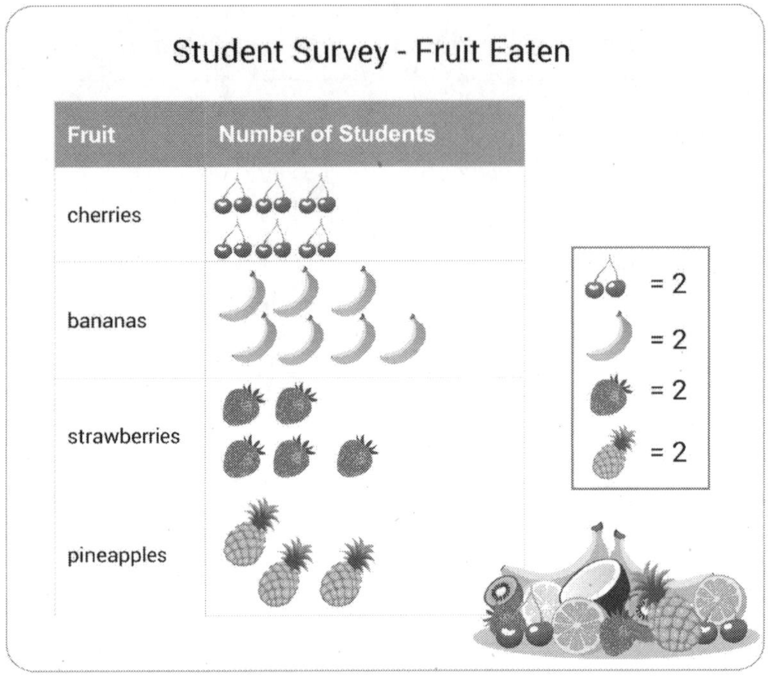

A circle graph, also called a pie chart, shows categorical data with each category representing a percentage of the whole data set. To make a circle graph, the percent of the data set for each category must be determined. To do so, the frequency of the category is divided by the total number of data points and converted to a percent. For example, if 80 people were asked what their favorite sport is and 20 responded basketball, basketball makes up 25% of the data ($\frac{20}{80} = 0.25 = 25\%$). Each category in a data set is represented by a **slice** of the circle proportionate to its percentage of the whole.

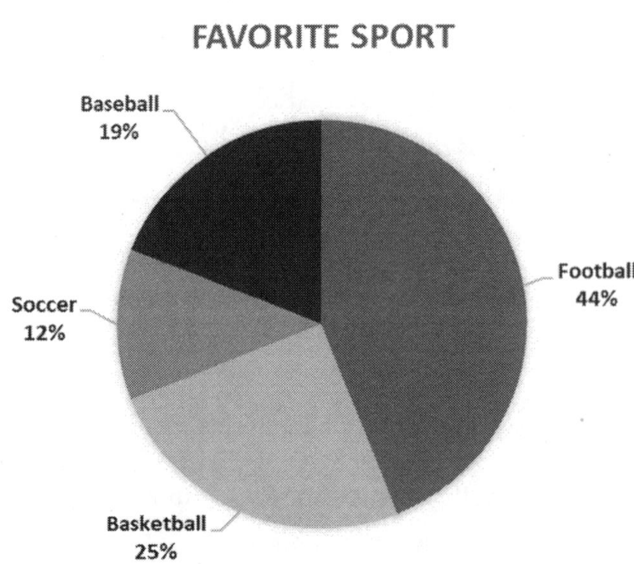

A scatter plot displays the relationship between two variables. Values for the independent variable, typically denoted by x, are paired with values for the dependent variable, typically denoted by y. Each set of corresponding values are written as an ordered pair (x, y). To construct the graph, a coordinate grid is labeled with the x-axis representing the independent variable and the y-axis representing the dependent variable. Each ordered pair is graphed.

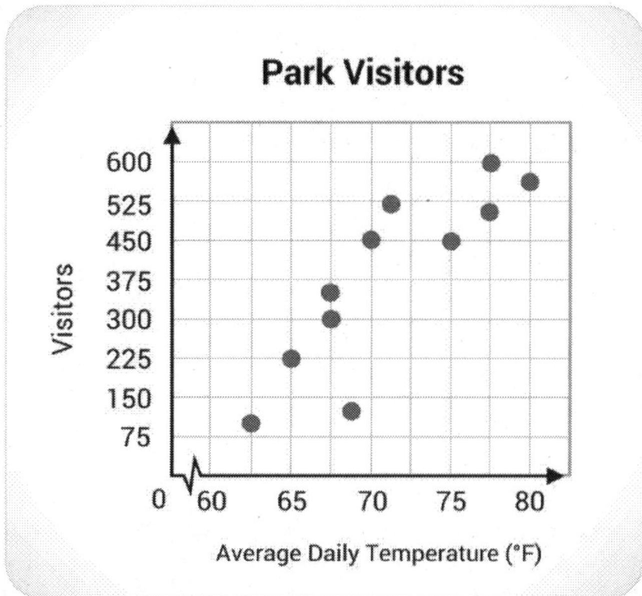

Like a scatter plot, a line graph compares two variables that change continuously, typically over time. Paired data values (ordered pairs) are plotted on a coordinate grid with the x- and y-axis representing the two variables. A line is drawn from each point to the next, going from left to right. A double line graph simply displays two sets of data that contain values for the same two variables. The double line graph below displays the profit for given years (two variables) for Company A and Company B (two data sets).

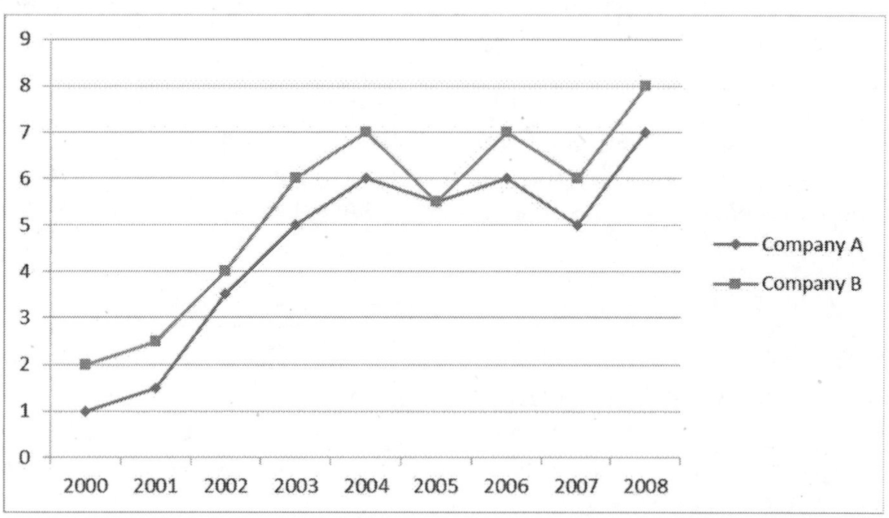

Choosing the appropriate graph to display a data set depends on what type of data is included in the set and what information must be shown.

Scatter plots and line graphs can be used to display data consisting of two variables. Examples include height and weight, or distance and time. A correlation between the variables is determined by examining the points on the graph. Line graphs are used if each value for one variable pairs with a distinct value for the other variable. Line graphs show relationships between variables.

Interpreting Competing Data

Be careful of questions with competing studies. These questions will ask the student to interpret which of two studies shows the greater amount or the higher rate of change between two results.

Here's an example. A research facility runs studies on two different antibiotics: Drug A and Drug B. The Drug A study includes 1,000 participants and cures 600 people. The Drug B study includes 200 participants and cures 150 people. Which drug is more successful?

The first step is to determine the percentage of each drug's rate of success. Drug A was successful in curing 60% of participants, while Drug B achieved a 75% success rate. Thus, Drug B is more successful based on these studies, even though it cured fewer people.

Sample size and experiment consistency should also be considered when answering questions based on competing studies. Is one study significantly larger than the other? In the antibiotics example, the Drug A study is five times larger than Drug B. Thus, Drug B's higher efficacy could be a result of the smaller sample size, rather than the quality of the drug.

Consistency between studies is directly related to sample size. Let's say the research facility elects to conduct more studies on Drug B. In the next study, there are 400 participants, and 200 are cured. The success rate of the second study is 50%. The results are clearly inconsistent with the first study, which means more testing is needed to determine the drug's efficacy. A hallmark of mathematical or scientific research is repeatability. Studies should be consistent and repeatable, with an appropriately large sample size, before drawing extensive conclusions.

Evaluate Data Sets, Tables, Charts, and Graphs Using Statistics

Mean, Median, and Mode

The center of a set of data (statistical values) can be represented by its mean, median, or mode. These are sometimes referred to as measures of central tendency.

Mean

The first property that can be defined for this set of data is the **mean**. This is the same as the average To find the mean, add up all the data points, then divide by the total number of data points. For example, suppose that in a class of 10 students, the scores on a test were 50, 60, 65, 65, 75, 80, 85, 85, 90, 100. Therefore, the average test score will be:

$$\frac{50+60+65+65+75+80+85+85+90+100}{10}=75.5$$

The mean is a useful number if the distribution of data is normal (more on this later), which means that the frequency of different outcomes has a single peak and is roughly equally distributed on both sides of that peak. However, it is less useful in some cases where the data might be split or where there are some **outliers**. Outliers are data points that are far from the rest of the data. For example, suppose there are 10 executives and 90 employees at a company. The executives make $1,000 per hour, and the employees make $10 per hour.

Therefore, the average pay rate will be:

$$\frac{\$1{,}000 \times 11 + \$10 \times 90}{100} = \$119 \text{ per hour}$$

In this case, this average is not very descriptive since it's not close to the actual pay of the executives *or* the employees.

Median

Another useful measurement is the **median**. In a data set, the median is the point in the middle. The middle refers to the point where half the data comes before it and half comes after, when the data is recorded in numerical order. For instance, these are the speeds of the fastball of a pitcher during the last inning that he pitched (in order from least to greatest):

90, 92, 93, 93, 95, 96, 97, 97, 97

There are nine total numbers, so the middle or **median** number is the 5th one, which is 95.

In cases where the number of data points is an even number, then the average of the two middle points is taken. In the previous example of test scores, the two middle points are 75 and 80. Since there is no single point, the average of these two scores needs to be found. The average is:

$$\frac{75 + 80}{2} = 77.5$$

The median is generally a good value to use if there are a few outliers in the data. It prevents those outliers from affecting the "middle" value as much as when using the mean.

Since an outlier is a data point that is far from most of the other data points in a data set, this means an outlier also is any point that is far from the median of the data set. The outliers can have a substantial effect on the mean of a data set, but they usually do not change the median or mode, or do not change them by a large quantity. For example, consider the data set (3, 5, 6, 6, 6, 8). This has a median of 6 and a mode of 6, with a mean of $\frac{34}{6} \approx 5.67$. Now, suppose a new data point of 1,000 is added so that the data set is now (3, 5, 6, 6, 6, 8, 1,000). The median and mode, which are both still 6, remain unchanged. However, the average is now $\frac{1034}{7}$, which is approximately 147.7. In this case, the median and mode will be better descriptions for most of the data points.

Outliers in a given data set are sometimes the result of an error by the experimenter, but oftentimes, they are perfectly valid data points that must be taken into consideration.

Mode

One additional measure to describe a set of data is the **mode**. This is the data point that appears most frequently. If two or more data points all tie for the most frequent appearance, then each of them is considered a mode. In the case of the test scores, where the numbers were 50, 60, 65, 65, 75, 80, 85, 85, 90, 100, there are two modes: 65 and 85.

Describing a Set of Data

A set of data can be described in terms of its center, spread, shape and any unusual features. To determine the range of a set of data, find the minimum and maximum value of the data points within the set. The range is calculated by subtracting the lowest value from the highest value in the set. Find the absolute value of the solution, as measuring the distance between the values must be a positive number.

The center of a data set can be measured by its mean, median, or mode. The spread of a data set refers to how far the data points are from the center (mean or median). A data set with all its data points clustered around the center will have a small spread. A data set covering a wide range of values will have a large spread.

When a data set is displayed as a graph like the one below, the shape indicates if a sample is normally distributed, symmetrical, or has measures of skewness. When graphed, a data set with a normal distribution will resemble a bell curve.

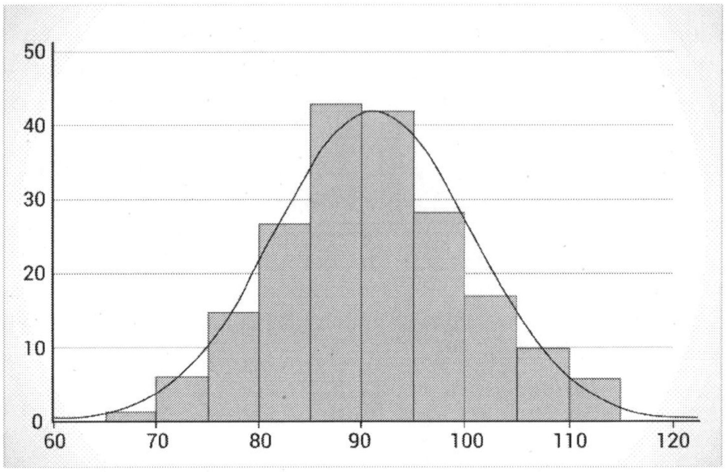

If the data set is symmetrical, each half of the graph when divided at the center is a mirror image of the other. If the graph has fewer data points to the right, the data is skewed right. If it has fewer data points to the left, the data is skewed left.

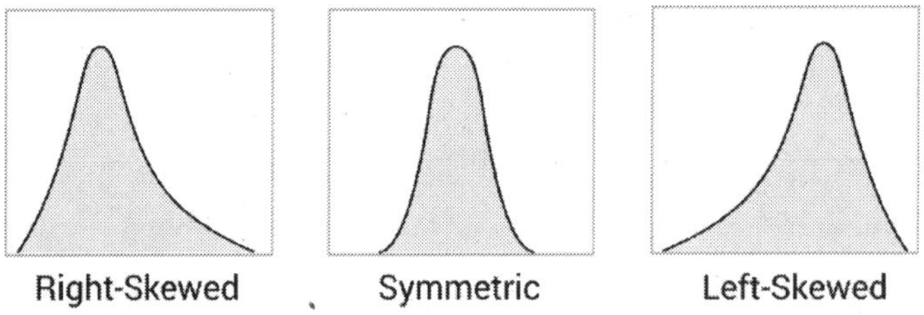

A description of a data set should include any unusual features such as gaps or outliers. A gap is a span within the range of the data set containing no data points. An outlier is a data point with a value either extremely large or extremely small when compared to the other values in the set.

The graphs above can be referred to as **unimodal** since they all have a single peak. In contrast to **bimodal** graph has two peaks.

Correlation

An **X-Y diagram**, also known as a scatter diagram, visually displays the relationship between two variables. The independent variable is placed on the ***x*-axis**, or **horizontal axis**, and the **dependent variable** is placed on the ***y*-axis**, or **vertical axis**.

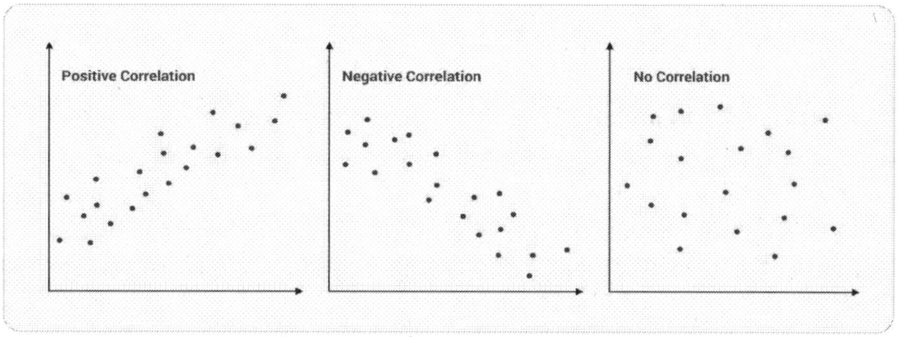

As shown in the figures above, an X-Y diagram may demonstrate a positive, negative, or no correlation between the two variables. In the first scatter plot, as the x increases, y increases as well. The opposite is true as well: as y increases, x also increases. Thus, there is a **positive correlation** (or **direct correlation**) because one variable appears to positively affect the other variable. If the line of best-fit has a negative slope (*y*-values decrease as *x*-values increase), then a **negative correlation** (or **inverse correlation**) exists. If a line of best-fit cannot be drawn, then no correlation exists. A positive or negative correlation can also be categorized as strong or weak, depending on how closely the points are grouped around the line of best fit.

It's important to note, however, that a positive correlation between two variables doesn't equate to a cause-and-effect relationship. For example, a positive correlation between labor hours and units produced may not equate to a cause-and-effect relationship between the two. Any instance of correlation only indicates how likely the presence of one variable is in the instance of another. The variables should be further analyzed to determine which, if any, other variables (i.e., quality of employee work) may contribute to the positive correlation.

Comparing Data

Comparing data sets within statistics can mean many things. The first way to compare data sets is by looking at the center and spread of each set. The center of a data set can mean two things: median or mean. The **median** is the halfway point of a data set, and it splits the data into two intervals. The **mean** is the average value of the data within a set. It's calculated by adding up all of the data in the set and dividing the total by the number of data points. Outliers can significantly impact the mean. Additionally, two completely different data sets can have the same mean. For example, a data set with values ranging from 0 to 100 and a data set with values ranging from 44 to 56 can both have means of 50. The first data set has a much wider range, which is known as the **spread** of the data. This measures how varied the data is within each set.

Calculating Probabilities to Determine the Likelihood of an Outcome

Given a set of possible outcomes *X*, a **probability distribution** on *X* is a function that assigns a probability to each possible outcome. The probability of a given outcome must be between zero and 1, while the total probability must be 1. If the outcomes are $(x_1, x_2, x_3, \dots x_n)$, and the probability distribution is *p*, then the following rules are applied.

- $0 \leq p(x_i) \leq 1$, for any i.
- $\sum_{i=1}^{n} p(x_i) = 1$.

If $p(x_i)$ is constant, then this is called a **uniform probability distribution**, and $p(x_i) = \frac{1}{n}$. For example, on a six-sided die, the probability of each of the six outcomes will be $\frac{1}{6}$.

If seeking the probability of an outcome occurring in some specific range *A* of possible outcomes, written $P(A)$, add up the probabilities for each outcome in that range. For example, consider if a word problem asked you to figure the probability of getting a 3 or lower when a six-sided die is rolled. The possible rolls are 1, 2, 3, 4, 5, and 6. So, to get a 3 or lower, a roll of 1, 2, or 3 must be completed. The probabilities of each of these is $\frac{1}{6}$, so add these to get:

$$p(1) + p(2) + p(3) = \frac{1}{6} + \frac{1}{6} + \frac{1}{6} = \frac{1}{2}$$

Explaining the Relationship Between Two Variables

Sometimes, when data are measured, it is not simply measuring the frequency of a given outcome, but rather measuring a relationship between two different quantities. In these cases, there is usually one variable that is controlled, the **independent variable**, and one that depends on this variable, the **dependent variable**. If there is a relationship between the two variables, then they are said to be **correlated**.

There are two caveats to these terms. First, the independent variable is not necessarily controlled by the experimenters. It is simply the one chosen to organize the data. In other words, the data are divided up based on the value of an independent variable. Second, finding a significant relationship between the dependent variable and the independent variable does not necessarily imply that there is a causal relationship between the two variables. It only means that once the independent variable is known, a fairly accurate prediction of the dependent variable can be made. This is often expressed with the phrase *correlation does not imply causation*. In other words, just because there is a relationship between two variables does not mean that one is the cause of the other. There could be other factors involved that are the real cause.

Consider some examples. An experimenter could do an experiment in which the independent variable is the number of hours that a student studies for a given test, and the dependent variable is the score the student receives when he or she actually takes the test. Such an experiment would attempt to measure whether there is a relationship between the time spent studying and the score a student receives when taking the test.

The expectation would be that the larger value of the independent variable would yield a larger value for the dependent variable. Another experimenter might do an experiment with runners, where the independent variable is the length of the runner's leg, and the dependent variable is the time it takes for the runner to run a fixed distance. In this experiment, as the independent variable increases, the dependent variable would be expected to decrease.

As an example of the phenomenon that correlation does not imply causation, consider an experiment where the independent variable is the value of a person's house, and the dependent variable is their income. Although people in more expensive houses are expected to make more money, it is clear that their expensive houses are not the cause of them making more money. This illustrates one example of why it is important for experimenters to be careful when drawing conclusions about causation from their data.

Correlation and Covariations

Covariance is a general term referring to how two variables move in relation to each other. Take for example an employee that gets paid by the hour. For them, hours worked and total pay have a positive covariance. As hours worked increases, so does pay.

The simplest type of correlation between two variables is a **linear correlation**. If the independent variable is *x* and the dependent variable is *y*, then a linear correlation means:

$$y = mx + b$$

If *m* is positive, then *y* will increase as *x* increases. If *m* is negative, then *y* will decrease while *x* increases. The variable *b* represents the value of *y* when *x* is 0.

As one example of such a correlation, consider a manufacturing plant. Suppose *x* is the number of units produced by the plant, and *y* is the cost to the company. In this example, *b* will be the cost of the plant itself. The plant will cost money even if it is never used, just by buying the machinery. For each unit produced, there will be a cost for the labor and the material. Let *m* represent this cost to produce one unit of the product.

For a more concrete example, suppose a computer factory costs \$100,000. It requires \$100 of parts and \$50 of labor to make one computer. How much will it cost for a company to make 1,000 computers? To figure this, let *y* be the amount of money the company spends, and let *x* be the number of computers. The cost of the factory is \$100,000, so $b = 100{,}000$. On the other hand, the cost of producing a computer is the parts plus labor, or \$150, so $m = 150$. Therefore:

$$y = 150x + 100{,}000$$

Substitute 1,000 for *x* and get:

$$y = 150 \times 1{,}000 + 100{,}000 = 150{,}000 + 100{,}000 = 250{,}000$$

It will cost the company \$250,000 to make 1,000 computers.

Calculating Geometric Quantities

Perimeter and Area

Length is the measurement of distance from a point to another point, often measured in units of feet, meters, or related units. **Perimeter** is the measurement of a distance around something or the sum of all side lengths of a polygon. Think of perimeter as the length of the boundary, like a fence. In contrast, **area** is the space occupied by a defined enclosure, like a field enclosed by a fence.

When thinking about perimeter, think about walking around the outside of something. When thinking about area, think about the amount of space or **surface area** something takes up.

Square

The perimeter of a square is measured by adding together all of the sides. Since a square has four equal sides, its perimeter can be calculated by multiplying the length of one side by 4. Thus, the formula is $P = 4 \times s$, where s equals one side. For example, the following square has side lengths of 5 meters:

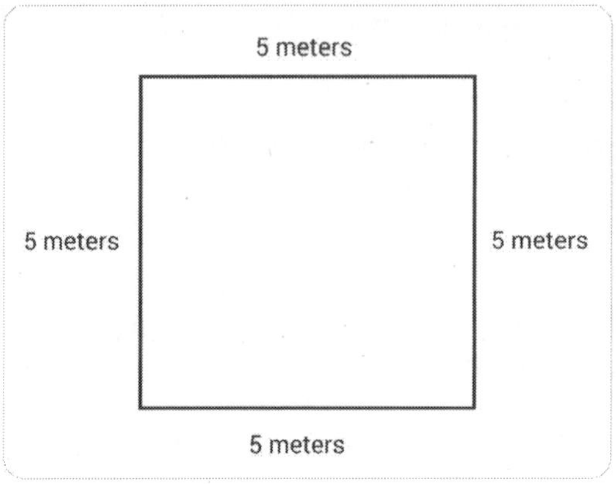

The perimeter is 20 meters because 4 times 5 is 20.

The area of a square is the length of a side squared. For example, if the side of a square is 5 centimeters, then the area is 25 square centimeters. The formula for this example is $A = s^2 = 5^2 = 25$ square centimeters.

$$A = lw = 6(7) = 42 \text{ square inches}$$

Rectangle

Like a square, a rectangle's perimeter is measured by adding together all of the sides. But as the sides are unequal, the formula is different. A rectangle has equal values for its lengths (long sides) and equal values for its widths (short sides), so the perimeter formula for a rectangle is:

$$P = l + l + w + w = 2l + 2w$$

l equals length
w equals width

The area is found by multiplying the length by the width, so the formula is $A = l \times w$.

For example, if the length of a rectangle is 10 inches and the width 8 inches, then the perimeter is 36 inches because:

$$P = 2l + 2w = 2(10) + 2(8)$$

$$20 + 16 = 36 \text{ inches}$$

Triangle

A triangle's perimeter is measured by adding together the three sides, so the formula is $P = a + b + c$, where a, b, and c are the values of the three sides. The area is the product of one-half the base and height so the formula is:

$$A = \frac{1}{2} \times b \times h$$

It can be simplified to:

$$A = \frac{bh}{2}$$

The base is the bottom of the triangle, and the height is the distance from the base to the peak. If a problem asks to calculate the area of a triangle, it will provide the base and height.

For example, if the base of the triangle is 2 feet and the height 4 feet, then the area is 4 square feet. The following equation shows the formula used to calculate the area of the triangle:

$$\mathrm{A} = \frac{1}{2}\mathrm{bh} = \frac{1}{2}(2)(4) = 4 \text{ square feet}$$

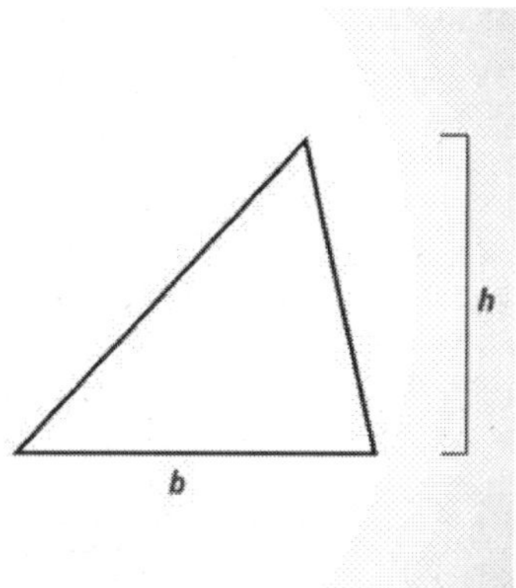

Circle

A circle's perimeter—also known as its **circumference**—is measured by multiplying the diameter by π. Diameter is the straight line measured from a point on one side of the circle to a point directly across on the opposite side of the circle. Diameter is the straight line measured from a point on one side of the circle to a point directly across on the opposite side of the circle. π is referred to as pi and is equal to 3.14 (with rounding). So, the formula is $\pi \times d$. This is sometimes expressed by the formula $C = 2 \times \pi \times r$, where r is the radius of the circle. These formulas are equivalent, as the radius equals half of the diameter.

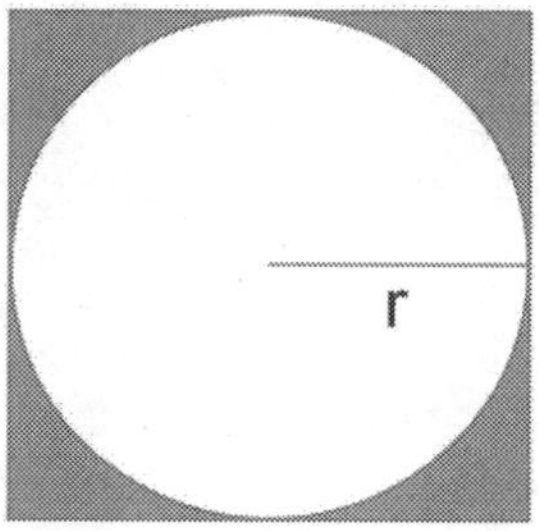

The area of a circle is calculated through the formula $A = \pi \times r^2$. The test will indicate either to leave the answer with π attached or to calculate to the nearest decimal place, which means multiplying by 3.14 for π.

Arc

The **arc of a circle** is the distance between two points on the circle. The length of the arc of a circle in terms of **degrees** is easily determined if the value of the central angle is known. The length of the arc is simply the value of the central angle. In this example, the length of the arc of the circle in degrees is 75°.

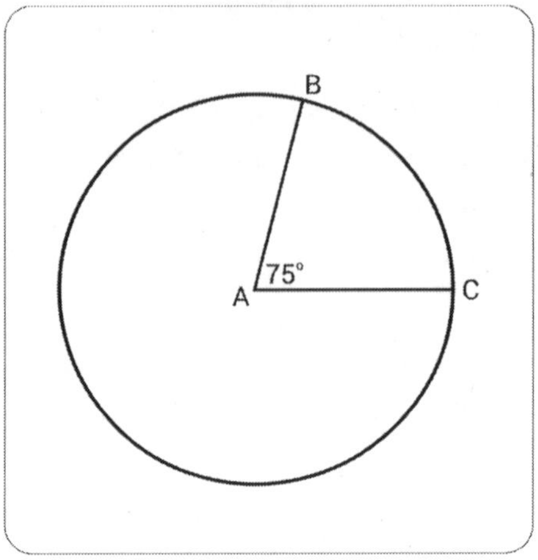

To determine the length of the arc of a circle in **distance**, the values for both the central angle and the radius must be known. This formula is:

$$\frac{central\ angle}{360°} = \frac{arc\ length}{2\pi r}$$

The equation is simplified by cross-multiplying to solve for the arc length.

In the following example, to solve for arc length, substitute the values of the central angle (75°) and the radius (10 inches) into the equation above

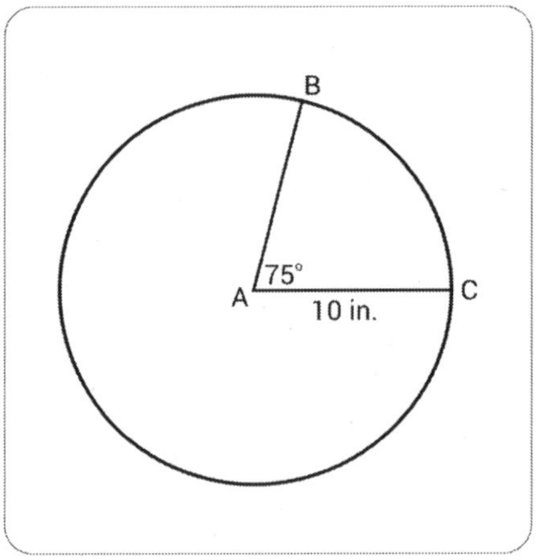

$$\frac{75°}{360°} = \frac{arc\ length}{2(3.14)(10in.)}$$

To solve the equation, first cross-multiply: $4710 = 360(arc\ length)$. Next, divide each side of the equation by 360. The result of the formula is that the arc length is 13.1 (rounded).

Irregular Shapes

The perimeter of an irregular polygon is found by adding the lengths of all of the sides. In cases where all of the sides are given, this will be very straightforward, as it will simply involve finding the sum of the provided lengths. Other times, a side length may be missing and must be determined before the perimeter can be calculated.

Consider the example below:

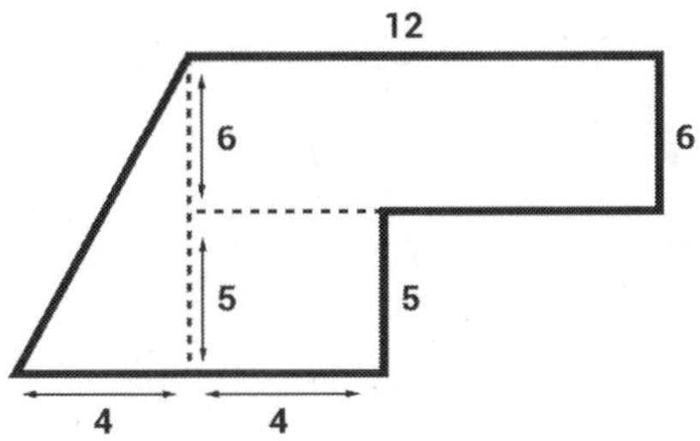

All of the side lengths are provided except for two: the horizontal line on the right between the vertical sides that measure 5 and 6, and the angled side on the left.

The horizontal side is easiest to solve, as test takers can identify that the length of the missing side, s, plus the length of the bottom horizontal side (4) are equal to the length of the top side (12). This could also be written as the formula $4 + s = 12$, and solved with an answer of 8.

Next, it's time to solve for the angled side on the left. Test takers should notice that this is the hypotenuse of a right triangle. The other two sides of the triangle are provided (the base is 4 and the height is 6 + 5 = 11). The Pythagorean Theorem can be used to find the length of the hypotenuse of a right triangle, using the equation $a^2 + b^2 = c^2$, where c represents the hypotenuse.

Substituting the side values provided yields:

$$(4)^2 + (11)^2 = c^2$$

Therefore, c = $\sqrt{16 + 121} = 11.7$

Finally, the perimeter can be found by adding this new side length with the other provided lengths to get the total length around the figure:

$$4 + 4 + 5 + 8 + 6 + 12 + 11.7 = 50.7$$

Although units are not provided in this figure, remember that reporting units with a measurement is important.

The area of an irregular polygon is found by decomposing, or breaking apart, the figure into smaller shapes. When the area of the smaller shapes is determined, these areas are added together to produce the total area of the area of the original figure. Consider the same example provided before:

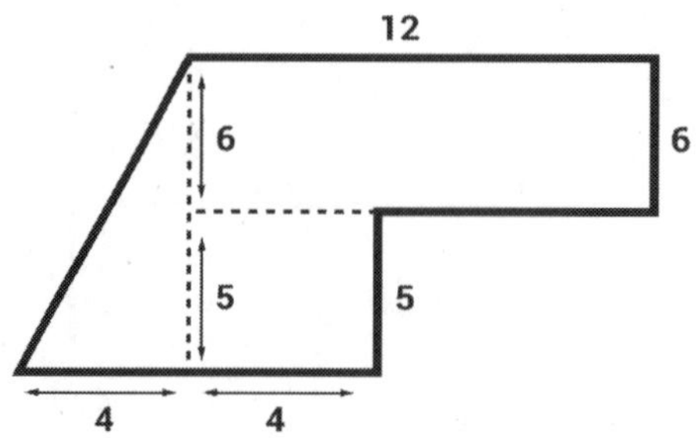

The irregular polygon is decomposed into two rectangles and a triangle. The area of the large rectangle ($A = l \times w \rightarrow A = 12 \times 6$) is 72 square units. The area of the small rectangle is 20 square units ($A = 4 \times 5$). The area of the triangle ($A = \frac{1}{2} \times b \times h \rightarrow A = \frac{1}{2} \times 4 \times 11$) is 22 square units. The sum of the areas of these figures produces the total area of the original polygon:

$$A = 72 + 20 + 22 \rightarrow A = \text{ 114 square units}$$

Volume as a Cubic Unit Measure

Geometry in three dimensions is similar to geometry in two dimensions. The main new feature is that three points now define a unique *plane* that passes through each of them. Three dimensional objects can be made by putting together two-dimensional figures in different surfaces. Below, some of the possible three-dimensional figures will be provided, along with formulas for their volumes and surface areas.

A rectangular prism is a box whose sides are all rectangles meeting at 90° angles. Such a box has three dimensions: length, width, and height. If the length is *x*, the width is *y*, and the height is *z*, then the volume is given by $V = xyz$.

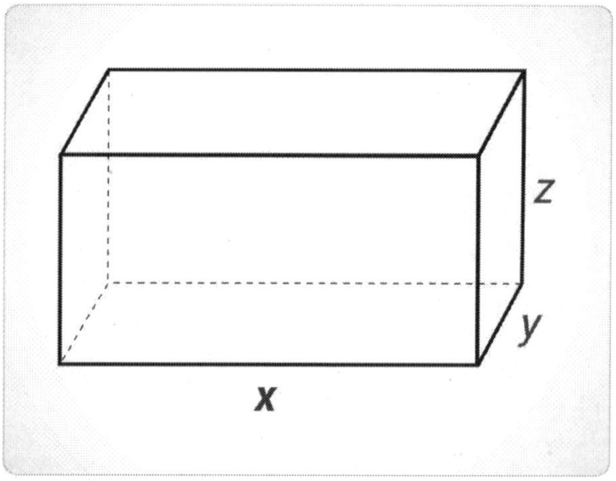

The surface area will be given by computing the surface area of each rectangle and adding them together. There are a total of six rectangles. Two of them have sides of length *x* and *y*, two have sides of length *y* and *z*, and two have sides of length *x* and *z*. Therefore, the total surface area will be given by:

$$SA = 2xy + 2yz + 2xz$$

A **rectangular pyramid** is a figure with a rectangular base and four triangular sides that meet at a single vertex. If the rectangle has sides of length *x* and *y*, then the volume will be given by:

$$V = \frac{1}{3}xyh$$

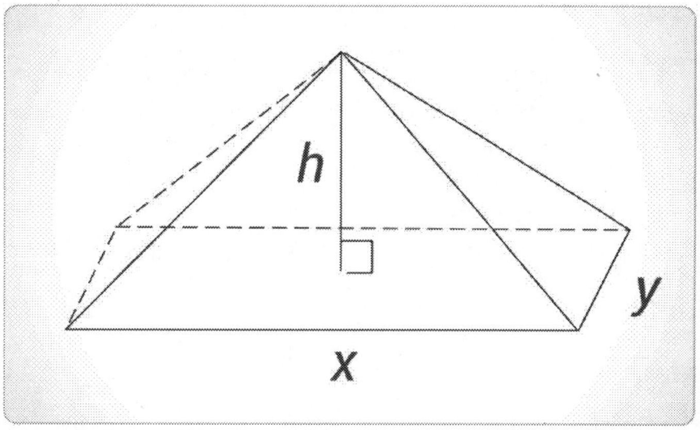

To find the surface area, the dimensions of each triangle need to be known. However, these dimensions can differ depending on the problem in question. Therefore, there is no general formula for calculating total surface area.

A **sphere** is a set of points all of which are equidistant from some central point. It is like a circle, but in three dimensions. The volume of a sphere of radius *r* is given by:

$$V = \frac{4}{3}\pi r^3$$

The surface area is given by:

$$A = 4\pi r^2$$

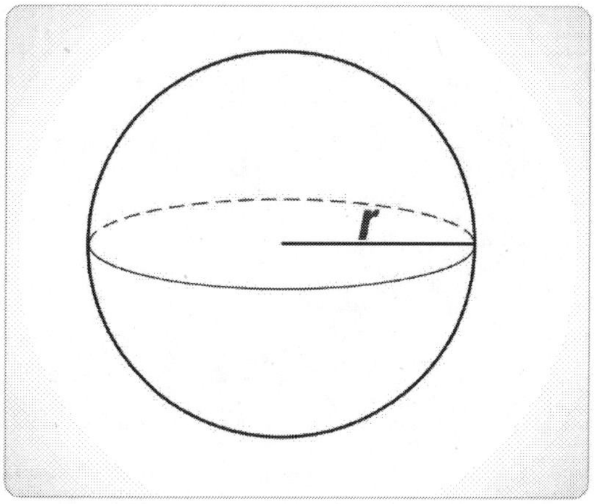

Converting Units

American Measuring System

The measuring system used today in the United States

developed from the British units of measurement during colonial times. The most typically used units in this customary system are those used to measure weight, liquid volume, and length, whose common units are found below. In the customary system, the basic unit for measuring weight is the ounce (oz); there are 16 ounces (oz) in 1 pound (lb) and 2000 pounds in 1 ton. The basic unit for measuring liquid volume is the ounce (oz); 1 ounce is equal to 2 tablespoons (tbsp) or 6 teaspoons (tsp), and there are 8 ounces in 1 cup, 2 cups in 1 pint (pt), 2 pints in 1 quart (qt), and 4 quarts in 1 gallon (gal). For measurements of length, the inch (in) is the base unit; 12 inches make up 1 foot (ft), 3 feet make up 1 yard (yd), and 5280 feet make up 1 mile (mi).

However, as there are only a set number of units in the customary system, with extremely large or extremely small amounts of material, the numbers can become awkward and difficult to compare. Here is a conversion chart for common customary measurements:

Common Customary Measurements		
Length	**Weight**	**Capacity**
1 foot = 12 inches	1 pound = 16 ounces	1 cup = 8 fluid ounces
1 yard = 3 feet	1 ton = 2,000 pounds	1 pint = 2 cups
1 yard = 36 inches		1 quart = 2 pints
1 mile = 1,760 yards		1 quart = 4 cups
1 mile = 5,280 feet		1 gallon = 4 quarts
		1 gallon = 16 cups

Metric System

Aside from the United States, most countries in the world have adopted the metric system embodied in the International System of Units (SI). The three main SI base units used in the metric system are the meter (m), the kilogram (kg), and the liter (L); meters measure length, kilograms measure mass, and liters measure volume.

These three units can use different prefixes, which indicate larger or smaller versions of the unit by powers of ten. This can be thought of as making a new unit, which is sized by multiplying the original unit in size by a factor.

These prefixes and associated factors are:

Metric Prefixes			
Prefix	**Symbol**	**Multiplier**	**Exponential**
kilo	k	1,000	10^3
hecto	h	100	10^2
deca	da	10	10^1
no prefix		1	10^0
deci	d	0.1	10^{-1}
centi	c	0.01	10^{-2}
milli	m	0.001	10^{-3}

The correct prefix is then attached to the base. Some examples:

1 milliliter equals .001 liters.
1 kilogram equals 1,000 grams.

Choosing the Appropriate Measuring Unit

Some units of measure are represented as square or cubic units depending on the solution. For example, perimeter is measured in linear units, area is measured in square units, and volume is measured in cubic units

Also be sure to use the most appropriate unit for the thing being measured. A building's height might be measured in feet or meters while the length of a nail might be measured in inches or centimeters. Additionally, for SI units, the prefix should be chosen to provide the most succinct available value. For example, the mass of a bag of fruit would likely be measured in kilograms rather than grams or milligrams, and the length of a bacteria cell would likely be measured in micrometers rather than centimeters or kilometers.

Conversion

Converting measurements in different units between the two systems can be difficult because they follow different rules. The best method is to look up an English to Metric system conversion factor and then use a series of equivalent fractions to set up an equation to convert the units of one of the measurements into those of the other.

The table below lists some common conversion values that are useful for problems involving measurements with units in both systems:

English System	**Metric System**
1 inch	2.54 cm
1 foot	0.3048 m
1 yard	0.914 m
1 mile	1.609 km
1 ounce	28.35 g
1 pound	0.454 kg
1 fluid ounce	29.574 mL
1 quart	0.946 L
1 gallon	3.785 L

Consider the example where a scientist wants to convert 6.8 inches to centimeters. The table above is used to find that there are 2.54 centimeters in every inch, so the following equation should be set up and solved:

$$\frac{6.8 \text{ in}}{1} \times \frac{2.54 \text{ cm}}{1 \text{ in}} = 17.272 \text{ cm}$$

Notice how the inches in the numerator of the initial figure and the denominator of the conversion factor cancel out. (This equation could have been written simply as $6.8 \text{ in} \times 2.54 \text{ cm} = 17.272 \text{ cm}$, but it was shown in detail to illustrate the steps). The goal in any conversion equation is to set up the fractions so that the units you are trying to convert from cancel out and the units you desire remain.

For a more complicated example, consider converting 2.15 kilograms into ounces. The first step is to convert kilograms into grams and then grams into ounces. Note that the measurement you begin with does not have to be put in a fraction.

So, in this case, 2.15 kg is by itself although it's technically the numerator of a fraction:

$$2.15\text{ kg} \times \frac{1{,}000\text{g}}{\text{kg}} = 2150\text{ g}$$

Then, use the conversion factor from the table to convert grams to ounces:

$$2{,}150\text{ g} \times \frac{1\text{ oz}}{28.35\text{ g}} = 75.8$$

Mathematics Practice Quiz

1. The graph of which function has an x—intercept of -2?
   a. $y = 2x - 3$
   b. $y = 4x + 2$
   c. $y = x^2 + 5x + 6$
   d. $y = 2x^2 + 3x - 1$

2. A train traveling 50 miles per hour takes a trip lasting 3 hours. If a map has a scale of 1 inch per 10 miles, how many inches apart are the train's starting point and ending point on the map?
   a. 14 inches
   b. 12 inches
   c. 13 inches
   d. 15 inches

3. The area of a given rectangle is $24\ square\ centimeters$. If the measure of each side is multiplied by 3, what is the area of the new figure?
   a. 48 cm
   b. 72 cm
   c. 216 cm
   d. $13{,}824$ cm

4. In the figure below, what is the area of the shaded region?

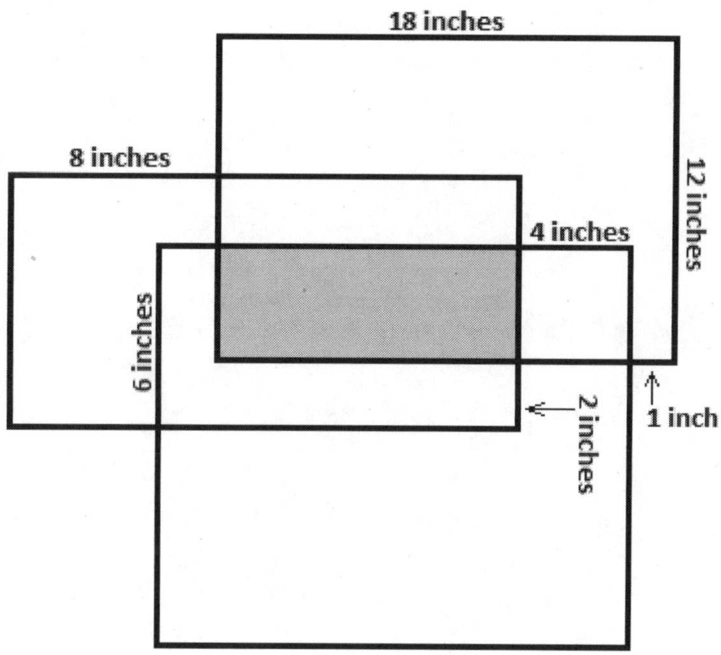

   a. 48 square inches
   b. 52 square inches
   c. 44 square inches
   d. 56 square inches

5. A couple buys a house for \$150,000. They sell it for \$165,000. By what percentage did the house's value increase?

a. 10%
b. 13%
c. 15%
d. 17%

See answers on the next page.

Answer Explanations

1. C: An x-intercept is a point where the graph crosses the x-axis. At this point, the value of y is 0. To determine if an equation has an x-intercept of –2, substitute –2 for x, and calculate the value of y. If the value of –2 for x corresponds with a y-value of 0, then the equation has an x-intercept of –2. The only answer choice that produces this result is Choice *C*.

$$0 = (-2)^2 + 5(-2) + 6$$

2. D: First, the train's journey in the real world is:

$$3\text{ h} \times 50\frac{\text{mi}}{\text{h}} = 150\text{ mi}$$

On the map, 1 inch corresponds to 10 miles, so that is equivalent to:

$$150\text{ mi} \times \frac{1\text{ in}}{10\text{ mi}} = 15\text{ in}$$

Therefore, the start and end points are 15 inches apart on the map.

3. C: 216 cm. Because area is a two-dimensional measurement, the dimensions are multiplied by a scale that is squared to determine the scale of the corresponding areas. The dimensions of the rectangle are multiplied by a scale of 3. Therefore, the area is multiplied by a scale of 3^2 (which is equal to 9):

$$24\text{ cm} \times 9 = 216\text{ cm}$$

4. B: This can be determined by finding the length and width of the shaded region. The length can be found using the length of the top rectangle, which is 18 inches, and then subtracting the extra lengths of 4 inches and 1 inch. This means the length of the shaded region is 13 inches. Next, the width can be determined using the 6-inch measurement and subtracting the 2-inch measurement. This means that the width is 4 inches. Thus, the area is:

$$13 \times 4 = 52\text{ sq. in.}$$

5. A: The value went up by $\$165{,}000 - \$150{,}000 = \$15{,}000$. Out of \$150,000, this is $\frac{15{,}000}{150{,}000} = \frac{1}{10}$. If we multiply the top and bottom by 10 to give us a denominator of 100, the result is $\frac{10}{100}$, or 10%.

Human Anatomy and Physiology

Demonstrate Knowledge of the General Orientation of Human Anatomy

Anatomy may be defined as the structural makeup of an organism. The study of anatomy may be divided into microscopic/fine anatomy and macroscopic/gross anatomy. Fine anatomy concerns itself with viewing the features of the body with the aid of a microscope, while gross anatomy concerns itself with viewing the features of the body with the naked eye. **Physiology** refers to the functions of an organism, and it examines the chemical or physical functions that help the body function appropriately.

Body Cavities

The body is partitioned into different hollow spaces that house organs. The human body contains the following cavities:

- **Cranial cavity**: The cranial cavity is surrounded by the skull and contains organs such as the brain and pituitary gland.
- **Thoracic cavity**: The thoracic cavity is encircled by the sternum (breastbone) and ribs. It contains organs such as the lungs, heart, trachea (windpipe), esophagus, and bronchial tubes.
- **Abdominal cavity**: The abdominal cavity is separated from the thoracic cavity by the diaphragm. It contains organs such as the stomach, gallbladder, liver, small intestines, and large intestines. The abdominal organs are held in place by a membrane called the peritoneum.
- **Pelvic cavity**: The pelvic cavity is enclosed by the pelvis, or bones of the hip. It contains organs such as the urinary bladder, urethra, ureters, anus, and rectum. It contains the reproductive organs as well. In females, the pelvic cavity also contains the uterus.
- **Spinal cavity**: The spinal cavity is surrounded by the vertebral column. The vertebral column has five regions: cervical, thoracic, lumbar, sacral, and coccygeal. The spinal cord runs through the middle of the spinal cavity.

Three Primary Body Planes

A plane is an imaginary flat surface. The three primary planes of the human body are frontal, sagittal, and transverse. The coronal plane is a vertical plane that divides the body or organ into front (anterior) and back (posterior) portions. The sagittal, or lateral, plane is a vertical plane divides the body or organ into right and left sides. The transverse plane is a horizontal plane that divides the body or organ into upper and lower portions. In medical imaging, computed tomography (CT) scans are oriented only in the transverse plane; while magnetic resonance imaging (MRI) scans may be oriented in any of the three planes.

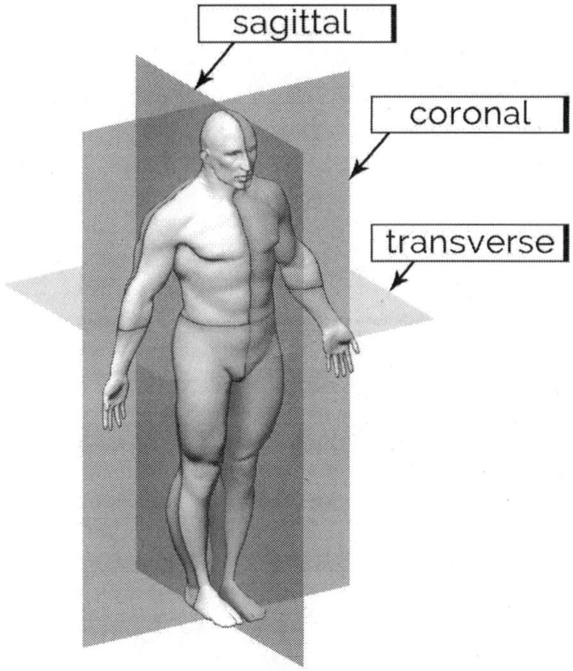

Terms of Direction

Medial refers to a structure being closer to the midline of the body. For example, the nose is medial to the eyes.

Lateral refers to a structure being farther from the midline of the body, and it is the opposite of **medial**. For example, the eyes are lateral to the nose.

Proximal refers to a structure or body part located near an attachment point. For example, the elbow is proximal to the wrist.

Distal refers to a structure or body part located far from an attachment point, and it is the opposite of **proximal**. For example, the wrist is distal to the elbow.

Anterior means toward the front in humans. For example, the lips are anterior to the teeth. The term **ventral** can be used in place of **anterior**.

Posterior means toward the back in humans, and it is the opposite of **anterior**. For example, the teeth are posterior to the lips. The term **dorsal** can be used in place of **posterior**.

Superior means above and refers to a structure closer to the head. For example, the head is superior to the neck. The terms **cephalic** or **cranial** may be used in place of **superior**.

Inferior means below and refers to a structure farther from the head, and it is the opposite of **superior**. For example, the neck is inferior to the head. The term **caudal** may be used in place of **inferior**.

Superficial refers to a structure closer to the surface. For example, the muscles are superficial because they are just beneath the surface of the skin.

Deep refers to a structure farther from the surface, and it is the opposite of **superficial**. For example, the femur is a deep structure lying beneath the muscles.

Body Regions

Terms for general locations on the body include:

- **Cervical**: relating to the neck (can also refer to the cervix, as in cervical cancer)
- Clavicular: relating to the clavicle, or collarbone
- Ocular: relating to the eyes
- Acromial: relating to the shoulder
- Cubital: relating to the elbow
- Brachial: relating to the arm
- Carpal: relating to the wrist
- Thoracic : relating to the chest
- Abdominal: relating to the abdomen
- Pubic: relating to the groin
- Pelvic: relating to the pelvis, or bones of the hip
- Femoral: relating to the femur, or thigh bone
- Geniculate: relating to the knee
- Pedal: relating to the foot
- Palmar: relating to the palm of the hand
- Plantar: relating to the sole of the foot

Abdominopelvic Regions and Quadrants

The abdominopelvic region may be defined as the combination of the abdominal and the pelvic cavities. The region's upper border is the breasts and its lower border is the groin region. The region is divided into the following nine sections:

- **Right hypochondriac**: region below the cartilage of the ribs
- **Epigastric**: region above the stomach between the hypochondriac regions
- **Left hypochondriac**: region below the cartilage of the ribs
- **Right lumbar**: region of the waist
- **Umbilical**: region between the lumbar regions where the umbilicus, or belly button (navel), is located
- **Left lumbar**: region of the waist
- **Right inguinal**: region of the groin
- **Hypogastric**: region below the stomach between the inguinal regions
- **Left inguinal**: region of the groin

A simpler way to describe the abdominopelvic area is to divide it into the following quadrants:

- **Right upper quadrant (RUQ)**: Encompasses the right hypochondriac, right lumbar, epigastric, and umbilical regions.
- **Right lower quadrant (RLQ)**: Encompasses the right lumbar, right inguinal, hypogastric, and umbilical regions.

- **Left upper quadrant (LUQ)**: Encompasses the left hypochondriac, left lumbar, epigastric, and umbilical regions.
- **Left lower quadrant (LLQ)**: Encompasses the left lumbar, left inguinal, hypogastric, and umbilical regions.

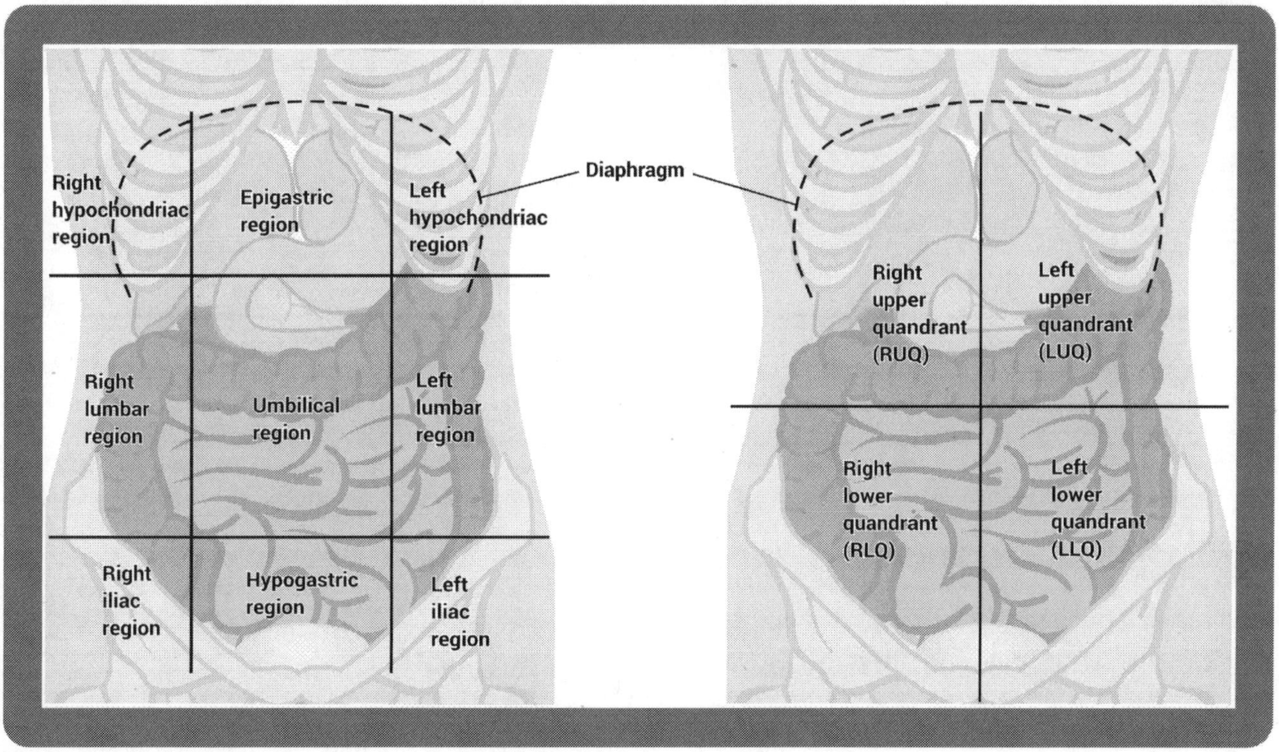

Levels of Organization of the Human Body

All the parts of the human body are built of individual units called **cells**. Groups of similar cells are arranged into **tissues,** different tissues are arranged into **organs,** and organs working together form entire **organ systems.** The human body has twelve organ systems that govern circulation, digestion, immunity, hormones, movement, support, coordination, urination & excretion, reproduction (male and female), respiration, and general protection.

Here are some of the systems of the body:

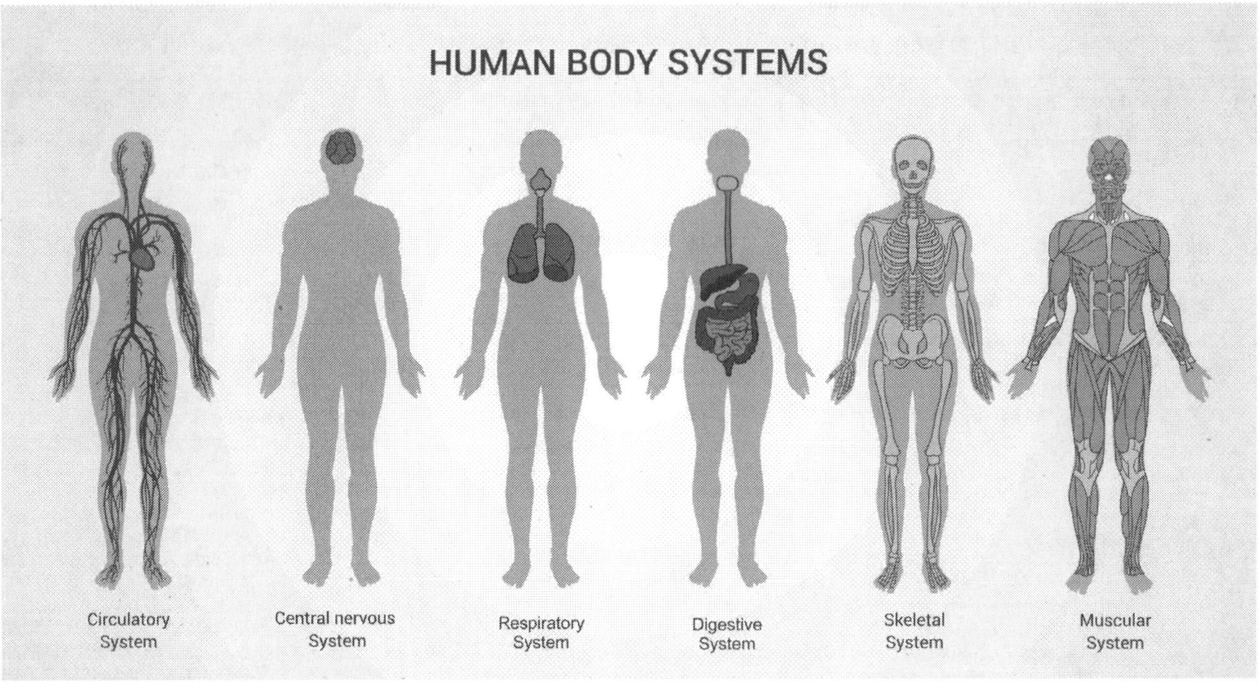

Describe the Anatomy and Physiology of the Respiratory System

The respiratory system enables breathing and supports the energy-making process in cells. The respiratory system transports an essential reactant, oxygen, to cells so that they can produce energy in their mitochondria via cellular respiration. The respiratory system also removes carbon dioxide, a waste product of cellular respiration.

This system is divided into the upper respiratory system and the lower respiratory system. The upper system comprises the nose, the nasal cavity and sinuses, and the pharynx. The lower respiratory system comprises the larynx (voice box), the trachea (windpipe), the small passageways leading to the lungs, and the lungs.

The pathway of oxygen to the bloodstream begins with the nose and the mouth. Upon inhalation, air enters the nose and mouth and passes into the sinuses where it gets warmed, filtered, and humidified. The throat, or the pharynx, allows the entry of both food and air; however, only air moves into the trachea, or windpipe, since the epiglottis covers the trachea during swallowing and prevents food from entering. The trachea contains mucus and cilia. The mucus traps many airborne pathogens while the cilia act as bristles that sweep the pathogens away toward the top of the trachea where they are either swallowed or coughed out.

The top of the trachea itself has two vocal cords, which make up the larynx. At its bottom, the trachea forks into two major bronchi—one for each lung. These bronchi continue to branch into smaller and smaller bronchioles before terminating in grape-like air sacs called alveoli; these alveoli are surrounded by capillaries and provide the body with an enormous amount of surface area to exchange oxygen and carbon dioxide gases, in a process called external respiration.

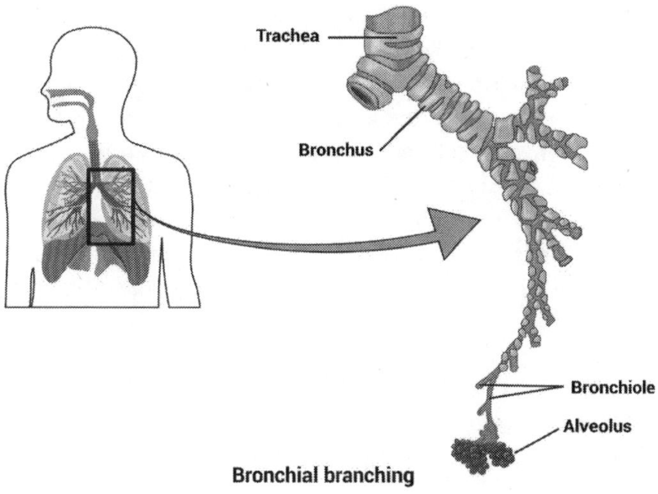

In total, the lungs contain about 1500 miles of airway passages. The right lung is divided into three lobes (superior, middle, and inferior), and the left lung is divided into two lobes (superior and inferior).

The left lung is smaller than the right lung, likely because it shares its space in the chest cavity with the heart.

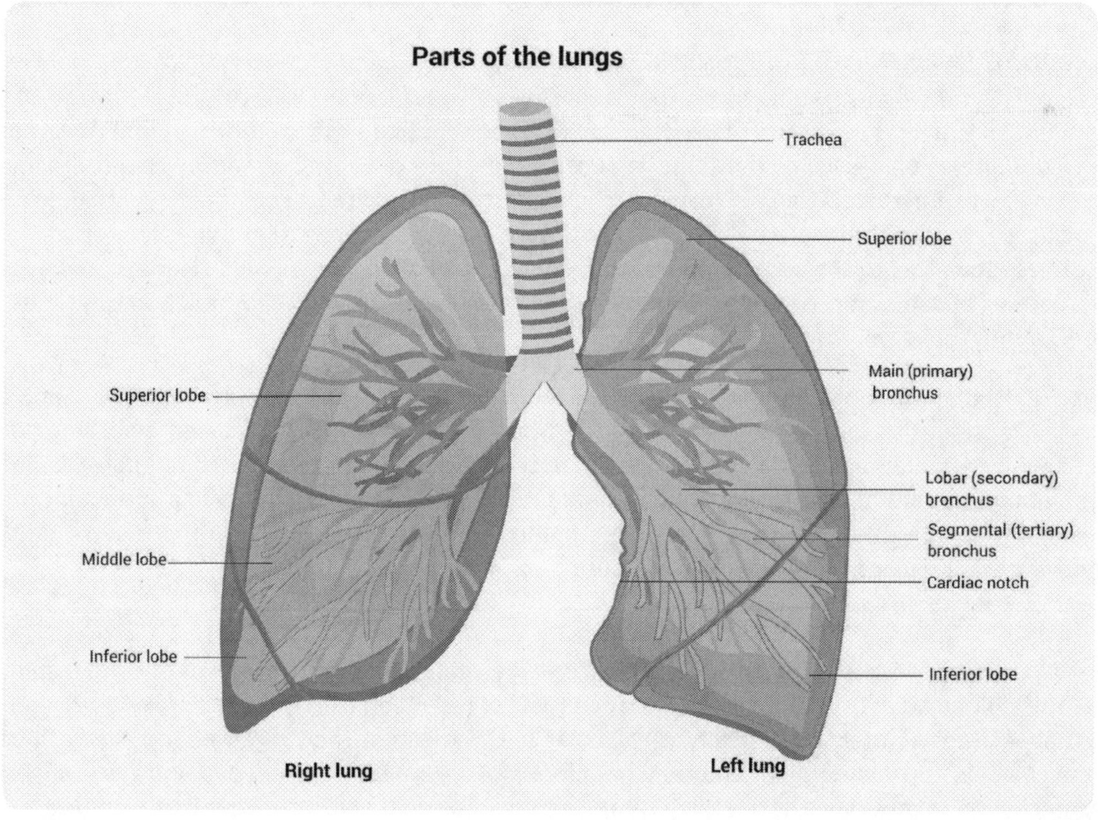

A flat muscle underneath the lungs called the diaphragm controls breathing. When the diaphragm contracts, the volume of the chest cavity increases and indirectly decreases its air pressure. This decrease in air pressure creates a vacuum, and the lungs pull in air to fill the space. This difference in air pressure pulls the air from outside of the body into the lungs in a process called negative pressure breathing.

Upon inhalation or inspiration, oxygen in the alveoli diffuses into the capillaries to be carried by blood to cells throughout the body, in a process called internal respiration. A protein called hemoglobin in red blood cells easily bonds with oxygen, removing it from the blood and allowing more oxygen to diffuse in. This protein allows the blood to take in 60 times more oxygen than the body could without it, and this explains how oxygen can become so concentrated in blood even though it is only 21% of the atmosphere. While oxygen diffuses from the alveoli into the capillaries, carbon dioxide diffuses from the capillaries into the alveoli. When the diaphragm relaxes, the elastic lungs snap back to their original shape; this decreases the volume of the chest cavity and increases the air pressure until it is back to normal. This increased air pressure pushes the carbon dioxide waste from the alveoli through exhalation or **expiration**.

The autonomic nervous system controls breathing. The medulla oblongata gets feedback regarding the carbon dioxide levels in the blood and will send a message to the diaphragm that it is time for a contraction. While breathing can be voluntary, it is mostly under autonomic control.

Functions of the Respiratory System

The respiratory system has many functions. Most importantly, it provides a large area for gas exchange between the air and the circulating blood. It protects the delicate respiratory surfaces from environmental variations and defends them against pathogens. It is responsible for producing the sounds that the body makes for speaking and singing, as well as for non-verbal communication. It also helps regulate blood volume and blood pressure by releasing vasopressin, and it is a regulator of blood pH due to its control over carbon dioxide release, as the aqueous form of carbon dioxide is the chief buffering agent in blood.

Factors Affecting Respiratory Function

The bronchiolar walls consist of smooth muscle that is sensitive to specific chemicals or neural controls of respiration. When an irritant is inhaled, a reflex of the nervous system (parasympathetic division) results in a constriction of the bronchioles, which significantly reduces the passage of air. Inflammatory chemicals and histamines during an asthma attack can also cause bronchoconstriction such that pulmonary ventilation ceases. On the other hand, the release of epinephrine via sympathetic nervous system activation can reduce airway resistance. Respiratory diseases can lead to the accumulation of infectious material or mucus, which leads to airway resistance. As a result, breathing becomes more difficult. When the bronchioles are obstructed, ventilation cannot be restored even during extreme respiratory efforts.

When the type II alveolar cells of the respiratory membrane do not produce enough surfactant (a genetic condition), the alveoli can collapse due to surface tension. Such a condition is called respiratory distress syndrome (RDS), which may be due to environmental causes or genetic factors. Consequently, the alveoli must be reinflated by mechanical ventilation. In Infant RDS (IRDS), infants that are born prematurely will have a deficiency in a surfactant protein B and cannot keep the alveoli inflated between each breath. IRDS can be treated with a synthetic surfactant and a mechanical device that provides positive airway pressure throughout respiration.

Gas Exchange

In the lungs, the alveolus consists of gas-filled air spaces called alveoli. Bordering the alveolus is the respiratory membrane, a thick blood air barrier (0.5 microns) that consists of red blood cells in a capillary endothelium, a type II alveolar cell that secretes a surfactant, and a type I alveolar cell epithelium. The capillaries and elastic fibers surround all the alveoli. The respiratory membrane has blood flowing on the capillary end and gas exchange in the alveolus. The exchange of gases such as oxygen (O_2) and carbon dioxide (CO_2) occurs by simple diffusion, whereby oxygen gas passes from the alveolus into the capillary (blood) and carbon dioxide exits the capillary into the alveolus.

Describe the Anatomy and Physiology of the Cardiovascular System

The cardiovascular system (also called the circulatory system) is a network of organs and tubes that transport blood, hormones, nutrients, oxygen, and other gases to cells and tissues throughout the body. The major components of the circulatory system are the blood vessels, blood, and heart.

Blood Vessels

In the circulatory system, blood vessels are responsible for transporting blood throughout the body. The three major types of blood vessels in the circulatory system are arteries, veins, and capillaries. Arteries carry blood from the heart to the rest of the body. Veins carry blood from the body back to the heart. Capillaries connect arteries to veins and form networks that exchange materials between the blood and the cells.

In general, arteries are stronger and thicker than veins, as they withstand high pressures exerted by the blood as the heart pumps it through the body. Arteries control blood flow through either vasoconstriction (narrowing of the blood vessel's diameter) or vasodilation (widening of the blood vessel's diameter). The blood in veins is under much lower pressures, so veins have valves to prevent the backflow of blood.

Most of the exchange between the blood and tissues takes place through the capillaries. There are three types of capillaries: continuous, fenestrated, and sinusoidal.

Continuous capillaries are made up of epithelial cells tightly connected together. As a result, they limit the types of materials that pass into and out of the blood. Continuous capillaries are the most common type of capillary. Fenestrated capillaries have openings that allow materials to be freely exchanged between the blood and tissues. They are commonly found in the digestive, endocrine, and urinary systems. Sinusoidal capillaries have larger openings and allow proteins and blood cells through. They are found primarily in the liver, bone marrow, and spleen.

Blood

Blood is vital to the human body. It is a liquid connective tissue that serves as a transport system for supplying cells with nutrients and carrying away their wastes. The average adult human has five to six quarts of blood circulating through their body. Approximately 55% of blood is plasma (the fluid portion), and the remaining 45% is composed of solid cells and cell parts. There are three major types of blood cells:

- **Red blood cells, or erythrocytes, transport oxygen throughout the body.** They contain a protein called hemoglobin that allows them to carry oxygen. The iron in the hemoglobin gives the cells and the blood their red colors.
- **White blood cells, or leukocytes, are responsible for fighting infectious diseases and maintaining the immune system.** There are five types of white blood cells: neutrophils, lymphocytes, eosinophils, monocytes, and basophils.
- **Platelets** are cell fragments that play a central role in the blood clotting process.

All blood cells in adults are produced in the bone marrow—red blood cells from red marrow and white blood cells from yellow marrow.

Heart

The heart is a two-part, muscular pump that forcefully pushes blood throughout the human body. The human heart has four chambers—two upper atria and two lower ventricles separated by a partition called the septum. There is a pair on the left and a pair on the right. Anatomically, **left** and **right** correspond to the sides of the body that the patient themselves would refer to as left and right.

Four valves help to section off the chambers from one another. Between the right atrium and ventricle, the three flaps of the tricuspid valve keep blood from backflowing from the ventricle to the atrium, similar to how the two flaps of the mitral valve work between the left atrium and ventricle. As these two valves lie between an atrium and a ventricle, they are referred to as atrioventricular (AV) valves. The other two valves are semilunar (SL) and control blood flow into the two great arteries leaving the ventricles. The pulmonary valve connects the right ventricle to the pulmonary artery, while the aortic valve connects the left ventricle to the aorta.

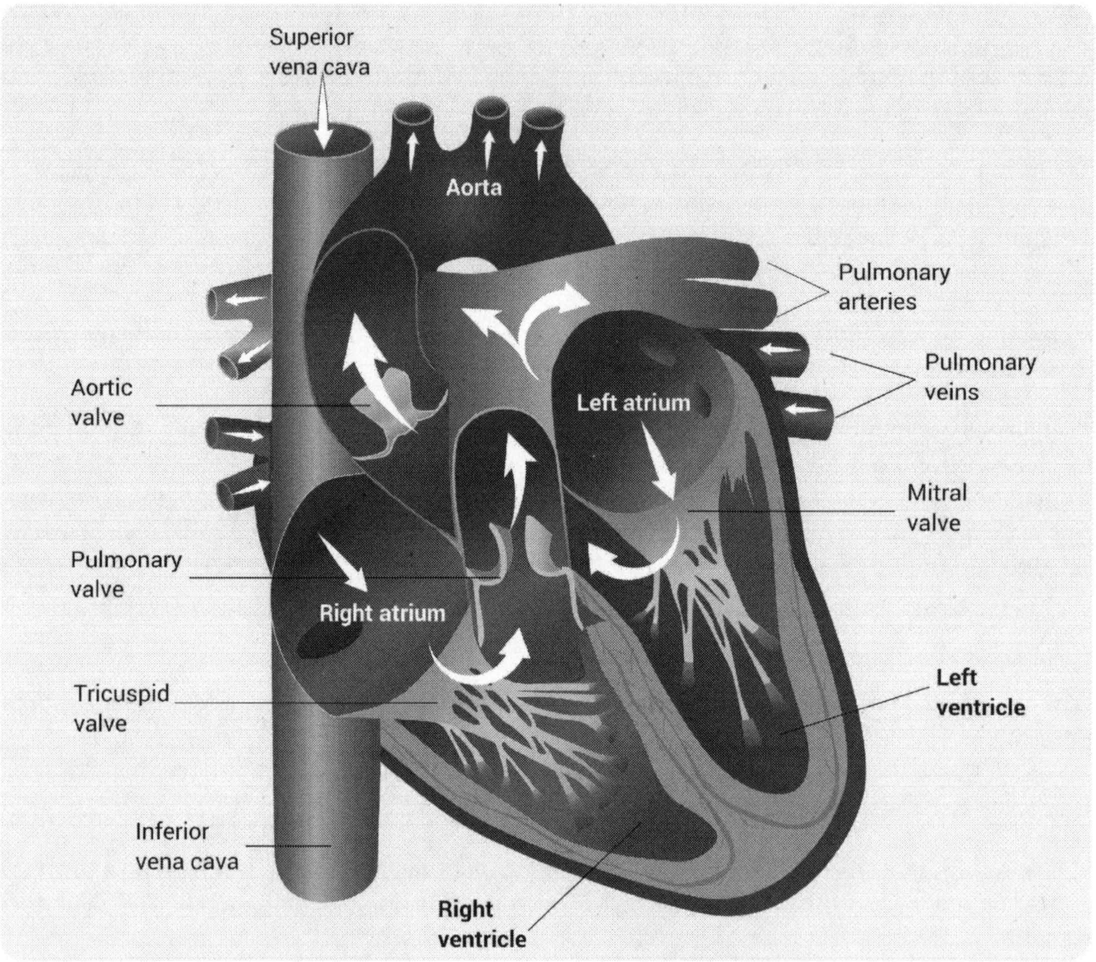

Cardiac Cycle

A cardiac cycle is one complete sequence of cardiac activity. The cardiac cycle represents the relaxation and contraction of the heart and can be divided into two phases: diastole and systole.

Diastole is the phase during which the heart relaxes and fills with blood. It gives rise to the diastolic blood pressure (DBP), which is the bottom number of a blood pressure reading. Systole is the phase during which the heart contracts and discharges blood. It gives rise to the systolic blood pressure (SBP), which is the top number of a blood pressure reading. The heart's electrical conduction system coordinates the cardiac cycle.

Types of Circulation

Five major blood vessels manage blood flow to and from the heart: the superior vena cava and inferior vena cava, the aorta, the pulmonary artery, and the pulmonary vein.

The superior vena cava is a large vein that drains blood from the head and the upper body. The inferior vena cava is a large vein that drains blood from the lower body. The aorta is the largest artery in the human body and carries blood from the heart to body tissues. The pulmonary arteries carry blood from the heart to the lungs. The pulmonary veins transport blood from the lungs to the heart.

In the human body, there are two types of circulation: pulmonary circulation and systemic circulation. Pulmonary circulation supplies blood to the lungs. Deoxygenated blood enters the right atrium of the heart and is routed through the tricuspid valve into the right ventricle. Deoxygenated blood then travels from the right ventricle of the heart through the pulmonary valve and into the pulmonary arteries. The pulmonary arteries carry the deoxygenated blood to the lungs. In the lungs, oxygen is absorbed, and carbon dioxide is released. The pulmonary veins carry oxygenated blood to the left atrium of the heart.

Systemic circulation supplies blood to all other parts of the body, except the lungs. Oxygenated blood flows from the left atrium of the heart through the mitral, or bicuspid, valve into the left ventricle of the heart. Oxygenated blood is then routed from the left ventricle of the heart through the aortic valve and into the aorta. The aorta delivers blood to the systemic arteries, which supply the body tissues. In the tissues, oxygen and nutrients are exchanged for carbon dioxide and other wastes. The deoxygenated blood along with carbon dioxide and wastes enter the systemic veins, where they are returned to the right atrium of the heart via the superior and inferior vena cava.

Describe the Anatomy and Physiology of the Digestive System

The human body relies completely on the digestive system to meet its nutritional needs. After food and drink are ingested, the digestive system breaks them down into their component nutrients and absorbs them so that the circulatory system can transport them to other cells to use for growth, energy, and cell repair. These nutrients may be classified as proteins, lipids, carbohydrates, vitamins, and minerals.

The digestive system is thought of chiefly in two parts: the digestive tract (also called the alimentary tract or gastrointestinal tract) and the accessory digestive organs. The digestive tract is the pathway in which food is ingested, digested, absorbed, and excreted. It is composed of the mouth, pharynx, esophagus, stomach, small and large intestines, rectum, and anus. **Peristalsis**, or wave-like contractions of smooth muscle, moves food and wastes through the digestive tract. The accessory digestive organs are the salivary glands, liver, gallbladder, and pancreas.

Mouth and Stomach

The mouth is the entrance to the digestive system. Here, the mechanical and chemical digestion of the food begins. The food is chewed mechanically by the teeth and shaped into a **bolus** by the tongue so that it can be more easily swallowed by the esophagus. The food also becomes more watery and pliable with the addition of saliva secreted from the salivary glands, the largest of which are the parotid glands. The glands also secrete amylase in the saliva, an enzyme which begins chemical digestion and breakdown of the carbohydrates and sugars in the food.

The food then moves through the pharynx and down the muscular esophagus to the stomach.

The stomach is a large, muscular sac-like organ at the distal end of the esophagus. Here, the bolus is subjected to more mechanical and chemical digestion. As it passes through the stomach, it is physically squeezed and crushed while additional secretions turn it into a watery nutrient-filled liquid that exits into the small intestine as **chyme**.

The stomach secretes a great many substances into the **lumen** of the digestive tract. Some cells produce gastrin, a hormone that prompts other cells in the stomach to secrete a gastric acid composed mostly of hydrochloric acid (HCl). The HCl is at such a high concentration and low pH that it denatures most proteins and degrades a lot of organic matter. The stomach also secretes mucous to form a protective film that keeps the corrosive acid from dissolving its own cells. Gaps in this mucous layer can lead to peptic ulcers. Finally, the stomach also uses digestive enzymes like proteases and lipases to break down proteins and fats; although there are some gastric lipases here, the stomach is most known for breaking down proteins.

Endocrine cells of the upper gastrointestinal tract—primarily the stomach—produce a hormone called ghrelin, which signals feelings of hunger to increase nutrient intake and affects energy spent on ATP production and lipid storage. In contrast, enterocytes in the small intestine produce a hormone called leptin, which signals feelings of satiety, or fullness. Leptin functions by acting against hunger-promoting hormones and promoting hunger suppression hormones. In a healthy system, these two hormones help balance the individual's hunger and satiety to help control nutrient intake.

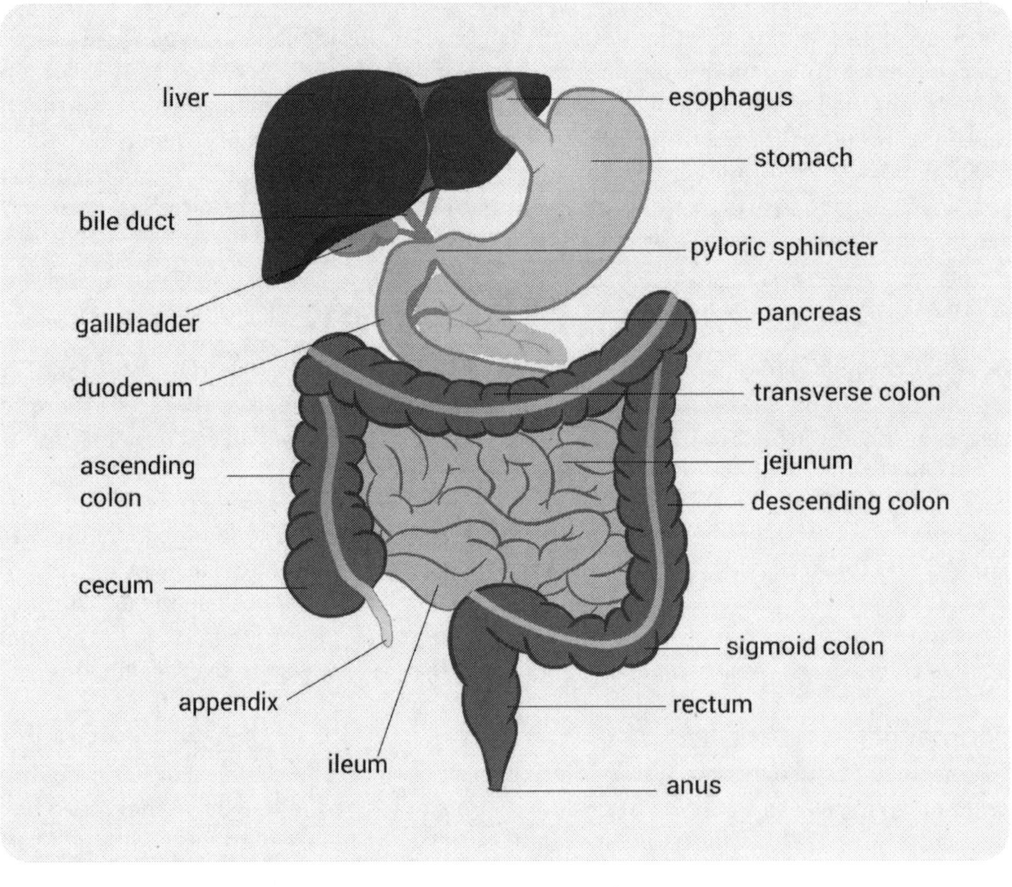

Small Intestine

The chyme from the stomach enters the first part of the small intestine, the **duodenum**, through the **pyloric sphincter**, and its extreme acidity is partly neutralized by sodium bicarbonate secreted along with mucous. The presence of chyme in the duodenum triggers the secretion of the hormones secretin and cholecystokinin (CCK). Secretin acts on the pancreas to dump more sodium bicarbonate into the small intestine so that the pH is kept at a reasonable level, while CCK acts on the pancreas to stimulate secretions and the gallbladder to release the **bile** that it has been storing. Bile, a substance produced by the liver and stored in the gallbladder, helps to **emulsify** or dissolve fats and lipids. Bile is composed primarily from water, bile salts (organic acid compounds), bilirubin, and lipids. The acids found in bile specifically aid in digestion.

Because of the bile (which aids in lipid absorption) and the secreted lipases (which break down fats), the duodenum is the chief site of fat digestion in the body. The duodenum also represents the last major site of chemical digestion in the digestive tract, as the other two sections of the small intestine (the **jejunum** and **ileum**) are instead heavily involved in absorption of nutrients.

The small intestine reaches 40 feet in length, and its cells are arranged in small finger-like projections called villi. This is due to its key role in the absorption of nearly all nutrients from the ingested and digested food, effectively transferring them from the lumen of the GI tract to the bloodstream, where they travel to the cells that need them. These nutrients include simple sugars like glucose from carbohydrates, amino acids from proteins, emulsified fats, electrolytes like sodium and potassium, minerals like iron and zinc, and vitamins like D and B12. Vitamin B12's absorption, though it takes place in the intestines, is actually aided by **intrinsic factor** that was released into the chyme back in the stomach.

Large Intestine

The leftover parts of food that remain unabsorbed or undigested in the lumen of the small intestine next travel through the large intestine, which is also referred to as the large bowel or colon. The large intestine is mainly responsible for water absorption. As the chyme at this stage no longer has anything useful that can be absorbed by the body, it is now referred to as **waste**, and it is stored in the large intestine until it can be excreted from the body. Removing the liquid from the waste transforms it from liquid to solid stool, or feces.

This waste first passes from the small intestine to the cecum, a pouch that forms the first part of the large intestine. In herbivores, it provides a place for bacteria to digest cellulose, but in humans most of it is vestigial and is known as the appendix. From the cecum, waste next travels up the ascending colon, across the transverse colon, down the descending colon, and through the sigmoid colon to the rectum. The rectum is responsible for the final storage of waste before it is expelled through the anus. The anal canal is a small portion of the rectum leading through to the anus and the outside of the body.

Pancreas

The pancreas has endocrine and exocrine functions. The endocrine function involves releasing the hormone insulin, which decreases blood sugar (glucose) levels, and glucagon, which increases blood sugar (glucose) levels, directly into the bloodstream. Both hormones are produced in the islets of Langerhans, insulin in the beta cells and glucagon in the alpha cells.

The exocrine function of the pancreas involves the secretion of inactive digestive enzymes (zymogens) from acinar cells into the main pancreatic duct. The main pancreatic duct joins the common bile duct, which empties into the small intestine (specifically the duodenum). The digestive enzymes are then activated and take part in the digestion of carbohydrates, proteins, and fats within chyme (the mixture of partially digested food and digestive juices).

Describe the Anatomy and Physiology of the Nervous System

Nervous System

The human nervous system coordinates the body's response to stimuli from inside and outside the body. There are two major types of nervous system cells: neurons and neuroglia. Neurons are the workhorses of the nervous system and form a complex communication network that transmits electrical impulses termed action potentials, while neuroglia connect and support the neurons.

Although some neurons monitor the senses, some control muscles, and some connect the brain to other neurons, all neurons have four common characteristics:

- Dendrites: These receive electrical signals from other neurons across small gaps called **synapses**.
- Nerve cell body: This is the hub of processing and protein manufacture for the neuron.
- Axon: This transmits the signal from the cell body to other neurons.
- Terminals: These bridge the neuron to dendrites of other neurons and deliver the signal via chemical messengers called neurotransmitters.

Here is an illustration of this:

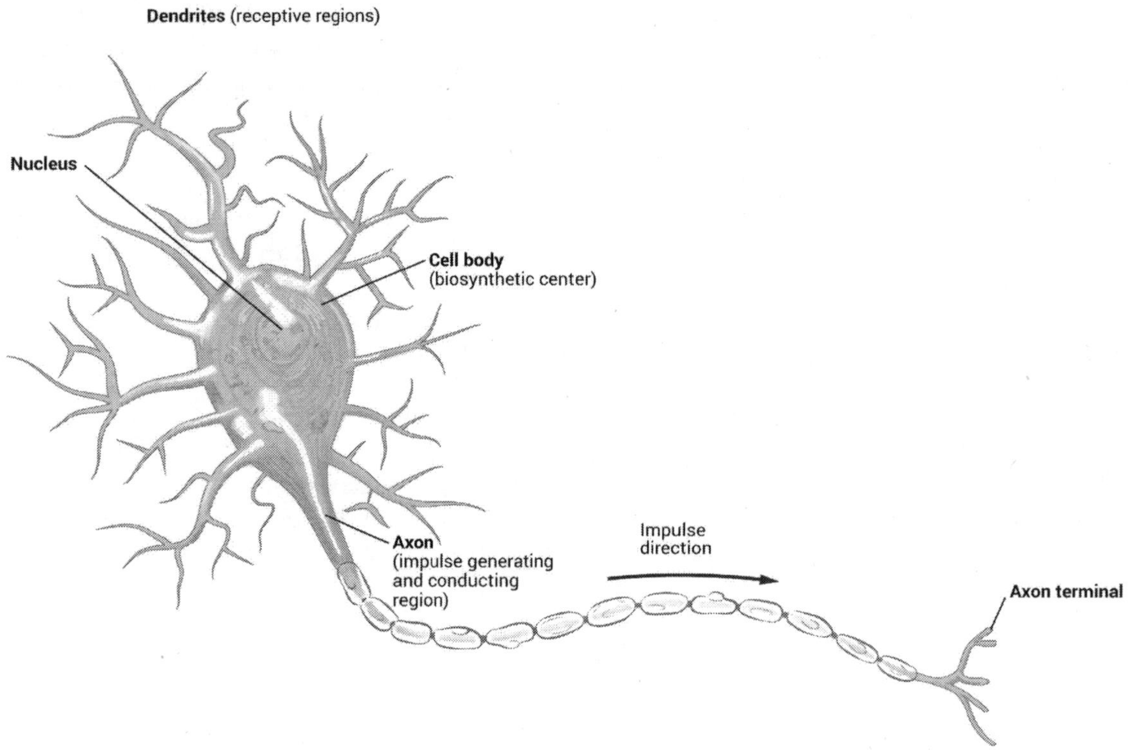

There are two major divisions of the nervous system, central and peripheral:

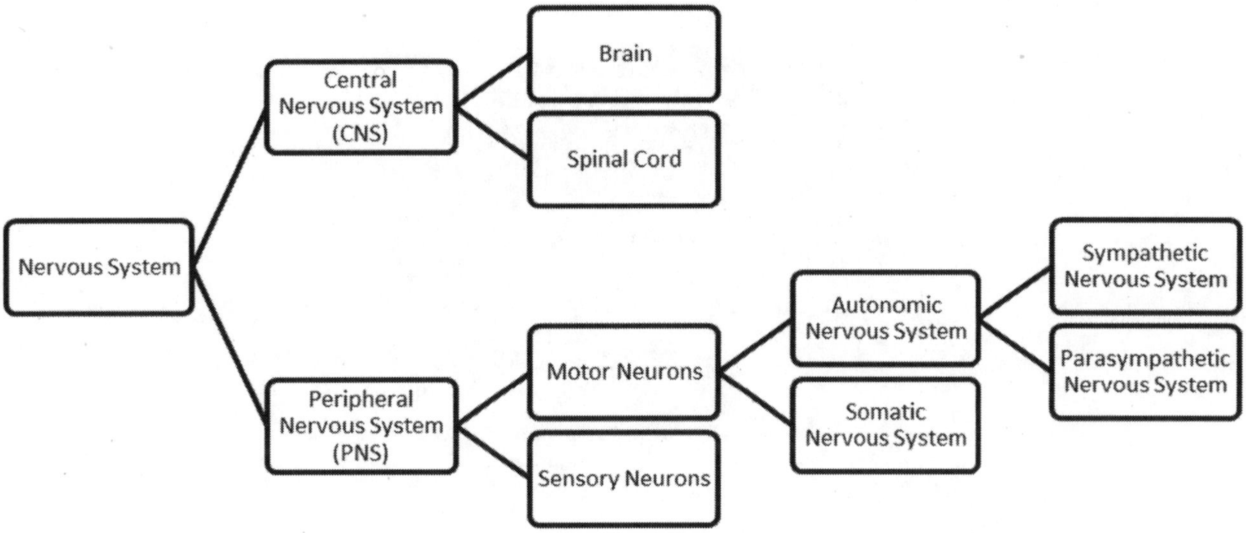

Central Nervous System

The central nervous system (CNS) consists of the brain and spinal cord. Three layers of membranes called the meninges cover and separate the CNS from the rest of the body.

The major divisions of the brain are the forebrain, the midbrain, and the hindbrain.

The forebrain consists of the cerebrum, the thalamus and hypothalamus, and the rest of the limbic system. The **cerebrum** is the largest part of the brain, and its most well-documented part is the outer cerebral cortex. The cerebrum is divided into right and left hemispheres, and each cerebral cortex hemisphere has four discrete areas, or lobes: frontal, temporal, parietal, and occipital. The frontal lobe governs duties such as voluntary movement, judgment, problem solving, and planning, while the other lobes are more sensory. The temporal lobe integrates hearing and language comprehension, the parietal lobe processes sensory input from the skin, and the occipital lobe processes visual input from the eyes. For completeness, the other two senses, smell and taste, are processed via the olfactory bulbs. The thalamus helps organize and coordinate all of this sensory input in a meaningful way for the brain to interpret.

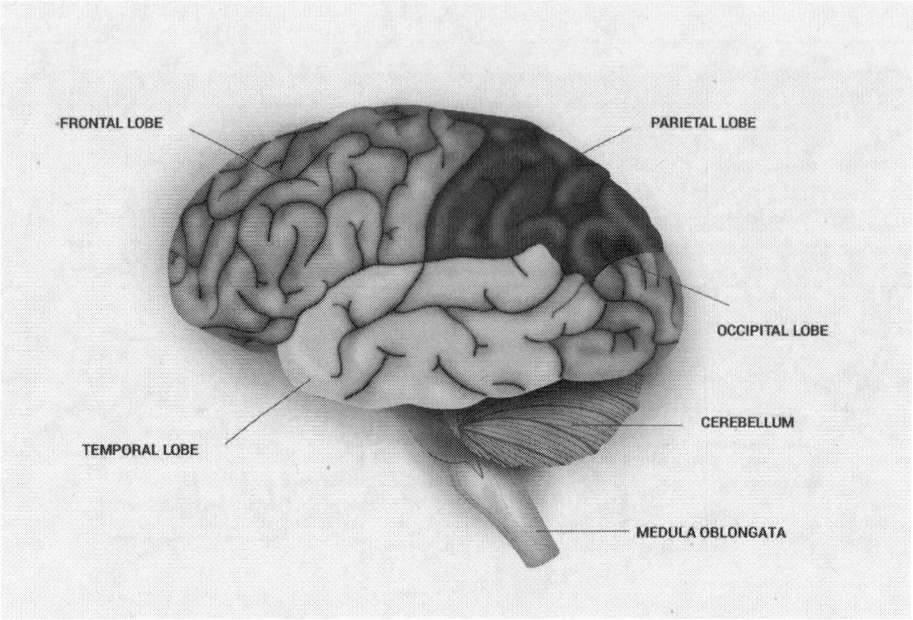

The hypothalamus controls the endocrine system and all of the hormones that govern long-term effects on the body. Each hemisphere of the limbic system includes a hippocampus (which plays a vital role in memory), an amygdala (which is involved with emotional responses like fear and anger), and other small bodies and nuclei associated with memory and pleasure.

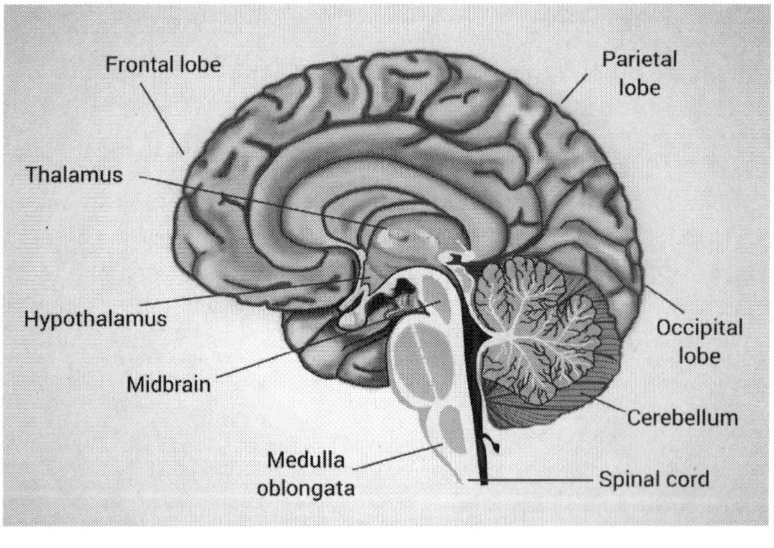

The midbrain is in charge of alertness, sleep/wake cycles, and temperature regulation, and it includes the substantia nigra, which produces dopamine and is involved with reward and movement. The notable components of the hindbrain include the medulla oblongata and cerebellum. The medulla oblongata is located just above the spinal cord and is responsible for crucial involuntary functions such as breathing, swallowing, and regulating heart rate and blood pressure. Together with other parts of the hindbrain, the midbrain and medulla oblongata form the brain stem. The brain stem connects the spinal cord to the rest of the brain. To the rear of the brain stem sits the cerebellum, which plays key roles in posture, balance, and muscular coordination. The spinal cord itself, which is encapsulated by the protective bony spinal column, carries sensory information to the brain and motor information to the body.

Peripheral Nervous System

The peripheral nervous system (PNS) includes all nervous tissue besides the brain and spinal cord. The PNS consists of the sets of cranial and spinal nerves and relays information between the CNS and the rest of the body. The PNS has two divisions: the autonomic nervous system and the somatic nervous system.

Autonomic Nervous System

The autonomic nervous system (ANS) governs involuntary, or reflexive, body functions. Ultimately, the autonomic nervous system controls functions such as breathing, heart rate, digestion, body temperature, and blood pressure.

The ANS is split between parasympathetic nerves and sympathetic nerves. These two nerve types are antagonistic, and have opposite effects on the body. Parasympathetic nerves predominate resting conditions, and decrease heart rate, decrease breathing rate, prepare digestion, and allow urination and excretion. Sympathetic nerves, on the other hand, become active when a person is under stress or excited, and they increase heart rate, increase breathing rates, and inhibit digestion, urination, and excretion.

Somatic Nervous System and the Reflex Arc

The somatic nervous system (SNS) governs the conscious, or voluntary, control of skeletal muscles and their corresponding body movements. The SNS contains afferent and efferent neurons. Afferent neurons carry sensory messages from the skeletal muscles, skin, or sensory organs to the CNS. Efferent neurons relay motor messages from the CNS to skeletal muscles, skin, or sensory organs.

The SNS also has a role in involuntary movements called reflexes. A reflex is defined as an involuntary response to a stimulus. They are transmitted via what is termed a **reflex arc**, where a stimulus is sensed by an affector and its afferent neuron, interpreted and rerouted by an interneuron, and delivered to effector muscles by an efferent neuron where they respond to the initial stimulus. A reflex is able to bypass the brain by being rerouted through the spinal cord; the interneuron decides the proper course of action rather than the brain. The reflex arc results in an instantaneous, involuntary response. For example, a physician tapping on the knee produces an involuntary knee jerk referred to as the patellar tendon reflex.

Neuron Form and Function

Nerve cells, or neurons, feature branchlike protrusions which receive and transmit electrochemical signals to somatic cells and other neurons. Nerve cells that signal other nerve cells are called interneurons, and are located in the central nervous system. Neurons that send information to the CNS are called sensory neurons, while those that send signals to the body's muscles and organs are motor neurons. There are several parts of neurons that are fairly unique from other cells in the body. The central body of the neuron is called the soma, where most of the neuron's proteins are produced and where the nucleus is located. From the soma, there are many types of protrusions that can extend out. Short, branching extensions of the cell called dendrites (named for their treelike appearance) are where most signals are received and processed along with inside the soma.

The most characteristic protrusion is called the axon; each neuron possesses no more than one axon. Each axon has microtubules running its length to support the axon's structure. The axon is wrapped in segments by layers of myelin from Schwann cells in the PNS, or oligodendrocytes in the CNS. These layers make what is called the myelin sheath and partially insulate the axon, increasing the speed of propagation of an action potential by leaving small, periodic gaps. Ions can only flow in and out of the axon at those gaps, called nodes of Ranvier, so the influx of positively charged sodium ions can only occur there.

Describe the Anatomy and Physiology of the Muscular System

The **muscular system** is responsible for involuntary and voluntary movement of the body. There are three types of muscle: skeletal, cardiac, and smooth.

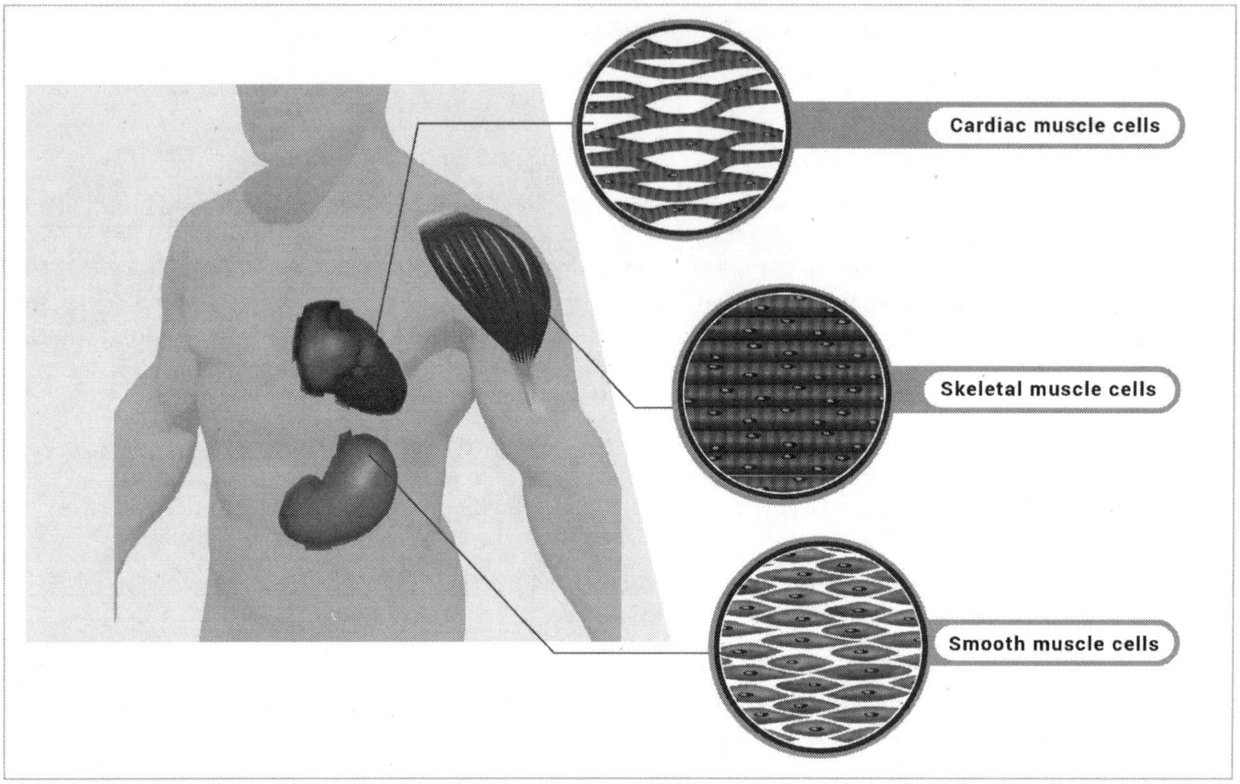

Skeletal Muscles

Skeletal muscles*, or voluntary muscles, are attached to bones by tendons and are responsible for voluntary movement.* The connecting tendons are made up of dense bands of connective tissue and have collagen fibers that firmly attach the muscle to the bone. Their fibers are actually woven into the coverings of the bone and muscle so that they can withstand pressure and tension. They usually work in opposing pairs like the biceps and triceps, for example.

Skeletal muscles are made of bundles of long fibers that are composed of cells with many nuclei due to their length. These fibers contain myofibrils, and myofibrils are made of alternating filaments. The thicker myosin filaments are in between the smaller actin filaments in a unit called a sarcomere, and the overlapping regions of these filaments give the muscle its characteristic striated, or striped, appearance. Actin filaments are attached to exterior Z lines, myosin filaments are attached to a central M line, and when a muscle is at rest, there is a gap between the Z line and the myosin filaments. Only when the muscle contracts and the actin filaments slide over the myosin filaments does the myosin reach the Z line, as illustrated in the picture below. This sliding-filament model of muscle contraction is dependent on myosin molecules forming and breaking cross-bridges with actin in order to pull the actin filaments closer to the M line.

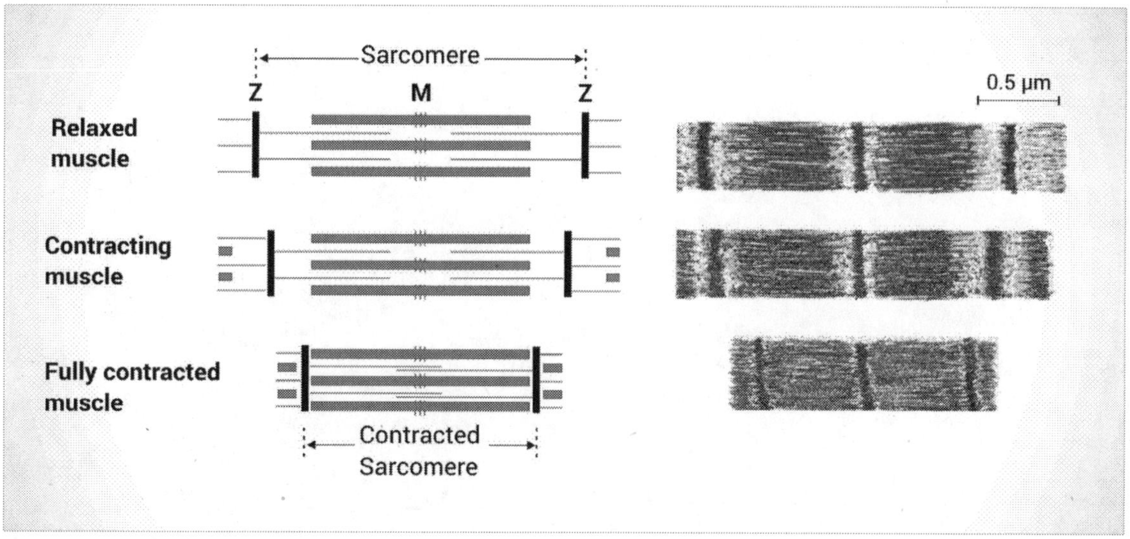

Skeletal muscles are controlled by the nervous system. Motor neurons connect to muscle fibers via neuromuscular junctions. Motor neurons must release the neurotransmitter acetylcholine, which causes the release of calcium ions from the sarcoplasmic reticulum to stimulate myosin cross-bridging and contraction. The sarcoplasmic reticulum is a network of structural tubules in the muscle fiber's cytoplasm that stores components needed for contraction. When acetylcholine is no longer released, calcium returns to the sarcoplasmic reticulum and contraction ends.

Smooth Muscles

Smooth muscles are responsible for involuntary movement, such as food moving through the digestive tract and blood moving through vessels. They have only one nucleus and do not have striations because actin and myosin filaments do not have an organized arrangement like skeletal muscles do. Unlike skeletal muscle, smooth muscle doesn't rely on neuromuscular junctions for intercellular communication. Instead, they operate via gap junctions, which send impulses directly from cell to cell.

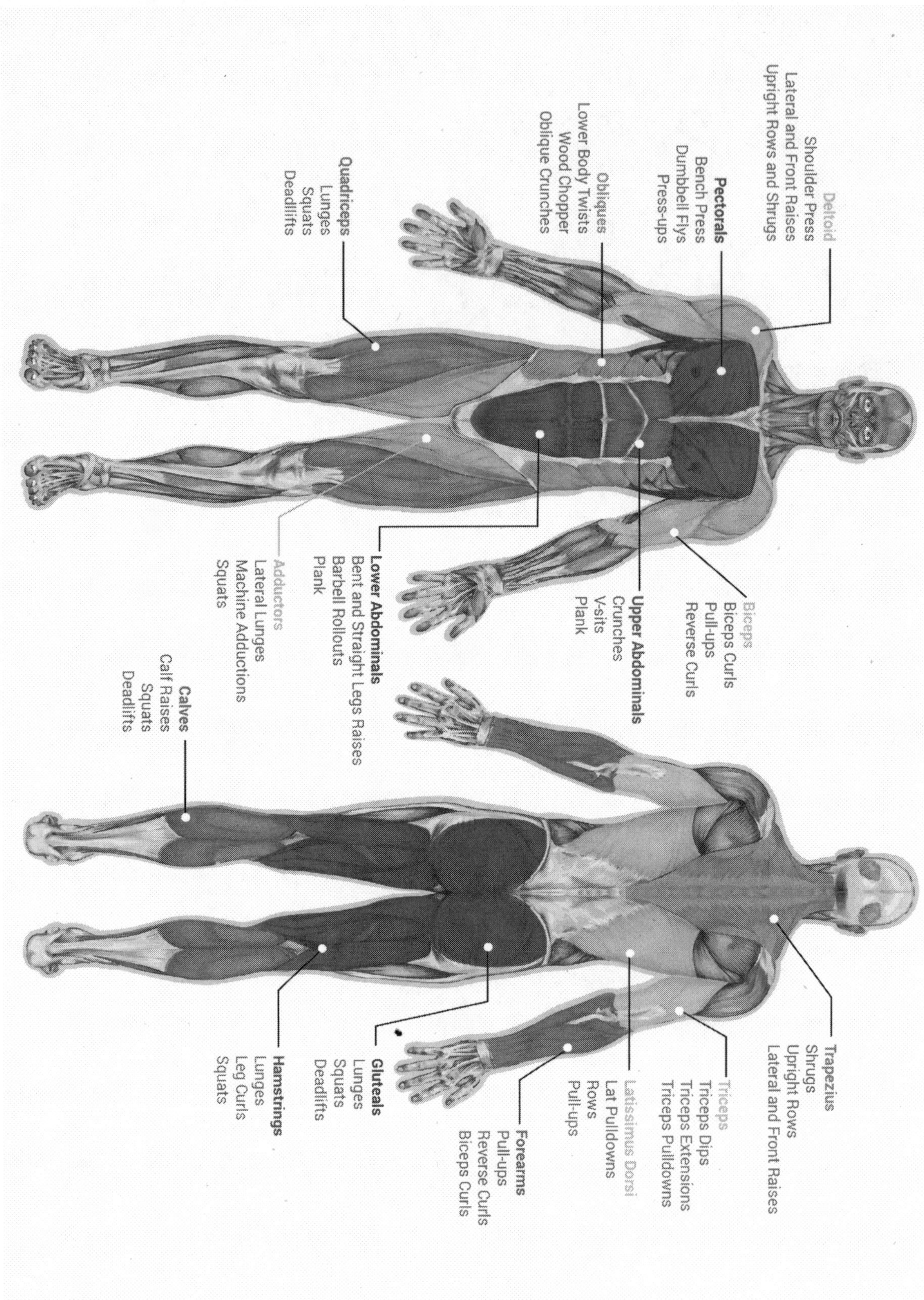
Deltoid
Shoulder Press
Lateral and Front Raises
Upright Rows and Shrugs
Pectorals
Bench Press
Dumbbell Flys
Press-ups
Obliques
Lower Body Twists
Wood Chopper
Oblique Crunches
Quadriceps
Lunges
Squats
Deadlifts
Biceps
Biceps Curls
Pull-ups
Reverse Curls
Upper Abdominals
Crunches
V-sits
Plank
Lower Abdominals
Bent and Straight Legs Raises
Barbell Rollouts
Plank
Adductors
Lateral Lunges
Machine Adductions
Squats
Calves
Calf Raises
Squats
Deadlifts
Trapezius
Shrugs
Upright Rows
Lateral and Front Raises
Triceps
Triceps Dips
Triceps Extensions
Triceps Pulldowns
Latissimus Dorsi
Lat Pulldowns
Rows
Pull-ups
Forearms
Pull-ups
Reverse Curls
Biceps Curls
Gluteals
Lunges
Squats
Deadlifts
Hamstrings
Lunges
Leg Curls
Squats

Cardiac Muscles

Cardiac muscle cells are found only in the heart, where they control the heart's rhythm and blood pressure. Like skeletal muscle, cardiac muscle has striations, but cardiac muscle cells are smaller than skeletal muscle cells, so they typically have only one nucleus. Like smooth muscle, cardiac muscles do not require neurotransmitter release by motor neurons to function, and they instead operate via gap junctions.

Describe the Anatomy and Physiology of the Male and Female Reproductive System

The reproductive system is responsible for producing, storing, nourishing, and transporting functional reproductive cells, or gametes, in the human body. It includes the reproductive organs, also known as **gonads**, the reproductive tract, the accessory glands and organs that secrete fluids into the reproductive tract, and the perineal structures, which are the external genitalia.

Reproduction involves the passing of genes from one generation to the next, and that is accomplished through haploid gametes. Gametes have gone through meiosis and have 23 chromosomes, half the normal number. The male gamete is sperm, and the female gamete is an egg or ovum. When a sperm fertilizes an egg, they create a zygote, which is the first cell of a new organism. The zygote has a full set of 46 chromosomes because it received 23 from each parent. Because of gene shuffling during sperm and egg development, sperm and egg chromosome sets are all different, which results in the variety seen in humans.

Zygotes are a type of stem cell, and thus are able to grow and change, or **differentiate**, into any other type of cell in the body. This ability to differentiate into other types of cells is an important quality known as **cell potency**. A cell that can only become one type of cell would be referred to as unipotent, while stem cells that can differentiate into any of the adult cells in the body would be called **pluripotent**. Cells like precursor T cells in the immune system are an example of **multipotent cells**—those with limited ability to differentiate.

Male Reproductive System

The entire male reproductive system is designed to generate sperm and produce semen that facilitate fertilization of eggs, the female gametes. The **testes** are the endocrine glands that secrete testosterone, a hormone that is important for secondary sex characteristics and sperm development, or **spermatogenesis**. Testosterone is in the androgen steroid-hormone family. The testes also produce and store 500 million **spermatocytes**, which are the male gametes, each day. Testes are housed in the scrotum, which is a sac that hangs outside the body so that spermatogenesis occurs at cooler and optimal conditions.

The seminiferous tubules within the testes produce spermatocytes, which then travel to the epididymis where they are stored as they mature. Then, the sperm move to the ejaculatory duct via the vas deferens. The ejaculatory duct contains more than just sperm. The seminal vesicles secrete an alkaline substance that will help sperm survive in the acidic vagina. The prostate gland secretes enzymes bathed in a milky white fluid, which is important for thinning semen after ejaculation to increase its likelihood of reaching the egg. The bulbourethral gland, or Cowper's gland, secretes an alkaline fluid that lubricates the urethra prior to ejaculation to neutralize any acidic urine residue.

The sperm, along with all the exocrine secretions, are collectively called semen. In order for sexual intercourse to successfully transfer sperm from the male to the female's egg, the penis must be erect, which occurs via arousal and increased circulation. During sexual intercourse, ejaculation will forcefully expel the contents of the semen up through the vagina and effectively deliver the sperm to the egg. The muscular prostate gland is important for ejaculation. Each ejaculation releases 2 to 6 million sperm. Sperm has a whip-like flagellum tail that facilitates movement.

Female Reproductive System

The vagina is the passageway that sperm must travel through to reach an egg, the female gamete. Surrounding the vagina are the labia minor and labia major, both of which are folds that protect the urethra, which is used for urination and is part of the urinary system, and the vaginal opening. The clitoris is rich in nerve-endings, making it sensitive and highly stimulated during sexual intercourse. It is above the vagina and urethra. An exocrine gland called the Bartholin's glands secretes a fluid during arousal that is important for lubrication.

The female gonads are the ovaries. Ovaries generally alternate producing one gamete, an egg or oocyte, per month. They are also responsible for secreting the hormones estrogen and progesterone. Fertilization cannot happen unless the ejaculated sperm finds the egg, which is only available at certain times of the month. Eggs, or ova, develop in the ovaries in clusters surrounded by follicles, and after puberty, they are delivered to the uterus once a month via the fallopian tubes. The 28-day average journey of the egg to the uterus is called the **menstrual cycle**, and it is highly regulated by the endocrine system. The regulatory hormones Gonadotropin releasing hormone (GnRH), luteinizing hormone (LH), and follicle-stimulating hormone (FSH) orchestrate the menstrual cycle. Ovarian hormones estrogen and progesterone are also important in timing as well as for vascularization of the uterus in preparation for pregnancy. Fertilization usually happens around **ovulation**, which is when the egg is inside the fallopian tube. The resulting zygote travels down the tube and implants into the uterine wall. The uterus protects and nourishes the developing embryo for nine months, until it is ready for the outside environment.

If the egg released is unfertilized, the uterine lining will slough off during menstruation. Should a fertilized egg, called a zygote, reach the uterus, it will embed itself into the uterine wall due to uterine vascularization that will deliver blood, nutrients, and antibodies to the developing embryo. The uterus is where the embryo will develop for the next nine months. Mammary glands are important female reproductive structures because they produce the milk provided for babies during lactation. Milk contains nutrients and antibodies that benefit the baby.

Describe the Anatomy and Physiology of the Integumentary System

The integumentary system includes skin, hair, nails, oil glands, and sweat glands. The largest organ of the integumentary system (and of the body), the skin, acts as a barrier and protects the body from mechanical impact, variations in temperature, microorganisms, chemicals, and UV radiation from the sun. It regulates body temperature, peripheral circulation, and excretes waste through sweat. It also contains a large network of nerve cells that relay changes in the external environment to the brain.

Layers of Skin

Skin consists of three layers, the surface epidermis, the inner dermis, and the subcutaneous hypodermis, located below the dermis and containing a layer of fat and connective tissue, which are both important for insulation.

The whole epidermis is composed of epithelial cells that lack blood vessels. The outer epidermis is composed of dead cells, which surround the living cells underneath. The most inner epidermal tissue is a single layer of cells called the stratum basale, which is composed of rapidly dividing cells that push old cells to the skin's surface. When being pushed out, the cells' organelles disappear, and they start producing a protein called keratin, which eventually forms a tough waterproof layer. This outer layer sloughs off every four to five weeks. The melanocytes in the stratum basale produce the pigment melanin, which absorbs UV rays and protects the skin. Skin also produces vitamin D if exposed to sunlight.

The dermis underneath the epidermis contains supporting collagen fibers peppered with nerves, blood vessels, hair follicles, sweat glands, oil glands, and smooth muscles.

Skin's Involvement in Temperature Homeostasis

The skin has a thermoregulatory role in the human body that is controlled by a negative feedback loop. The control center of temperature regulation is the hypothalamus in the brain. When the hypothalamus is alerted by receptors from the dermis, it secretes hormones that activate effectors to keep internal temperature at a set point of 98.6°F (37°C). If the environment is too cold, the hypothalamus will initiate a pathway that induces muscle shivering to release heat energy as well as constrict blood vessels to limit heat loss. In hot conditions, the hypothalamus will initiate a pathway that vasodilates blood vessels to increase heat loss and stimulate sweating for evaporative cooling. Evaporative cooling occurs when the hottest water particles evaporate and leave behind the coolest ones. This cools down the body.

Sebaceous Glands vs. Sweat Glands

The skin also contains oil glands, or sebaceous glands, and sweat glands that are exocrine because their substances are secreted through ducts. Endocrine glands secrete substances into the bloodstream instead. Oil glands are attached to hair follicles. They secrete sebum, an oily substance that moisturizes the skin, protecting it from water loss. Sebum also keeps the skin elastic. Also, sebum's slight acidity provides a chemical defense against bacterial and fungal infections.

Sweat glands not attached to hair follicles are called eccrine glands. They are all over the body, and are the sweat glands responsible for thermoregulation. They also remove bodily waste by secreting water and electrolytes. Sweat glands attached to hair follicles are apocrine glands, and there are far fewer apocrine sweat glands than eccrine sweat glands in the body. Apocrine glands are only active post-puberty. They secrete a thicker, viscous substance that is attractive to bacteria, leading to the unpleasant smell in armpits, feet, and the groin. They are stimulated during stress and arousal.

Integumentary System (Skin)

Skin consists of three layers: epidermis, dermis, and the hypodermis. There are four types of cells that make up the keratinized stratified squamous epithelium in the epidermis. They are keratinocytes, melanocytes, Merkel cells, and Langerhans cells. Skin is composed of many layers, starting with a basement membrane. On top of that sits the stratum germinativum, the stratum spinosum, the stratum granulosum, the stratum lucidum, and then the stratum corneum at the outer surface. Skin can be classified as thick or thin. These descriptions refer to the epidermis layer. Most of the body is covered with thin skin, but areas such as the palms are covered with thick skin. The dermis consists of a superficial papillary layer and a deeper reticular layer. The papillary layer is made of loose connective tissue, containing capillaries and the axons of sensory neurons. The reticular layer is a meshwork of tightly packed irregular connective tissue, containing blood vessels, hair follicles, nerves, sweat glands, and sebaceous glands. The hypodermis is a loose layer of fat and connective tissue. Since it is the third layer, if a burn reaches this third degree, it has caused serious damage.

Sweat glands and sebaceous glands are important exocrine glands found in the skin. Sweat glands regulate temperature, and remove bodily waste by secreting water, nitrogenous waste, and sodium salts to the surface of the body. Some sweat glands are classified as apocrine glands. Sebaceous glands are holocrine glands that secrete sebum, which is an oily mixture of lipids and proteins. Sebum protects the skin from water loss, as well as bacterial and fungal infections.

The three major functions of skin are protection, regulation, and sensation. Skin acts as a barrier and protects the body from mechanical impacts, variations in temperature, microorganisms, and chemicals. It regulates body temperature, peripheral circulation, and fluid balance by secreting sweat. It also contains a large network of nerve cells that relay changes in the external environment to the body.

Describe the Anatomy and Physiology of the Endocrine System

The endocrine system is made up of the ductless tissues and glands that secrete hormones directly into the bloodstream. It is similar to the nervous system in that it controls various functions of the body, but it does so via secretion of hormones in the bloodstream as opposed to nerve impulses. The endocrine system is also different because its effects last longer than that of the nervous system. Nerve impulses are immediate while hormone responses can last for minutes or even days.

The endocrine system works closely with the nervous system to regulate the physiological activities of the other systems of the body in order to maintain homeostasis. Hormone secretions are controlled by tight feedback loops that are generally regulated by the hypothalamus, the bridge between the nervous and endocrine systems. The hypothalamus receives sensory input via the nervous system and responds by stimulating or inhibiting the pituitary gland, which, in turn, stimulates or inhibits several other glands. The tight control is due to hormone secretions.

Hormones are chemicals that bind to specific target cells. Each hormone will only bind to a target cell that has a specific receptor that has the correct shape. For example, testosterone will not attach to skin cells because skin cells have no receptor that recognizes testosterone.

There are two types of hormones: steroid and protein. Steroid hormones are lipid, nonpolar substances, and most are able to diffuse across cell membranes. Once they do, they bind to a receptor that initiates a signal transduction cascade that affects gene expression. Non-steroid hormones bind to receptors on cell membranes that also initiate a signal transduction cascade that affects enzyme activity and chemical reactions.

Major Endocrine Glands

Hypothalamus: This gland is a part of the brain. It connects the nervous system to the endocrine system because it receives sensory information through nerves, and it sends instructions via hormones delivered to the pituitary gland.

Pituitary Gland: This gland is pea-sized and is found at the bottom of the hypothalamus. It has two lobes called the anterior and posterior lobes. It plays an important role in regulating other endocrine glands. For example, it secretes growth hormone, which regulates growth. Other hormones that are released by this gland control the reproductive system, childbirth, nursing, blood osmolarity, and metabolism.

The hormones and glands respond to each other via feedback loops, and a typical feedback loop is illustrated in the picture below. The hypothalamus and pituitary gland are master controllers of most of the other glands.

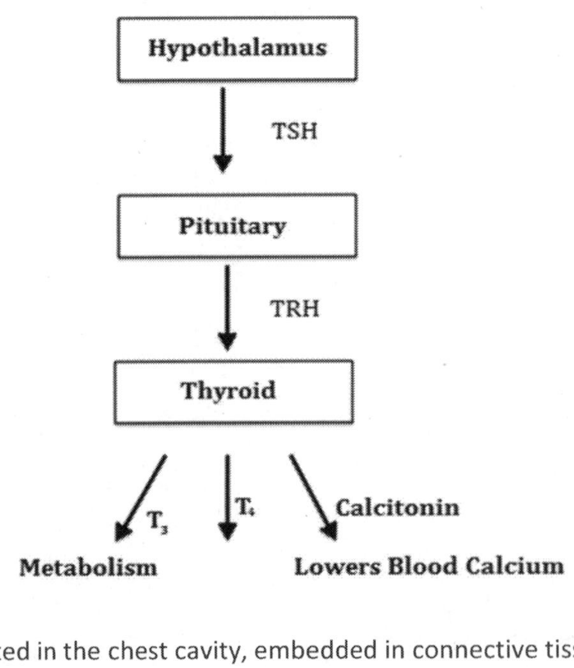

Thymus Gland: This gland is located in the chest cavity, embedded in connective tissue. It produces several hormones that are important for development and maintenance of T lymphocytes, which are important cells for immunity.

Adrenal Gland: One adrenal gland is attached to the top of each kidney. It produces epinephrine and norepinephrine which cause the "fight or flight" response in the face of danger or stress. These hormones raise heart rate, blood pressure, dilate bronchioles, and deliver blood to the muscles. All of these actions increase circulation and release glucose so that the body has an energy burst.

Pineal Gland: The pineal gland secretes melatonin, which is a hormone that regulates the body's circadian rhythm, which governs the natural wake-sleep cycle.

Testes and Ovaries: They secrete testosterone and both estrogen and progesterone, respectively. They are responsible for secondary sex characteristics, gamete development, and female hormones are important for embryonic development.

Thyroid Gland: This gland releases hormones like thyroxine and calcitonin. Thyroxine stimulates metabolism, and calcitonin monitors the amount of circulating calcium. Calcitonin signals the body to regulating calcium from bone reserves as well as kidney reabsorption of calcium.

Parathyroid Glands: These are four pea-sized glands located on the posterior surface of the thyroid. The main hormone that is secreted is called parathyroid hormone (PTH) which influences calcium levels like calcitonin, except it is antagonistic. PTH increases extracellular levels of calcium while calcitonin decreases it.

Pancreas: The pancreas is an organ that has both endocrine and exocrine functions. It functions outside of a typical feedback loop in that blood sugar seems to signal the pancreas itself. The endocrine functions are controlled by the pancreatic islets of Langerhans, which are groups of beta cells scattered throughout the gland that secrete insulin to lower blood sugar levels in the body. Neighboring alpha cells secrete glucagon to raise blood sugar. These complementary hormones keep blood sugar in check.

Feedback

Positive and Negative Feedback

Feedback loops are complex regulators that keep a balance between energy expenditure and energy conservation. One example of a feedback loop includes the complex mechanisms that maintain a human's optimal body temperature. This intricate feedback loop is controlled by the hypothalamus – the link between the nervous system and endocrine system in the brain. Upon receiving a neural stimulus, the hypothalamus stimulates or inhibits the pituitary gland based on nervous system input, which is how it regulates hormone levels that have specific physiological effects.

When body temperature is too low, the body is prompted to shiver, which releases energy from the muscles and warms the body. When body temperature is too high, the body initiates sweating, which regulates temperature through a process known as evaporative cooling. Evaporative cooling occurs because the water droplets heated by the body and released by sweat glands are the ones with the highest kinetic energy. The high kinetic energy results in the evaporation of the hottest water molecules, which leaves the cooler ones behind. Other endotherms, or organisms that regulate their temperature internally, have different mechanisms to cool down. Dogs, for example, only have sweat glands in their paws and nose, so they pant to use evaporative cooling by drawing moisture from their lungs.

Feedback Mechanisms

Organisms regulate cellular processes through feedback loops to fine-tune many other processes, including water osmolarity.

In blood, osmolarity refers to the concentration of the collective solutes and water in the blood, and it is regulated by the hypothalamus. The hypothalamus is the bridge between the nervous and endocrine systems via the pituitary gland, and it contains osmoreceptors that sense blood osmolarity. If blood has a low percentage of water, then an individual is dehydrated and has high blood osmolarity. If osmolarity is high, the hypothalamus stimulates the pituitary gland to release stored antidiuretic hormone (ADH). ADH stimulates the kidneys to increase water permeability in the collecting ducts, which increases reabsorption of water and reduces urine volume, meaning less water is lost through urination. This water-retaining mechanism will eventually lower the osmolarity, and when it falls below its set point, osmoreceptors will inhibit the hypothalamus from initiating reabsorption.

This is an example of a negative feedback loop because the stimulus feeds back to the regulator in order to change the production in the opposite direction. If production is too high, the system turns off, and if production is too low, the system turns on. Negative feedback loops respond to environmental conditions to keep them at a "set point."

Positive Feedback Loops

Positive feedback loops also exist to amplify responses in the presence of production, such as with intracellular signaling cascades or recruitment of cells in the immune system. They do not necessarily ensure cellular homeostasis, but rather they ensure functionality. For example, the production of oxytocin during childbirth is a critical positive feedback loop. In the case of childbirth, the initial stimulus is pressure on the cervix, which sends a message to the brain that causes the pituitary gland to secrete oxytocin, which acts on the uterus to stimulate contractions. As the pressure on the cervix increases, more oxytocin is produced in a positive feedback cycle. Once the baby and placenta are delivered, pressure on the cervix disappears, the pituitary stops producing oxytocin, and uterine contractions stop. Without this positive feedback loop, it would be impossible to provide the force necessary to deliver babies vaginally.

Malfunctions in Feedback Loops

Non-functional feedback loops can be deadly. The classic example is type I diabetes, in which there is an autoimmune response against the beta cells of the pancreas, the insulin-producing cells.

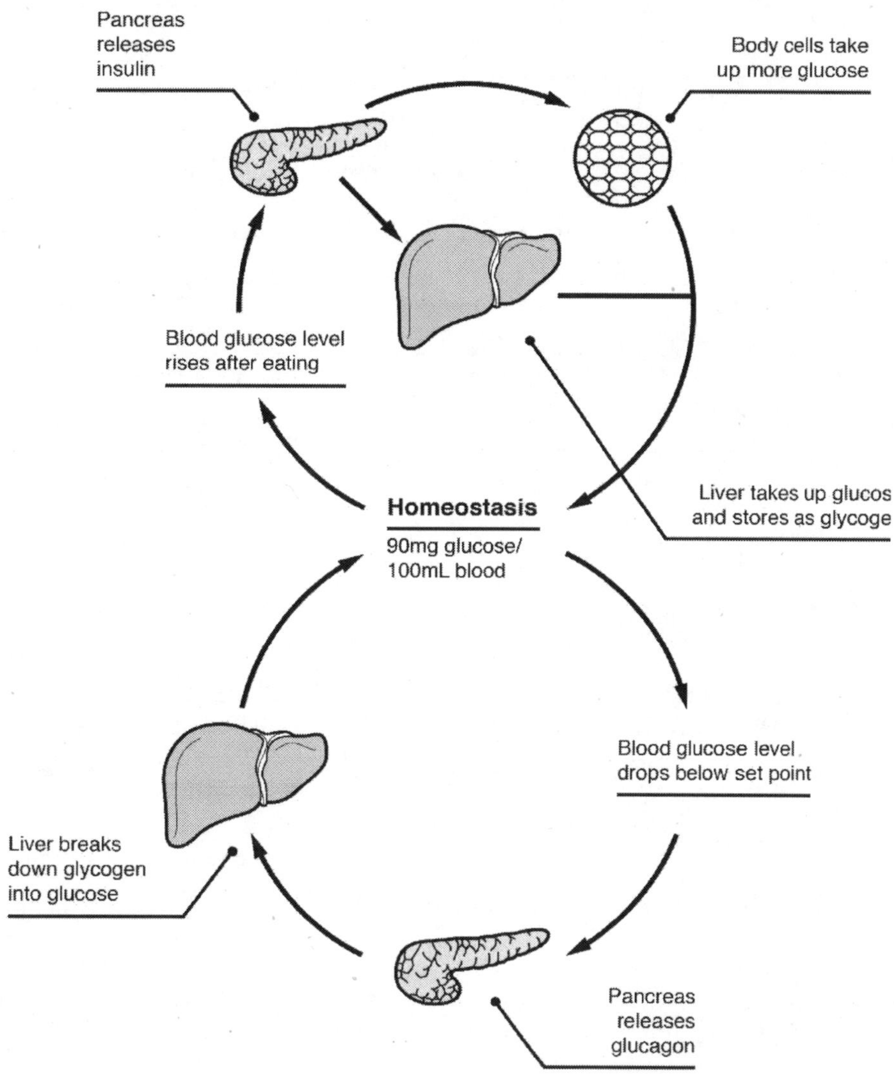

The balance between insulin and glucagon is disrupted when the pancreas can't produce insulin. Insulin serves to open the carrier proteins on cellular membranes, allowing glucose entry. In the absence of insulin, the carrier proteins in cells are not signaled to take in glucose, causing blood sugar to rise. In normal, healthy conditions, in response to high blood sugar, the pancreas is stimulated to produce more insulin from the beta cells (specialized insulin-producing cells). In diabetics, the beta cells have been destroyed by the autoimmune system. The whole bottom portion of the feedback loop is bypassed, and as a result, diabetics become severely hyperglycemic without artificial insulin administration. Severe hyperglycemia can result in coma and death.

Hormone Secretion and Function

The human body produces dozens of hormones in a variety of organs, each signaling action in a different part of the body, with either different or overlapping functions. The table below lists several common hormones listed according to the gland or organ they originate from, their chemical class, and their main functions.

Hormone	Gland	Class	Function
Aldosterone	Adrenal cortex	Amine	Promotes reabsorption of sodium and excretion of potassium in the kidneys
Glucocorticoids	Adrenal cortex	Steroid	Raises blood glucose level
Mineralocorticoids	Adrenal cortex	Steroid	Promotes reabsorption of sodium and excretion of potassium in the kidneys
Antidiuretic hormone (vasopressin)	Posterior pituitary gland	Peptide	Promotes water retention in the kidneys
Oxytocin	Posterior pituitary gland	Peptide	Stimulates contraction of uterus and mammary gland cells
Adrenocorticotropic hormone (ACTH)	Anterior pituitary gland	Peptide	Stimulates glucocorticoid steroid hormone secretion
Growth hormone (GH)	Anterior pituitary gland	Protein	Stimulates growth and metabolism
Luteinizing hormone (LH)	Anterior pituitary gland	Glycoprotein	Stimulates gonads to produce androgens
Follicle-stimulating hormone (FSH)	Anterior pituitary gland	Glycoprotein	Stimulates gamete production
Thyroid-stimulating hormone	Anterior pituitary gland	Glycoprotein	Stimulates thyroid gland to produce thyroxine, leading to stimulated metabolism
Prolactin	Anterior pituitary gland	Protein	Stimulates production and secretion of milk
Renin	Kidney	Peptide	Part of the renin-angiotensin system. Converts angiotensinogen to angiotensin I
Angiotensin	Liver	Peptide	Part of the renin-angiotensin system. Stimulates vasoconstriction
Erythropoietin	Kidney	Peptide	Stimulates erythrocyte production in bone marrow
Glucagon	Pancreas	Peptide	Promotes conversion of glycogen to glucose
Insulin	Pancreas	Peptide	Promotes absorption of glucose
Androgens	Testes	Steroid	Supports sperm formation and promotes development and maintenance of secondary sex characteristics in males
Estrogens	Ovaries	Steroid	Stimulates growth of uterine lining and promotes development and maintenance of secondary sex characteristics in females
Progestogens	Ovaries	Steroid	Promotes growth of uterine lining
Parathyroid hormone	Parathyroid glands	Peptide	Regulates blood calcium level
Thyroid hormones T_3 and T_4	Thyroid gland	Amine	Promotes and stimulates metabolism
Epinephrine	Adrenal gland	Amine	Increases blood glucose level, raising heart rate and stimulating metabolism Constricts minor blood vessels while dilating vessels in skeletal muscles
Norepinephrine	Adrenal gland	Amine	Increases blood glucose level and heart rate
Melatonin	Pineal gland	Amine	Involved in regulation of circadian rhythm
Growth hormone releasing hormone	Hypothalamus	Peptide	Stimulates growth hormone production and secretion

Hormone	Gland	Class	Function
Thyrotropin releasing hormone	Hypothalamus	Peptide	Stimulates thyrotropin production and secretion
Gonadotropin releasing hormone	Hypothalamus	Peptide	Stimulates FSH and LH production and secretion
Corticotropin releasing hormone	Hypothalamus	Peptide	Stimulates adrenocorticotropin secretion

Describe the Anatomy and Physiology of the Urinary System

The urinary system is made up of the kidneys, ureters, urinary bladder, and the urethra. It is the system responsible for removing waste products and balancing water and electrolyte concentrations in the blood. The urinary system has many important functions related to waste excretion. It regulates the concentrations of sodium, potassium, chloride, calcium, and other ions in the filtrate by controlling the amount of each that is reabsorbed during filtration. The reabsorption or secretion of hydrogen ions and bicarbonate contributes to the maintenance of blood pH. Certain kidney cells can detect any reductions in blood volume and pressure. If that happens, they secrete renin, which activates a hormone that causes increased reabsorption of sodium ions and water, raising volume and pressure. Under hypoxic conditions, kidney cells will secrete erythropoietin in order to stimulate red blood cell production. Kidney cells also synthesize calcitriol, which is a hormone derivative of vitamin D3 that aids in calcium ion absorption by the intestinal epithelium.

Under normal circumstances, humans have two functioning kidneys in the lower back and on either side of the spinal cord. They are the main organs that are responsible for filtering waste products out of the blood and regulating blood water and electrolyte levels. Blood enters the kidney through the renal artery, and urea and wastes are removed, while water and the acidity/alkalinity of the blood is adjusted. Toxic substances and drugs are also filtered. Blood exits through the renal vein, and the urine waste travels through the ureter to the bladder, where it is stored until it is eliminated through the urethra.

The kidneys have an outer renal cortex and an inner renal medulla that contain millions of tiny filtering units called nephrons. Nephrons have two parts: a glomerulus, which is the filter, and a tubule. The glomerulus is a network of capillaries covered by the Bowman's capsule, which is the entrance to the tubule. As blood enters the kidneys via the renal artery, the glomerulus allows for fluid and waste products to pass through it and enter the tubule. Blood cells and large molecules, such as proteins, do not pass through and remain in the blood. The filtrate passes through the tubule, which has several parts.

The proximal tubule comes first, and then the descending and ascending limbs of the loop of Henle dip into the medulla, followed by the distal tubule and collecting duct. The journey through the tubule involves exchanging materials between the tubule and bloodstream to regulate blood osmolarity, pH, and electrolyte concentrations. The final product at the collecting tubule is called **urine**, and it is delivered to the bladder by the ureter. The most central part of the kidney is the renal pelvis, and it acts as a funnel by delivering the urine from the millions of the collecting tubules to the ureters. The filtered blood exits through the renal vein and is returned to circulation.

Here's a look at the genitourinary system:

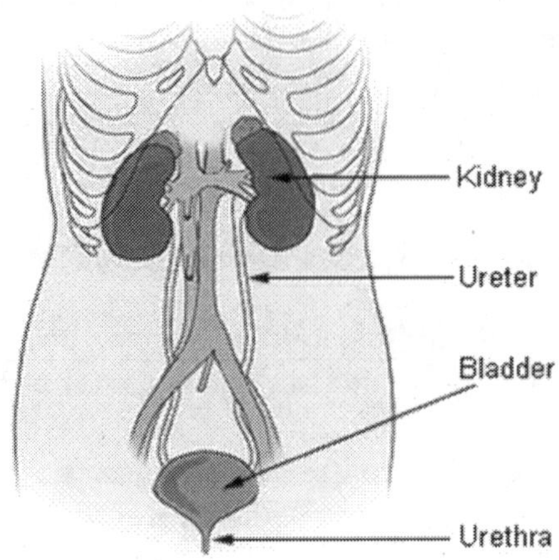

Here's a close up look at the kidney:

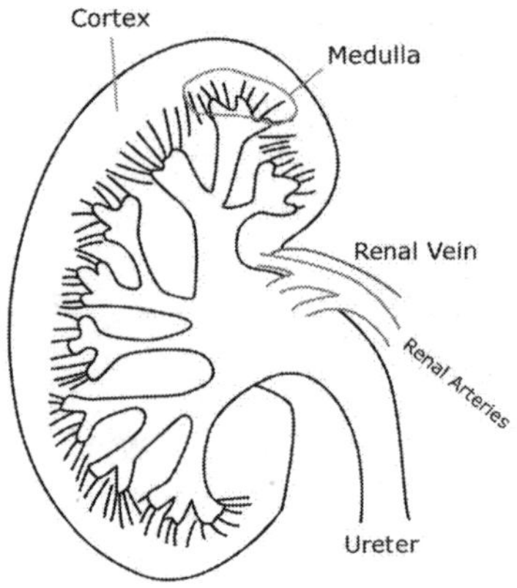

Nephron Form and Function

The kidney contains many small, conical or U-shaped units that make up the kidney. Most of them reside high in the cortex, though some start low in the cortex, closer to the medulla, and penetrate deep into the medulla. These many nodes are called nephrons where blood is first filtered through networks of capillaries called glomeruli, allowing dissolved blood components to diffuse with water across a thin membrane into what is called Bowman's capsule, leading to the next part of renal filtration, called the proximal tubule. The proximal tubule lies in the cortex and consists of two parts, the proximal convoluted tubule (PCT) and proximal straight tubule (PST). This section largely reabsorbs water, sodium, potassium, glucose, amino acids, phosphate, and citrate. The surface area for resorption is increased by microvilli on the cell surface.

The proximal tubule drains into the loop of Henle. The loop of Henle consists of a few portions, termed the descending limb, thin ascending limb, ascending limb, and cortical thick ascending limb, in order from proximal to distal end. The loop of Henle is responsible for roughly a quarter of the ions reabsorbed by the kidneys and a fifth of the water retained by the kidneys. Following the loop of Henle is the distal convoluted tubule (DCT). Here the blood's pH is regulated by absorbing bicarbonate and secreting hydrogen ions into the DCT or vice versa. Sodium and potassium levels are balanced again in the DCT—Potassium is secreted into the DCT and more sodium is reabsorbed in response to aldosterone, which is regulated by WNK kinases. Parathyroid hormone signals reabsorption of calcium ions. Following the DCT comes the connecting tubule and collecting ducts. The connecting tubule is the end of the renal tubule, and the levels of water and electrolytes in the filtrate prior to draining into the collecting ducts.

Waste Excretion

Once urine accumulates, it leaves the kidneys. The urine travels through the ureters into the urinary bladder, a muscular organ that is hollow and elastic. As more urine enters the urinary bladder, its walls stretch and become thinner so there is no significant difference in internal pressure. The urinary bladder stores the urine until the body is ready for urination, at which time, the muscles contract and force the urine through the urethra and out of the body.

Describe the Anatomy and Physiology of the Immune System

The immune system is the body's defense against invading microorganisms (bacteria, viruses, fungi, and parasites) and other harmful, foreign substances. It is capable of limiting or preventing infection.

There are two general types of immunity: innate immunity and acquired immunity. **Innate immunity** uses physical and chemical barriers to block microorganism entry into the body. The biggest barrier is the skin; it forms a physical barrier that blocks microorganisms from entering underlying tissues. Mucous membranes in the digestive, respiratory, and urinary systems secrete mucus to block and remove invading microorganisms. Other natural defenses include saliva, tears, and stomach acids, which are all chemical barriers intended to block infection with microorganisms. Acid is inhospitable to pathogens, as are tears, mucus, and saliva, which all contain a natural antibiotic called lysozyme. The respiratory passages contain microscopic cilia, which are like bristles that sweep out pathogens. In addition, macrophages and other white blood cells can recognize and eliminate foreign objects through phagocytosis or toxic secretions.

Acquired immunity refers to a specific set of events used by the body to fight a particular infection. Essentially, the body accumulates and stores information about the nature of an invading microorganism. As a result, the body can mount a specific attack that is much more effective than innate immunity. It also provides a way for the body to prevent future infections by the same microorganism.

Acquired immunity is divided into a primary response and a secondary response. The **primary immune response** occurs the first time a particular microorganism enters the body, where macrophages engulf the microorganism and travel to the lymph nodes. In the lymph nodes, macrophages present the invader to helper T lymphocytes, which then activate humoral and cellular immunity. **Humoral immunity** refers to immunity resulting from antibody production by B lymphocytes. After being activated by helper T lymphocytes, B lymphocytes multiply and divide into plasma cells and memory cells. Plasma cells are B lymphocytes that produce immune proteins called antibodies, or immunoglobulins. Antibodies then bind the microorganism to flag it for destruction by other white blood cells. **Cellular immunity** refers to the immune response coordinated by T lymphocytes. After being activated by helper T lymphocytes, other T lymphocytes attack and kill cells that cause infection or disease.

The **secondary immune response** takes place during subsequent encounters with a known microorganism. Memory cells respond to the previously encountered microorganism by immediately producing antibodies. Memory cells are B lymphocytes that store information to produce antibodies. The secondary immune response is swift and powerful because it eliminates the need for the time-consuming macrophage activation of the primary immune response. Suppressor T lymphocytes also take part to inhibit the immune response as an overactive immune response could cause damage to healthy cells.

Inflammation occurs if a pathogen evades the barriers and chemical defenses. It stimulates pain receptors, alerting the individual that something is wrong. It also elevates body temperature to speed up chemical reactions, although if a fever goes unchecked it can be dangerous due to the fact that extreme heat unfolds proteins. Histamine is secreted which dilates blood vessels and recruits white blood cells that destroy invaders non-specifically. The immune system is tied to the lymphatic system. The thymus, one of the lymphatic system organs, is the site of maturation of T-cells, a type of white blood cell. The lymphatic system is important in the inflammatory response because lymph vessels deliver leukocytes and collect debris that will be filtered in the lymph nodes and the spleen.

Antigen and Typical Immune Response

Should a pathogen evade barriers and survive through inflammation, an antigen-specific adaptive immune response will begin. Immune cells recognize these foreign particles by their antigens, which are their unique and identifying surface proteins. Drugs, toxins, and transplanted cells can also act as antigens. The body even recognizes its own cells as potential threats in autoimmune diseases.

When a macrophage engulfs a pathogen and presents its antigens, helper T cells recognize the signal and secrete cytokines to signal T lymphocytes and B lymphocytes so that they launch the cell-mediated and humoral response, respectively. The cell-mediated response occurs when the T lymphocytes kill infected cells by secreting cytotoxins. The humoral response occurs when B lymphocytes proliferate into plasma and memory cells. The plasma cells secrete antigen-specific antibodies, which bind to the pathogens so that they cannot bind to host cells. Macrophages and other phagocytic cells called neutrophils engulf and degrade the antibody/pathogen complex. The memory cells remain in circulation and initiate a secondary immune response, should the pathogen dare enter the host again.

Active and Passive Immunity

Acquired immunity occurs after the first antigen encounter. The first time the body mounts this immune response is called the primary immune response. Because the memory B cells store information about the antigen's structure, any subsequent immune response causes a secondary immune response, which is much faster and produces substantially more antibodies due to the presence of memory B cells. If the secondary immune response is strong and fast enough, it will fight off the pathogen before an individual becomes symptomatic. This is a natural means of acquiring immunity.

Vaccination is the process of inducing immunity. **Active immunization** refers to immunity gained by exposure to infectious microorganisms or viruses and can be **natural** or **artificial**. Natural immunization refers to an individual being exposed to an infectious organism as a part of daily life. For example, it was once common for parents to expose their children to childhood diseases such as measles or chicken pox. Artificial immunization refers to therapeutic exposure to an infectious organism as a way of protecting an individual from disease. Today, the medical community relies on artificial immunization as a way to induce immunity.

Vaccines are used for the development of active immunity. A vaccine contains a killed, weakened, or inactivated microorganism or virus that is administered through injection, by mouth, or by aerosol. Vaccinations are administered to prevent an infectious disease but do not always guarantee immunity. Due to circulating memory B cells after administration, the secondary response will fight off the pathogen should it be encountered again in many cases. Both illnesses and vaccinations cause active immune responses.

Passive immunity refers to immunity gained by the introduction of antibodies. This introduction can also be natural or artificial. The process occurs when antibodies from the mother's bloodstream are passed on to the bloodstream of the developing fetus. Breast milk can also transmit antibodies to a baby. Babies are born with passive immunity, which provides protection against general infection for approximately the first six months of its life.

Types of Leukocytes

There are many leukocytes, or white blood cells, involved in both innate and adaptive immunity. All are developed in bone marrow. Many have been mentioned in the text above, but a comprehensive list is included here for reference.

- Monocytes are large phagocytic cells.
    - Macrophages engulf pathogens and present their antigen. Some circulate, but others reside in lymphatic organs like the spleen and lymph nodes.
    - Dendritic cells are also phagocytic and antigen-presenting.
- Granulocytes are cells that contain secretory granules.
    - Neutrophils are the most abundant type of white blood cell. They are circulating and aggressive phagocytic cells that are part of innate immunity. They also secrete substances that are toxic to pathogens.
    - Basophils and mast cells secrete histamine, which stimulates the inflammatory response.
    - Eosinophils are found underneath mucous membranes and defend against multicellular parasites like worms. They have low phagocytic activity and primarily secrete destructive enzymes.
- T lymphocytes mature in the thymus.
    - Helper T cells recognize antigens presented by macrophages and dendritic cells and secrete cytokines, which mount the humoral and cell-mediated immune response.
    - Killer T cells are cytotoxic cells involved in the cell-mediated response by recognizing and poisoning infected cells.
    - Suppressor T cells suppress the adaptive immune response when there is no threat to conserve resources and energy.
    - Memory T cells remain in circulation to aid in the secondary immune response.
- B lymphocytes mature in bone marrow.
    - Plasma B cells secrete antigen-specific antibodies when signaled by Helper T cells and are degraded after the immune response.
    - Memory B cells store antigen-specific antibody making instructions and remain circulating after the immune response is over.

Natural killer cells are part of innate immunity and patrol and identify suspect-material. They respond by secreting cytotoxic substances.

Lymphatic System

The lymphatic system includes the spleen, thymus, tonsils, lymph nodes, lymphatic vessels, and the lymph. The spleen is located below the diaphragm and to the rear of the stomach. The thymus consists of specialized lymphatic tissue and lies in the mediastinum behind the sternum. The tonsils are globules of lymphoid tissue located in the oropharynx. The lymphatic vessels are very small and contain valves to prevent backflow in the system vessels. The vessels that lie in close proximity to the capillaries circulate the lymph. Lymph is composed of infectious substances and cellular waste products in addition to hormones and oxygen.

The main function of the lymphatic system is protection against infection. The system also conserves body fluids and proteins and absorbs vitamins from the digestive system.

The spleen filters the blood in order to remove toxic agents and is also a reservoir for blood that can be released into systemic circulation as needed. The thymus is the site of the development and regulation of white blood cells (WBCs). The tonsils trap and destroy infectious agents as they enter the body through the mouth. The lymphatic vessels circulate the lymph, and the lymph carries toxins and cellular waste products from the cell to the heart for filtration.

There is rapid growth of the thymus gland from birth to ten years. The action of the entire system declines from adulthood to old age, which means that the elderly are less able to respond to infection.

Describe the Anatomy and Physiology of the Skeletal System

Axial Skeleton and Appendicular Skeleton

The skeletal system is composed of 206 bones interconnected by tough connective tissue called ligaments. The **axial skeleton** can be considered the north-south axis of the skeleton. It includes the spinal column, sternum, ribs, and skull. There are 80 bones in the axial skeleton, and 33 of them are vertebrae. The ribs make up 12 of the bones in the axial skeleton.

The remaining 126 bones are in the **appendicular skeleton**, which contains bones of the appendages like the collarbone (clavicle), shoulders (scapula), arms, hands, hips, legs, and feet. The arm bones consist of the upper humerus, with the radius and ulna that attach to the hands. The wrists, hands, and fingers are composed of the carpals, metacarpals, and phalanges, respectively. The femur attaches to the hips. The patella or kneecap connects the femur to the fibula and tibia. The ankles, feet, and toes are composed of the tarsals, metatarsals, and phalanges, respectively.

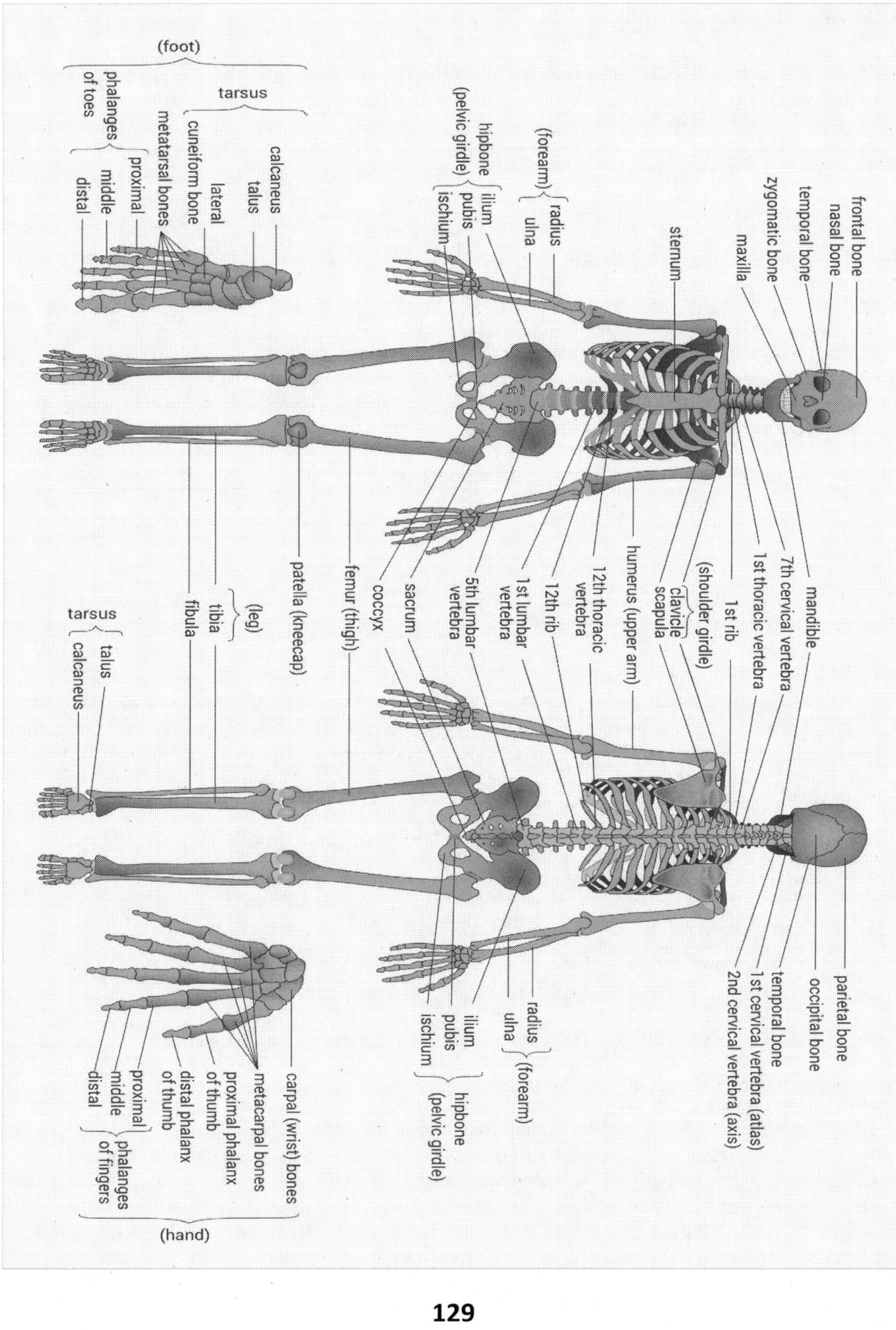
frontal bone
nasal bone
temporal bone
zygomatic bone
maxilla
sternum
(forearm)
radius
ulna
hipbone
(pelvic girdle)
ilium
pubis
ischium
(foot)
tarsus
calcaneus
talus
lateral
cuneiform bone
metatarsal bones
phalanges
of toes
proximal
middle
distal
mandible
7th cervical vertebra
1st thoracic vertebra
1st rib
(shoulder girdle)
clavicle
scapula
humerus (upper arm)
12th thoracic
vertebra
12th rib
1st lumbar
vertebra
5th lumbar
vertebra
sacrum
coccyx
femur (thigh)
patella (kneecap)
(leg)
tibia
fibula
tarsus
talus
calcaneus
parietal bone
occipital bone
temporal bone
1st cervical vertebra (atlas)
2nd cervical vertebra (axis)
radius
ulna
(forearm)
ilium
pubis
ischium
hipbone
(pelvic girdle)
carpal (wrist) bones
metacarpal bones
proximal phalanx
of thumb
distal phalanx
of thumb
proximal
middle
distal
phalanges
of fingers
(hand)

Functions of the Skeletal System

One of the skeletal system's most important functions is to protect vital internal organs. The skull protects the brain, the ribs protect the lungs and heart, the vertebrae protect the spinal column, and the pelvis protects the uterus and other reproductive organs. Red bone marrow produces red and white blood cells as well as platelets in a process known as hemopoiesis. As humans age, the red bone marrow produces fewer red blood cells and stores more lipids, and is termed yellow bone marrow due to the relative prevalence of fat cells. In adults, yellow marrow is dominant in the long bones of the arms and legs, while red marrow is mostly in the bones of the torso. The bones themselves store the essential minerals calcium and phosphorus. The organization of the skeleton allows us to stand upright and acts as a foundation for organs and tissues to attach and maintain their location. This is similar to how the wooden frame of a house has room partitions to designate the type of room and floors that furniture can attach to.

The skeletal system and the muscular system are physically interconnected and allow for voluntary movement. Strong connective tissues called tendons attach bones to muscles. Most muscles work in opposing pairs and act as levers. For example, flexing the biceps brings the upper arm and lower arm closer together and flexing the triceps moves them apart. Synovial joints are movable joints, and they are rich with cartilage, connective tissue, and synovial fluid, which acts as a lubricant. The majority of joints are synovial joints, and they include hinge joints, like the one at the elbow, which permits flexion and extension.

The vertebrae are cartilaginous joints, which have spaces between them filled with cushion-like intervertebral discs that act as shock absorbers. The tight fit between the vertebrae and the intervertebral discs helps to protect the spinal cord inside by limiting the movement between two adjacent vertebrae. However, because there are so many vertebrae, the backbone as a whole is somewhat flexible.

Fibrous joints like those in the skull have fibrous tissue between the bones and no cavity between them. These are fixed joints that are immobile.

Compact and Spongy Bone

Osteoclasts, osteoblasts, and osteocytes are the three types of bone cells. Osteoclasts break down old bone, osteoblasts make new bone, and osteocytes are the mature functional bone cells. Bone is constantly regenerating due to the osteoblasts/osteoclasts that line all types of bones and the blood vessels inside them. The cells exist within a matrix of collagen fibers and minerals. The collagen fibers provide resistance to tension and the minerals provide resistance to compression. Because of the collagen and mineral matrix, bones have ample reinforcement to collectively support the entire human body.

Bones can be classified as any of the following:

- Long bones include tube-like rods like the arm and leg bones.
- Short bones are tube-like rods that are smaller than long bones, like the fingers and toes.
- Flat bones are thin and flat like the ribs and breastbone.
- Irregular bones, like the vertebrae, are compact and don't fit into the other categories.

The outer tissue of the bone is surrounded by connective tissue known as periosteum. It appears shiny, smooth, and white. It protects the bone, anchors the bone to the connective tissue that surrounds muscles, and links the bone to the circulatory and nervous system. Compact bone is underneath the periosteum and is made of a dense blend of tightly packed osteocytes. It serves as a mineral reservoir of calcium and phosphorus. Compact bones have a Haversian system, which is composed of embedded blood vessels, lymph vessels, and nerve bundles that span the interior of the bone from one end to the other. Branching from the central canal to the surface of the bone are the canals of Volkmann, which deliver materials to peripheral osteocytes. Concentric circles surround the central Haversian canal, and these lamellae have gaps between them called lacunae where osteocytes are embedded.

In contrast, spongy bone is very porous and more flexible than compact bone. It is at the ends of long bones and the central part of flat bones. It looks like a honeycomb, and the open spaces are connected by trabeculae which are beams of tissue that add support. They add strength without adding excess mass.

Cartilage is a very flexible connective tissue made of collagen and flexible elastin. It has no blood vessels and obtains materials via diffusion. It is replaced by bone starting in infancy in a process called **ossification**.

Biology

Describe Cell Structure, Function, and Organization

Cell Structure and Function

The cell is the main functional and structural component of all living organisms. Robert Hooke, an English scientist, coined the term "cell" in 1665. Hooke's discovery laid the groundwork for the cell theory, which is composed of three principals:

1. All organisms are composed of cells.
2. All existing cells are created from other living cells.
3. The cell is the most fundamental unit of life.

Organisms can be unicellular (composed of one cell) or multicellular (composed of many cells). All cells must be bounded by a cell membrane, be filled with cytoplasm of some sort, and be coded by a genetic sequence.

The cell membrane separates a cell's internal and external environments. It is a selectively permeable membrane, which usually only allows the passage of certain molecules by diffusion. Phospholipids and proteins are crucial components of all cell membranes. The cytoplasm is the cell's internal environment and is aqueous, or water-based. The genome represents the genetic material inside the cell that is passed on from generation to generation.

Prokaryotes and Eukaryotes

Prokaryotic cells are much smaller than eukaryotic cells. The majority of prokaryotes are unicellular, while the majority of eukaryotes are multicellular. Prokaryotic cells have no nucleus, and their genome is found in an area known as the nucleoid. They also do not have membrane-bound organelles, which are "little organs" that perform specific functions within a cell.

Eukaryotic cells have a proper nucleus containing the genome. They also have numerous membrane-bound organelles such as lysosomes, endoplasmic reticula (rough and smooth), Golgi complexes, and mitochondria. The majority of prokaryotic cells have cell walls, while most eukaryotic cells do not have cell walls. The DNA of prokaryotic cells is contained in a single circular chromosome, while the DNA of eukaryotic cells is contained in multiple linear chromosomes. Prokaryotic cells divide using binary fission, while eukaryotic cells divide using mitosis. Examples of prokaryotes are bacteria and archaea while examples of eukaryotes are animals and plants.

Nuclear Parts of a Cell

Nucleus (plural nuclei): Houses a cell's genetic material, deoxyribonucleic acid (DNA), which is used to form chromosomes. A single nucleus is the defining characteristic of eukaryotic cells. The nucleus of a cell controls gene expression. It ensures genetic material is transmitted from one generation to the next.

Chromosomes: Complex thread-like arrangements composed of DNA that is found in a cell's nucleus. Humans have 23 pairs of chromosomes for a total of 46.

Chromatin: An aggregate of genetic material consisting of DNA and proteins called histones that forms chromosomes during cell division.

Histones: Octameric (eight-part) proteins that enable condensing of DNA. The complex of DNA and histones is known as a **nucleosome**, the most basic unit of chromatin, and it forms a 10-nanometer-wide structure resembling "beads on a string" due to DNA winding around histones looking like beads in electron microscopy. Further winding of DNA with histones forms a denser 30-nm fiber.

Nucleolus (plural nucleoli): The largest component of the nucleus of a eukaryotic cell. With no membrane, the primary function of the nucleolus is the production of ribosomes, which are crucial to the synthesis of proteins.

Cell Membranes

Cell membranes encircle the cell's cytoplasm, separating the intracellular environment from the extracellular environment. They are selectively permeable, which enables them to control molecular traffic entering and exiting cells. Cell membranes are made of a double layer of phospholipids studded with proteins. Cholesterol is also dispersed in the phospholipid bilayer of cell membranes to provide stability. The proteins in the phospholipid bilayer aid the transport of molecules across cell membranes.

Scientists use the term "fluid mosaic model" to refer to the arrangement of phospholipids and proteins in cell membranes. In that model, phospholipids have a head region and a tail region. The head region of the phospholipids is attracted to water (hydrophilic), while the tail region is repelled by it (hydrophobic). Because they are hydrophilic, the heads of the phospholipids are facing the water, pointing inside and outside of the cell. Because they are hydrophobic, the tails of the phospholipids are oriented inward between both head regions. This orientation constructs the phospholipid bilayer.

Cell membranes have the distinct trait of selective permeability. The fact that cell membranes are amphiphilic (having hydrophilic and hydrophobic zones) contributes to this trait. As a result, cell membranes are able to regulate the flow of molecules in and out of the cell.

Factors relating to molecules such as size, polarity, and solubility determine their likelihood of passage across cell membranes. Small molecules are able to diffuse easily across cell membranes compared to large molecules. Polarity refers to the charge present in a molecule. Polar molecules have regions, or poles, of positive and negative charge and are water soluble, while nonpolar molecules have no charge and are fat-soluble. Solubility refers to the ability of a substance, called a solute, to dissolve in a solvent. A soluble substance can be dissolved in a solvent, while an insoluble substance cannot be dissolved in a solvent. Nonpolar, fat-soluble substances have a much easier time passing through cell membranes compared to polar, water-soluble substances.

Active Transport Mechanisms

Active transport refers to the energy-requiring migration of molecules across a cell membrane. It's a useful way to move molecules from an area of low concentration to an area of high concentration. Adenosine triphosphate (ATP), the currency of cellular energy, is needed to work against the concentration gradient.

Active transport can involve carrier proteins that cross the cell membrane to pump molecules and ions across the membrane, like in facilitated diffusion. The difference is that active transport uses the energy from ATP to drive this transport, as typically the ions or molecules are going against their concentration gradient. For example, glucose pumps in the kidney pump all of the glucose into the cells from the lumen of the nephron even though there is a higher concentration of glucose in the cell than in the lumen. This is because glucose is a precious fuel source, and the body wants to conserve as much as possible. Pumps can either send a molecule in one direction, multiple molecules in the same direction (symports), or multiple molecules in different directions (antiports).

Active transport can also involve the movement of membrane-bound particles, either into a cell (endocytosis) or out of a cell (exocytosis). The three major forms of endocytosis are: **pinocytosis**, where the cell is **drinking** and intakes only small molecules; **phagocytosis**, where the cell is **eating** and intakes large particles or small organisms; and **receptor-mediated endocytosis**, where the cell's membrane splits off to form an internal vesicle as a response to molecules activating receptors on its surface. Exocytosis is the inverse of endocytosis, and the membranes of the vesicle join to that of the cell's surface while the molecules inside the vesicle are released outside. This is common in nervous and muscle tissue for the release of neurotransmitters and in endocrine cells for the release of hormones. The two major categories of exocytosis are excretion and secretion. Excretion is defined as the removal of waste from a cell. Secretion is defined as the transport of molecules, such as hormones or enzymes, from a cell.

Structure and Function of Cellular Organelles

Organelles are specialized structures that perform specific tasks in a cell. The term literally means "little organ." Most organelles are membrane bound and serve as sites for the production or degradation of chemicals. The following are organelles found in eukaryotic cells:

Nucleus: A cell's nucleus contains genetic information in the form of DNA. The nucleus is surrounded by the nuclear envelope. A single nucleus is the defining characteristic of eukaryotic cells. The nucleus is also the most important organelle of the cell. It contains the nucleolus, which manufactures ribosomes (another organelle) that are crucial in protein synthesis (also called gene expression).

Mitochondria: Mitochondria are oval-shaped and have a double membrane. The inner membrane has multiple folds called cristae. Mitochondria are responsible for the production of a cell's energy in the form of adenosine triphosphate (ATP). ATP is the principal energy transfer molecule in eukaryotic cells. Mitochondria also participate in cellular respiration.

Rough Endoplasmic Reticulum: The rough endoplasmic reticulum (RER) is composed of linked membranous sacs called cisternae with ribosomes attached to their external surfaces. The RER is responsible for the production of proteins that will eventually get shipped out of the cell.

Smooth Endoplasmic Reticulum: The smooth endoplasmic reticulum (SER) is composed of linked membranous sacs called cisternae without ribosomes, which distinguishes it from the RER. The SER's main function is the production of carbohydrates and lipids, which can be created expressly for the cell, or to modify the proteins from the RER that will eventually get shipped out of the cell.

Golgi Apparatus: The Golgi apparatus is located next to the SER. Its main function is the final modification, storage, and shipping of products (proteins, carbohydrates, and lipids) from the endoplasmic reticulum.

Lysosomes: Lysosomes are specialized vesicles that contain enzymes capable of digesting food, surplus organelles, and foreign invaders such as bacteria and viruses. They often destroy dead cells in order to recycle cellular components. Lysosomes are found only in animal cells.

Secretory Vesicles: Secretory vesicles transport and deliver molecules into or out of the cell via the cell membrane. Endocytosis refers to the movement of molecules into a cell via secretory vesicles. Exocytosis refers to the movement of molecules out of a cell via secretory vesicles.

Ribosomes: Ribosomes are not membrane bound. They are responsible for the production of proteins as specified from DNA instructions. Ribosomes can be free or bound.

Cilia and Flagella: Cilia are specialized hair-like projections on some eukaryotic cells that aid in movement, while flagella are long, whip-like projections that are used in the same capacity.

Here is an illustration of the cell:

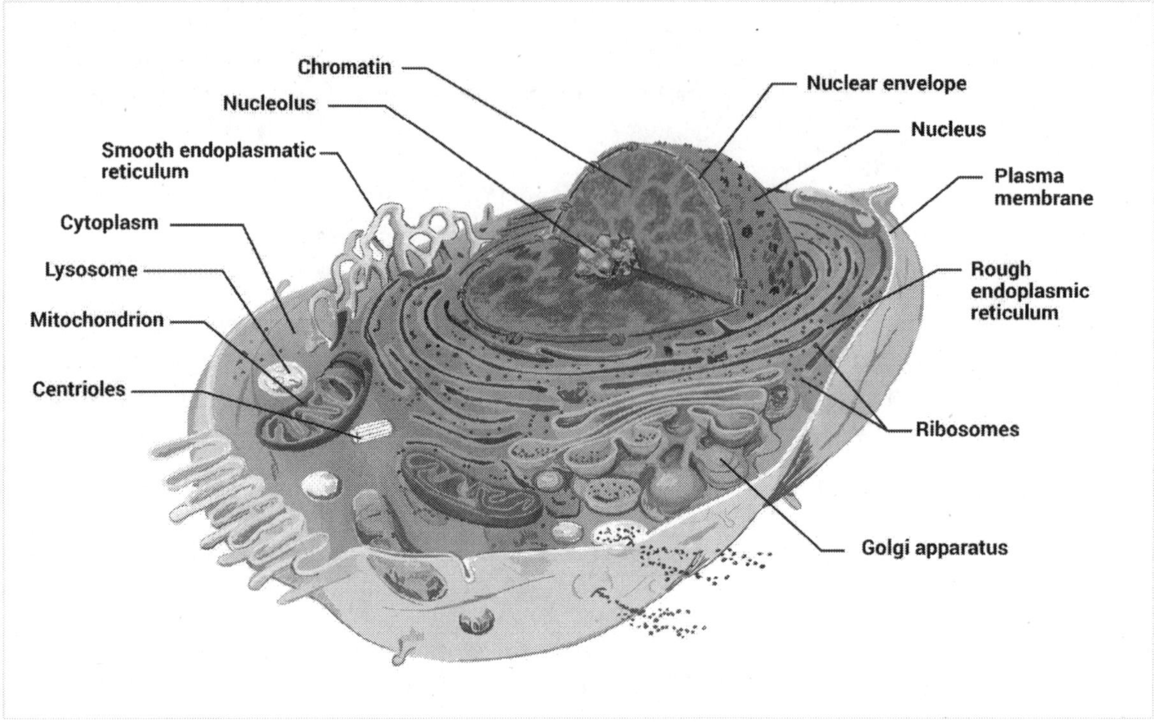

The following organelles are not found in animal cells:

Cell Walls: Cell walls can be found in plants, bacteria, and fungi, and are made of cellulose, peptidoglycan, and lignin, depending on the organism it surrounds. Each of these materials is a type of sugar recognized as a structural carbohydrate. The carbohydrates form rigid structures located outside of the cell membrane. Cell walls protect the cell, help maintain a cell's shape, and provide structural support.

Vacuoles: Plant cells have central vacuoles, which are essentially a membrane surrounding a body of water. They may store nutrients or waste products. Since vacuoles are large, they also help to support the structure of plant cells.

Chloroplasts: Chloroplasts are membrane-bound organelles that perform photosynthesis. They contain structural units called thylakoids. Chlorophyll, a green pigment that circulates within the thylakoids, harnesses light energy (sunlight) and helps convert it into chemical energy (glucose).

Cell Cycle

Events in the Cell Cycle

Cell Division and Transmitting Genetic Information

Cell division in eukaryotes occurs in two main stages: mitosis and cytokinesis. Before cell division, all the DNA must be present in the new cells. DNA replication occurs and ensures that each daughter cell will receive a complete genome. Even the cell's organelles are duplicated prior to cell division. Cell division takes place at the end of the cell cycle. The mitotic phase is the shortest part of the cell division cycle. The first step in cell division is mitosis, a process in which eukaryotic cells undergo nuclear division that results in the parent cell's dividing into two identical daughter cells. Mitosis can be broken down into five stages: prophase, prometaphase, metaphase, anaphase, and telophase. During mitosis, the nuclear membrane breaks down in the mitosis stage but later reforms. Chromosomes are arranged and separated so that each daughter cell receives a diploid of chromosomes. Humans have 46 chromosomes (23 pairs). The second main stage of cell division is called cytokinesis, and during this stage (late telophase), the cytoplasm divides into two genetically identical daughter cells. For animal cells, cytokinesis results in the formation of a cleavage furrow.

Stages of the Cell Cycle

A human cell may undergo cell division in about 24 hours. About 90% of the cell cycle is in a stage called interphase. Metabolic activity and growth occur throughout interphase. There are three primary phases in interphase called G1 (first gap), S (synthesis), and G2 (second gap). In all three phases, the cell grows as it is producing proteins and cytoplasmic organelles such as endoplasmic reticulum and mitochondria. The cell grows during the G1 phase and occupies about 5-6 hours of the cell cycle. In the S phase, the chromosomes are duplicated. About half the cell cycle, 12 hours, is spent in the S phase. In the G2 phase, the cell also continues to grow and prepares for cell division for about 4-6 hours. During the mitotic (M) phase, which involves mitosis and cytokinesis, the cell divides within 1 hour. During mitosis, the daughter chromosomes are distributed to the daughter nuclei. Cytokinesis divide the cytoplasm to produce each daughter cell.

Certain cells in a multicellular organism do not divide, or they do undergo division but less frequently than usual. Animal cells contain built-in stop signals that can stop the cell cycle at specific checkpoints, but these stop signals can be overridden with "go-ahead" signals. These cell types spend their time in a G0 phase performing a specific task. The G0 phase is related to the G1 phase. There are three main checkpoints in the G1, G2, and M phases; however, the most important one for cells is the G1 checkpoint. A go-ahead signal at G1 allows the cell to undergo the S, G2, and M phases. If the cell does not receive a go-ahead signal, it will exit the cycle and enter the G0 phase, a nondividing state. Most of the cells in our body are in the G0 phase. For example, muscle and nerve cells never divide. But nondividing liver cells can be called back from G0 to re-enter the cell cycle based on external cues such as the release of growth factors due to an injury. A growth factor is a type of protein released by specific cells that stimulate other cells to undergo division.

Mitosis

Mitosis is the process of cell division and replication in which the cell (mother) produces two identical copies of itself into daughter cells (except in rare mutations). This occurs because the DNA within the cell's nucleus is cleaved into two equal sets of chromosomes — the gene-carrying strands made of nucleic acids and proteins. Mitosis occurs throughout an organism's lifetime, producing cells during growth and development, and also replacing those lost through injury or apoptosis.

M Phase

Following DNA synthesis is the G2 phase, where the cell assembles the machinery necessary for cell division. Cell division then occurs in several stages:

PHASE	PHASE EVENTS	ANIMAL CELL DIAGRAM	PLANT CELL DIAGRAM
Prophase	Nucleus disappears and DNA condenses into chromosomes. DNA is already wrapped around histone proteins, and it continues to supercoil until it looks like the letter X. Sister chromatids on either side of the X are identical.	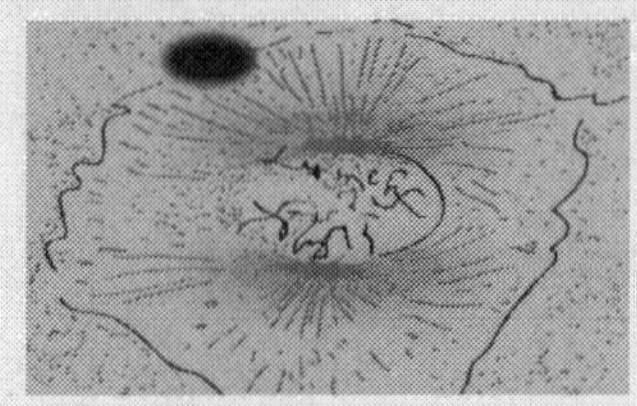	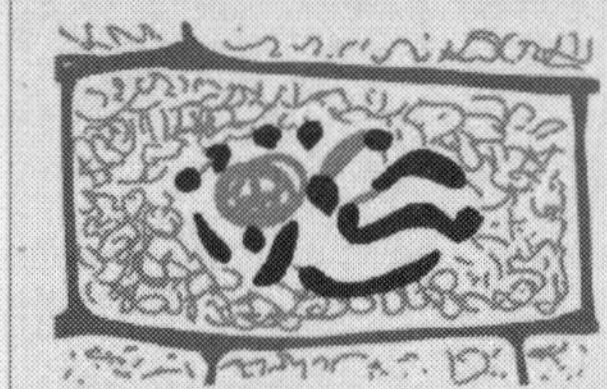
Metaphase	Chromosomes line up in the cell's center. Kinetochore microtubules extend from animal centrosomes that contain centrioles (organizing centers) on either side of the cell and attach to the centromeres (repeating sequences in the middle of the chromosomes). Nonkinetochore proteins elongate animal cells. This massive protein orchestra is collectively called the spindle apparatus. Plants lack centrioles but have microtubule organizing centers.	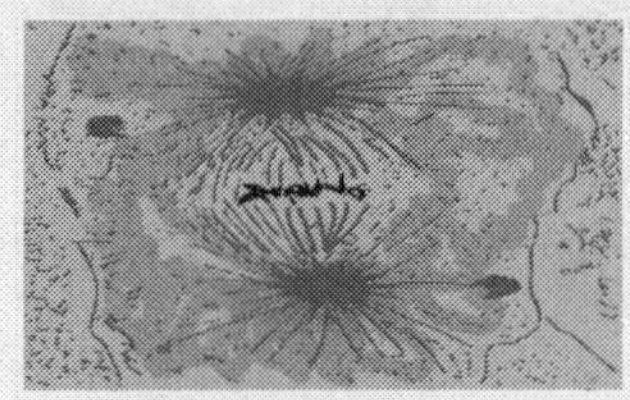	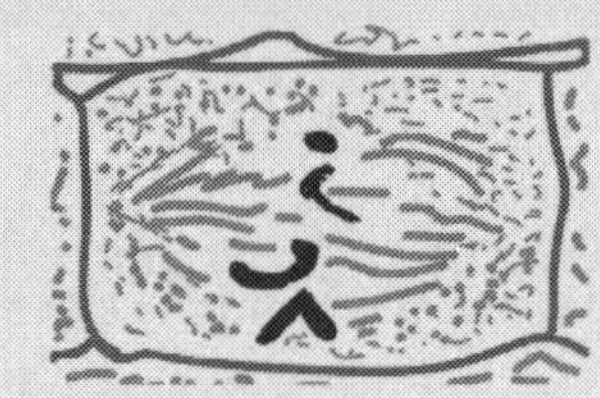
Anaphase	Kinetochore microtubules shorten/are pulled in and sister chromatids are separated and move to each daughter cell.	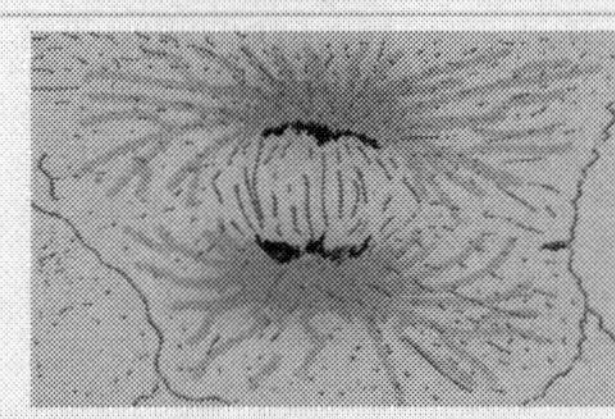	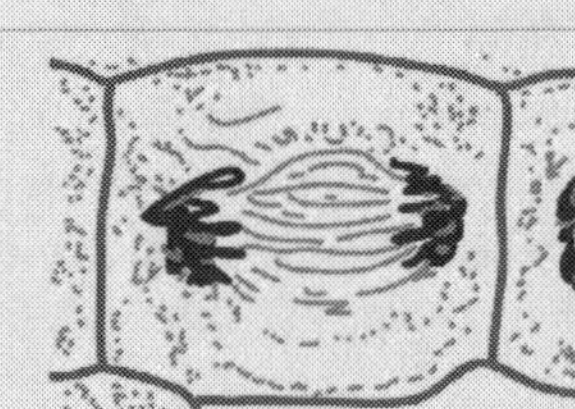
Telophase and Cytokinesis	Nuclei reform and chromosomes decondense within them. **Animals:** actin and myosin microfilaments pinch off the cytoplasm at the cleavage furrow to form two new cells **Plants:** cell plate (new cell wall) forms between daughter cells and extends to divide into two new cells	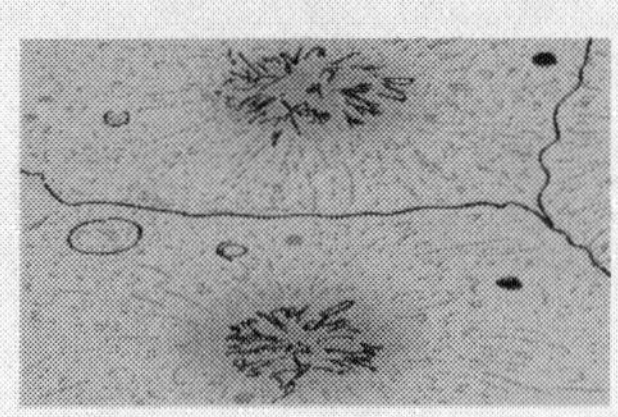	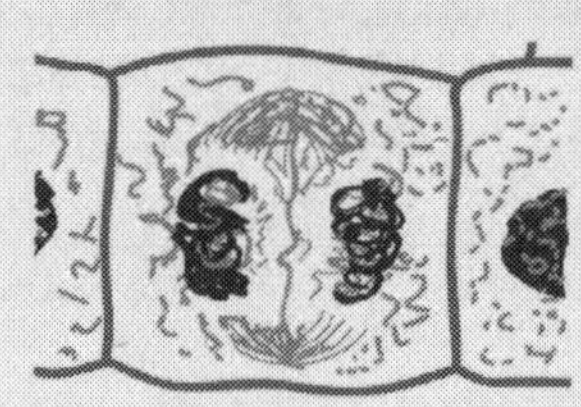

Mitosis occurs for many reasons:

- Development and growth of an organism
- Differentiation and specialization in multicellular organisms
- Replacement of cells with damage or rapid turnover

Cancer cells are the result of inappropriate cell division and occur when cells are unresponsive to checkpoint regulation and growth factor signals. Normal cells are density dependent and anchorage dependent, but cancer cells lose these properties.

Cellular Respiration

Cellular Respiration

Cellular respiration is the catabolic process of breaking down the bonds in glucose and releasing its potential energy in the form of ATP, or adenosine triphosphate. ATP harnesses small amounts of energy and uses it for processes in cellular metabolism. Each glucose molecule can produce about 32 ATP molecules. Breaking glucose and storing its energy in smaller molecules enables the cells to distribute energy across many metabolic reactions instead of just one.

ATP holds energy in the bonds between its phosphates. It also cycles back and forth between harnessing and distributing energy by forming and breaking a phosphate bond, as shown in the figure below.

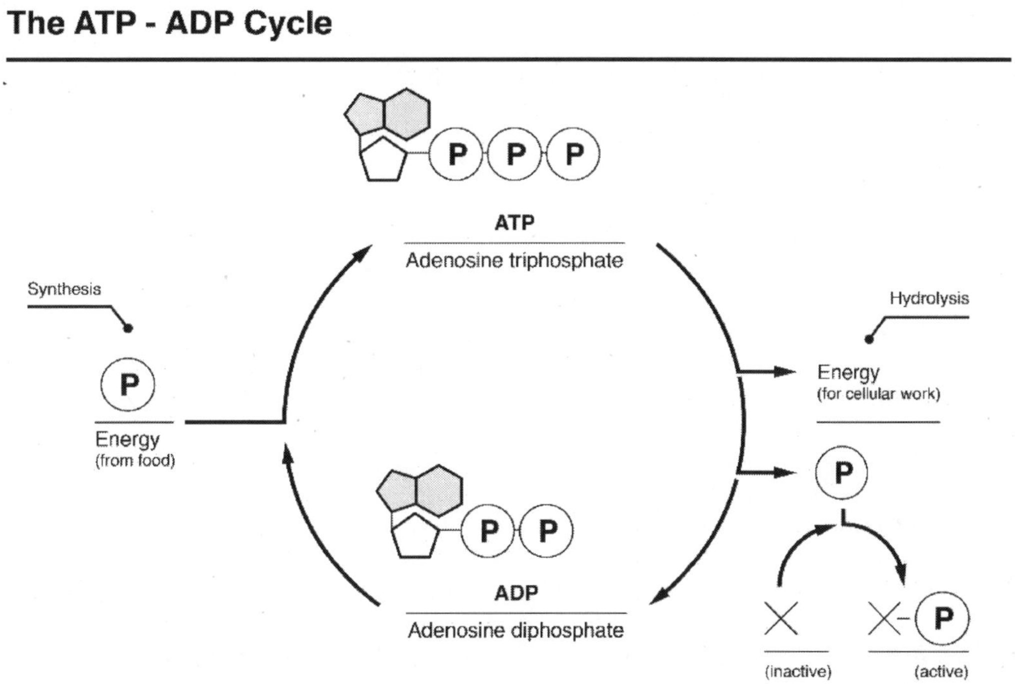

Cellular Respiration in Eukaryotes

All organisms, whether autotrophic or heterotrophic, use food to produce ATP in a process called respiration. Cellular respiration is the metabolic process that converts energy from nutrients into ATP and waste products. This will be explained in detail later. Prokaryotes use proteins on their cell membrane to perform respiration, while eukaryotes have specialized structures called mitochondria to do it.

Chloroplasts and mitochondria are the organelles responsible for all energy conversion in eukaryotic cells. All eukaryotes have mitochondria, but only plants and green algae have chloroplasts as well.

Electron Transport Chain

The energy source for oxidative phosphorylation (also known as the electron transport chain) are the electrons traveling through the membrane of the mitochondrial cristae in a redox reaction-driven electron transport chain. Their high energy is coupled with the active transport of the protons, and as they are passed down the chain in a series of redox reactions, oxygen becomes the final electron pair acceptor. The electrons and the hydrogen ions join an electronegative oxygen to form water.

Respiration

The chloroplast and mitochondria are key players in energy conversions (respiration and photosynthesis) in eukaryotes. In autotrophs, the energy products created through photosynthesis are used in cellular respiration. In heterotrophs, the energy needed for cellular respiration is obtained through food. The reactants and products of each cycle are listed below:

1a. Autotrophs only: Photosynthesis in the chloroplast makes glucose and oxygen to be used in cellular respiration:

$$6CO_2 + 6H_2O \rightarrow C_6H_{12}O_6 + 6O_2$$

1b. Heterotrophs only: consume glucose and pass its energy along the food chain

2. Both autotrophs and heterotrophs: Aerobic respiration occurs in the mitochondria, producing water, carbon dioxide, and energy.

$$C_6H_{12}O_6 + 6O_2 \rightarrow 6H_2O + 6CO_2 + 32ATP$$

3. Both autotrophs and heterotrophs: Organisms die, decompose, and their essential elements are re-used, and then the cycle repeats.

Energy Extraction from Cellular Respiration

Aerobic respiration uses oxygen and produces 30-32 ATP molecules using the mitochondria. Only a few of the ATP are generated via substrate-level phosphorylation in glycolysis and the Krebs cycle; the vast majority of ATP is generated through the electron transport chain and chemiosmosis.

The exact number of ATP molecules made per glucose molecule varies. Glycolysis and the Krebs cycle each produce a net gain of 2 ATP/GTP via substrate-level phosphorylation. Oxidative phosphorylation is more difficult to calculate. Each electron carrier NADH produces around 2.5 ATP, while $FADH_2$ produces around 1.5 ATP. These are not whole numbers because there is not a direct relationship between electron transport and phosphorylation — they are two different processes. One has to do with electrons traveling down the chain to the final electron acceptor: oxygen. The other has to do with the movement of hydrogen ions. Finally, some of the work done by oxidative phosphorylation might be distributed to other cellular processes because respiration does not exist in a vacuum.

Another example of the flexibility of energy production by respiration is seen in thermoregulation. Endothermic organisms have ways to regulate body heat, including shivering and sweating. Another is by using an uncoupling protein in the cristae during hibernation. A mitochondrial protein called uncoupling protein 1 (UCP1) in brown fat cells hijacks the proton motive force by preventing them from entering the ATP synthase and creating ATP. Instead, UCP1 moves the protons by increasing the permeability of the inner mitochondrial membrane, using energy from the proton gradient to be dissipated as heat. This helps keep hibernating animals warm without creating unneeded ATP, which helps animals conserve energy and keep their metabolic rates low.

In addition to two pyruvate molecules produced by glycolysis, six molecules of NADH and two molecules of flavin adenine dinucleotide ($FADH_2$) are produced and used by the ETC. Hydrogen atoms, transported by NADH and $FADH_2$ to the ETC, are used to produce ATP from ADP. The hydrogen atoms form a proton concentration gradient down the ETC that produces energy required to produce ATP. NADH and $FADH_2$ molecules rephosphorylate ADP to ATP via the ETC with each NADH producing three ATP molecules and $FADH_2$ producing two ATP molecules.

Glycolysis

The first step of breaking down glucose to make energy is called glycolysis (literally "glucose-splitter"), and it occurs in the cytosol of cells.

$$C_6H_{12}O_6 + 2ATP \rightarrow 2C_3H_4O_3 + 4ATP + 2NADH$$

$$\text{Glucose} + \text{activation energy} \rightarrow 2\ \text{Pyruvate} + \text{energy} + 2\ \text{electron carriers}$$

As shown in the previous formula, the overall goal of glycolysis is to break glucose in half and into 2 pyruvate molecules. In doing so, it peels off high-energy electrons that were contained in glucose. Two pairs of electrons (stored in phosphate groups) and two hydrogen atoms are invested into the electron carrier NAD+ that behaves just like the electron carrier in photosynthesis by shuttling electrons from one process to the next.

Glycolysis requires a 2ATP energy investment to proceed to completion, and it produces 4ATP via substrate level phosphorylation. This net gain of 2ATP is a small percentage of the total energy produced in aerobic respiration.

In the absence of oxygen, the 2ATP produced in glycolysis is the only energy gain there is, and fermentation, or anaerobic respiration, will initiate to recycle the electron carrier NAD^+. The two chief types of anaerobic respiration/fermentation are lactic acid fermentation and alcohol fermentation. When muscle cells have exceeded their aerobic capacity, they go into anaerobic respiration, which produces lactic acid and 2 net ATP. Yeast undergoes alcohol fermentation, producing carbon dioxide, ethyl alcohol, and 2 net ATP.

Glycolysis is performed via the following steps:

- Glucose is converted into Glucose-6-Phosphate (G6P) via the enzyme hexokinase (note that any enzyme ending in -kinase indicates that a phosphate group is going to be donated). Energy is lost because ATP loses a phosphate group and is converted into ADP in the process of creating G6P.
- G6P is then rearranged, turning from a hexagonal figure to a pentagonal figure, and is configured into Fructose-6-Phosphate (F6P) by an enzyme called phosphoglucose isomerase.
- F6P is converted into Fructose-1,6-Bisphosphate (F1,6BP) by phosphofructokinase, donating a phosphate group from ATP and turning it into ADP, losing energy.
- F1,6BP is then broken down into two 3-carbon molecules by the enzyme aldolase. These molecules are DHAP (dihydroxyacetone phosphate) and G3P (glucose-3-phosphate). DHAP acts as a kind of brake on glycolysis. If there is too much energy in the body, this reaction favors DHAP. However, if there is not enough energy in the body, this reaction favors G3P to go on to continue glycolysis.
- G3P is then converted into 1,3-Bisphosphoglycerate (1,3-BPG) via glyceraldehyde phosphate dehydrogenase. During this conversion, NADP+ is converted into NADPH.
- 1,3-BPG becomes 3-Phosphoglycerate (3-PG) via the enzyme phosphoglycerate kinase). Energy here is gained in the form of ATP, in which ADP gains a phosphate group through this enzyme.
- 3-PG is then mutated by phosphoglyceromutase into 2-Phosphoglycerate (2-PG).
- 2-PG is converted into phosphoenolpyruvate (PEP) via the enzyme enolase. Water is created via this process.
- Finally, PEP is converted into pyruvate through the enzyme pyruvate kinase, in which energy is again gained by the donation of a phosphate group to ADP to create ATP. Pyruvate is then entered into the Krebs cycle.

The Krebs Cycle

If oxygen is present in a eukaryotic organism, the remainder of the process of respiration will occur inside the mitochondria via the Krebs cycle and oxidative phosphorylation. The main goal of the Krebs cycle is to take pyruvate and break it down, producing NADH and $FADH_2$.

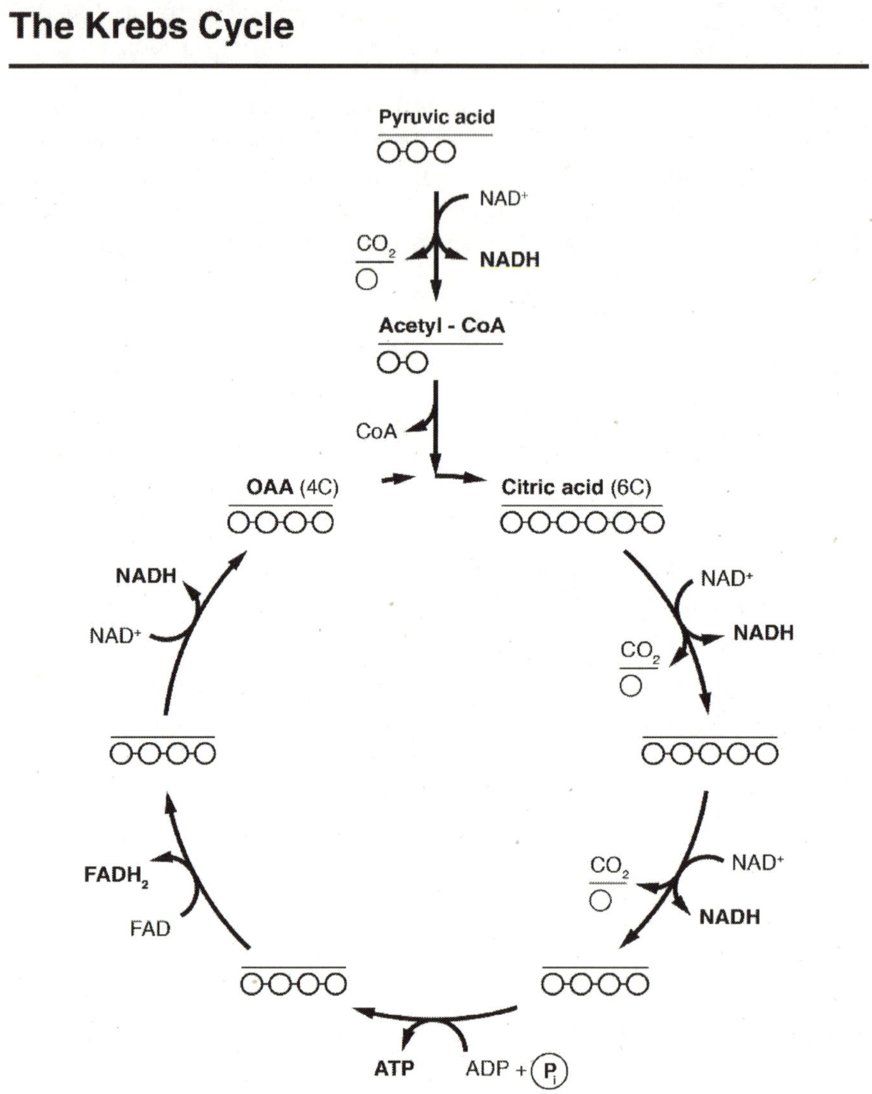

Upon entering the mitochondria, the pyruvate releases a pair of high-energy electrons, and a proton (H^+) to the electron carrier NAD^+, plus a carbon dioxide molecule. This happens while it is being converted into a two-carbon molecule attached to Coenzyme A, formally called Acetyl CoA. This step is called pyruvate oxidation. Acetyl CoA is used as fuel for the following citric acid (Krebs) cycle.

Including the intermediate stage, where pyruvate enters, two spins of the cycle (one for each pyruvate) produces the following:

- 2 CO_2 (from intermediate)
- 2 NADH (from intermediate)
- 4 CO2
- 6 NADH

- 2 FADH2
- 2 ATP (or GTP) via substrate-level phosphorylation. GTP is guanosine tri-phosphate, which is analogous to ATP.

NADH and $FADH_2$ are electron carriers, meaning they donate electrons to the electron transport chain. NADH donates two high-energy electrons and one proton (H+), while $FADH_2$ donates two electrons and two protons ($2\ H^+$). These high-energy electron and proton carriers then go through the process of oxidative phosphorylation, where many ATP molecules are made. Using the energy supplied by the electron transport chain, protons are transported through the integral protein complexes I, III, and IV along the inner mitochondrial membrane. The pumping of these protons out of the mitochondrial matrix across the cristae to the inner membrane space, establishes a concentration gradient. Just like in photosynthesis, this gradient provides the proton motive force to generate ATP when the hydrogen ion later passes through ATP synthase, causing it to spin and convert ADP to ATP.

Membrane Permeability

Selective Permeability

All cells contain a cell membrane, which is selectively permeable. Selective permeability means that it acts as a gatekeeper, allowing certain molecules and ions in and out while keeping unwanted ones at bay, at least until they are ready for use. This is achieved through active and passive transport, actively allowing molecules and ions through the opening and closing of cell membranes embedded within the phospholipid bilayer (using energy), or passively via a concentration gradient.

The cell membrane, or plasma membrane, has selective permeability with regard to size, charge, and solubility. With regard to molecule size, the cell membrane allows only small molecules to diffuse through it. Oxygen and water molecules are small and typically can pass through the cell membrane. The charge of the ions on the cell's surface also either attracts or repels ions. Ions with like charges are repelled, and ions with opposite charges are attracted to the cell's surface. Molecules that are soluble in phospholipids can usually pass through the cell membrane. Many molecules are not able to diffuse the cell membrane, and, if needed, those molecules must be moved through by active transport and vesicles.

Water is polar because of the bent shape of the molecule — one side of the molecule (the oxygen side) has a negative charge, and the other side (the hydrogen side) has a positive charge. Oxygen, though more negative than hydrogen, has a more positively charged *nucleus,* causing it to pull the two hydrogen molecules' electrons closer to itself. This results in a partial positive charge of the hydrogen side and makes oxygen more electronegative (see the following figure). The molecule is bent because the electrons pulled from hydrogen are not bonded to any other atoms and are termed "lone" electrons. Further, the two hydrogen atoms on the opposite side of the oxygen are repelled by their own positive forces, and the lone electrons are also repelled by their similar charges. Therefore, they stay as far away from each other as possible while still being held in place by oxygen.

Polar substances dissolve other polar substances. For example, when table salt (NaCl) is placed in water, the molecule is split into Na^+ and Cl^- because Na^+ is attracted to $O2^-$, and Cl^- is attracted to the H^+, essentially "tearing" the molecules apart. Polar substances are said to be hydrophilic (water-loving), and non-polar substance are said to be hydrophobic (water-fearing).

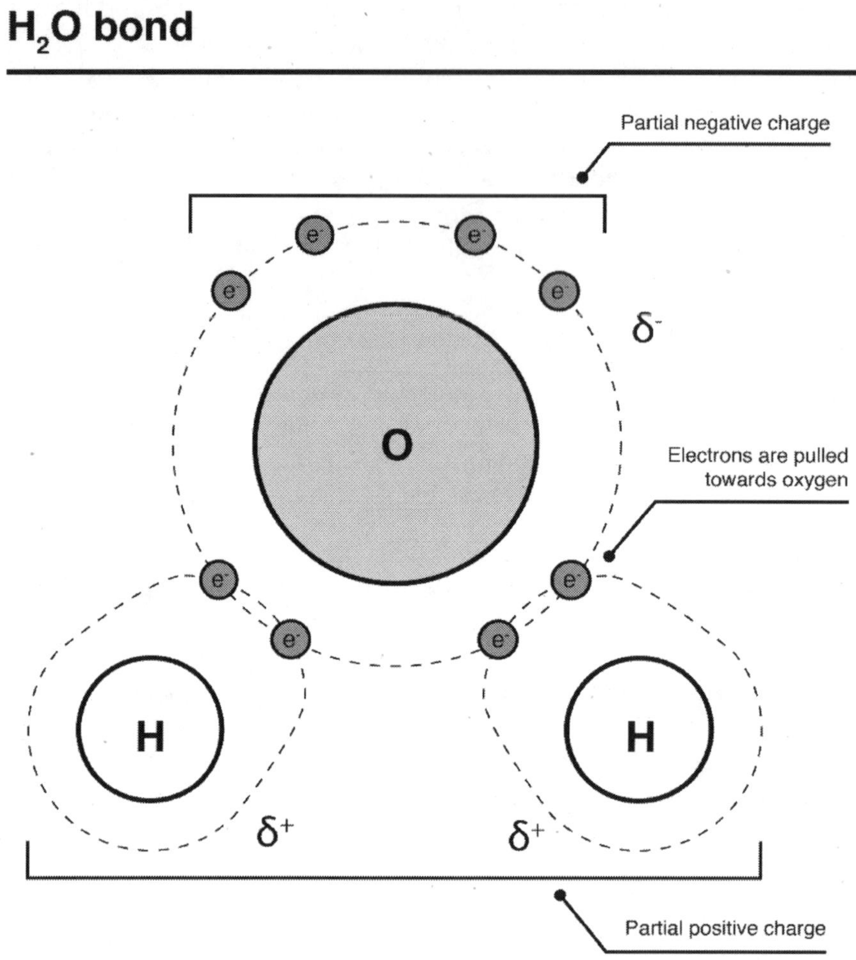

Role of the Cell Wall

Cholesterol is a hydrophobic steroid lipid. It embeds itself in animal cells' lipid bilayers between hydrophobic tails and regulates membrane fluidity. At high temperatures, the embedded cholesterol prevents melting because there is strength in numbers. Squeezing in an extra non-polar molecule provides for many more hydrophobic interactions to contribute to the "glue" that holds it together. In cold temperatures, on the other hand, cholesterol prevents freezing because its ringed structure interrupts adjacent phospholipids. This makes it more difficult for the hydrophobic tails to line up perfectly and freeze, which is similar to how adding electrolytes to water lowers its freezing point.

Plant cell walls are made of a polysaccharide called *cellulose* that offers structural support and protection to the plant. Prokaryotes, fungi, and some protists also have cell walls, although they are not necessarily made of cellulose. Chitin is the structural component of fungi, and bacteria have a cell wall made of peptidoglycan. Cell walls allow movement through channels called plasmodesmata.

Membrane Transport

Maintenance of Solute and Water Balance

Passive Transport

Passive transport is the movement of substances from high concentration to low concentration without the use of energy. This occurs because of the universe's tendency to achieve a state of equilibrium, or balance. For example, when food coloring is dropped into a cup of water, it spreads to the rest of the water until equilibrium is reached and there is a homologous solution. Passive transport comes in the following three varieties:

- Diffusion: When particles move from high concentration to low concentration, like when hot chocolate powder dissolves in water to form a tasty treat.
- Osmosis: When water moves from high concentration to low concentration via a permeable membrane. Water moves to the higher concentration of solutes in order to achieve a more equal water to solute ratio.
- Facilitated diffusion: When particles diffuse through a channel protein due to the membrane's selective permeability

Active Transport

Some transport requires energy for molecules to cross the membrane. Protein pumps are transmembrane proteins that use ATP to change their conformations so that they can force substances against their concentration gradient. For example, the sodium-potassium pump uses ATP to move three sodium (Na+) ions out of the cell and two potassium (K+) ions into the cell. This maintains the steep voltage gradient across the membrane in neurons and muscle cells so that the intracellular environment is more negative than the extracellular one. This membrane potential, along with the concentration gradient, creates an electrochemical gradient.

Another type of active transport, the proton pump, is critical to photosynthesis and respiration through its maintenance of proton gradients across the thylakoid and cristae, respectively.

Transport Across the Plasma Membrane

Endocytosis and exocytosis are examples of active transport required for the bulk movement of substances. They require vesicles, which are plasma membrane-bound delivery sacs. The different types of endocytosis are all similar in that the membrane folds inward so that it pinches off to create a vesicle that carries substances into the cell. The contents then travel to the lysosome, which is an acidic organelle that contains digestive enzymes. The lysosome breaks down the materials so that the cell can use them. Types of endocytosis include:

- Phagocytosis, or "cellular eating," occurs when a cell engulfs large particles and internalizes them by using vacuoles. This only happens in specialized cells such as immune cells.
- Pinocytosis, or "cellular drinking," occurs when a cell engulfs droplets of extracellular fluid and surrounds them with vesicles. This happens routinely in animal cells.
- Receptor-mediated endocytosis occurs when a ligand binds to a receptor protein that initiates a signal transduction cascade.

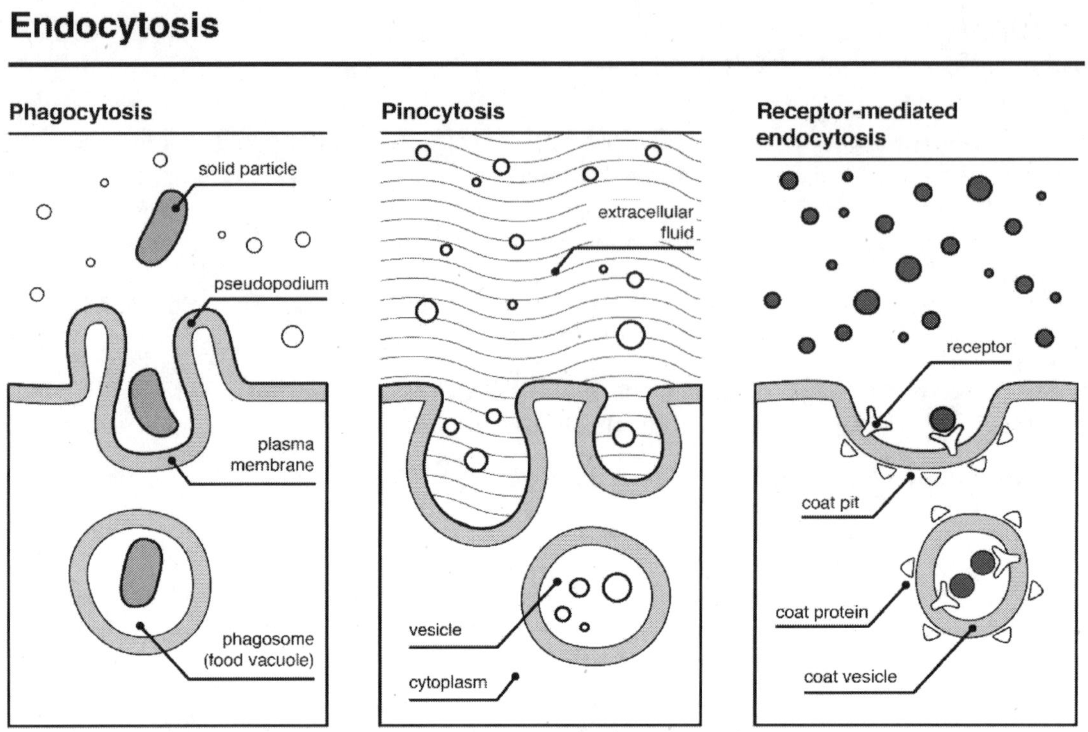

Exocytosis is the excretion of substances via vesicles. Neurotransmitters are excreted via exocytosis at synapses between neurons. Vesicles also release digestive enzymes, hormones, and cellular wastes. Exocytosis is also used when membrane proteins processed in the Golgi apparatus attach to vesicles that deliver the proteins to their membrane destination.

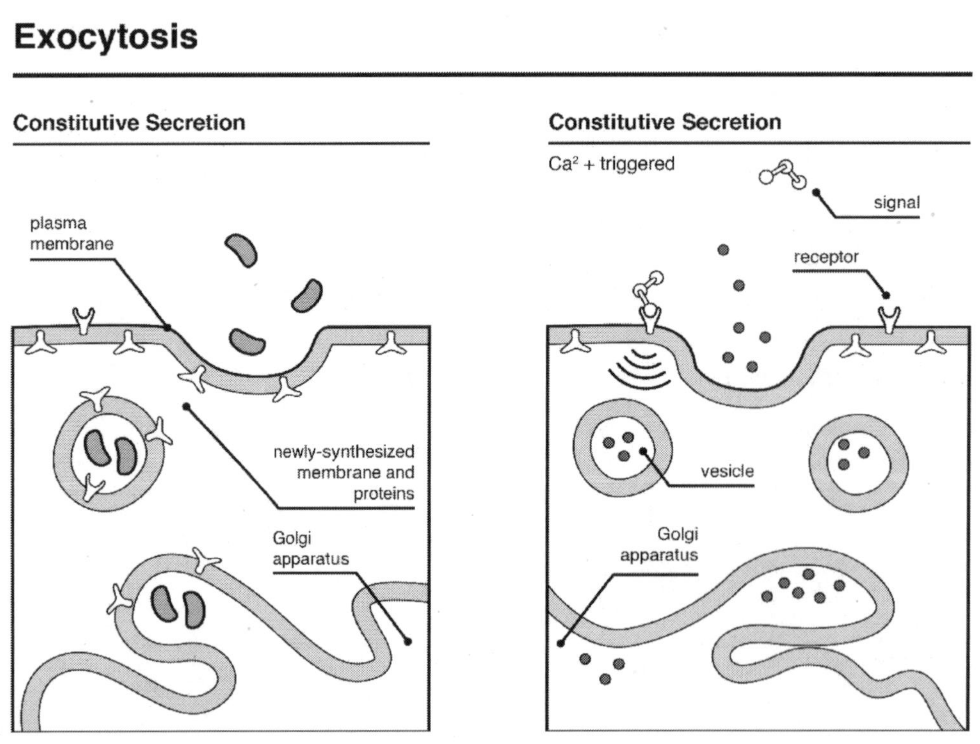

Facilitated Diffusion

Plasma Membrane Pass Through

Diffusions of Charged and Large Polar Molecules

Charged hydrogen ions diffuse or move from one side of a membrane to the other side such that the ions are randomly distributed, thereby increasing entropy. Diffusion moves from a high-concentration area to a low one. Entropy is a measure of disorder or disorganization. Every cellular process that occurs in a cell increases the total entropy. Oxygen, a nonpolar molecule, tends to diffuse into a cell since its concentration inside the cell is low. Carbon dioxide, a nonpolar molecular, diffuses outward because its concentration is low outside the cell.

Polar molecules and specific ions cannot move across a membrane on their own. Polar molecules are considered hydrophilic since they are polar like water. Polar or hydrophilic substances generally avoid contact with the phospholipid bilayer. However, these substances may pass through the lipid bilayer by passing through a transport protein that is found along the cell membrane. These transport proteins may be referred to as channel proteins; they function by allowing specific ions or molecules to tunnel across the membrane. The channel made up of these proteins through which ions or molecules travel may be called a hydrophilic channel.

Aquaporins

A specific channel protein called an aquaporin facilitates a hydrophilic channel of water molecules that pass through a cell membrane. An aquaporin may allow the passage of three billion water molecules for every second. Ten water molecules can fit in an aquaporin, and without the channel protein, only a small fraction of water molecules can pass through the same area in a second. Therefore, aquaporins increase the rate at which water molecules pass through cell membranes. Aquaporins will not allow the passage of hydronium ions (H_3O^+), but some of the channel proteins will allow the passage of glycerol.

Water passes through the semipermeable cell membrane through aquaporins, while small, uncharged substances, such as oxygen and carbon dioxide, diffuse freely. Water's passage is an example of channel-mediated facilitated diffusion, which is simply diffusing across the cell membrane with the help of a tunnel-like protein. In addition to channel-mediated diffusion, there is also carrier-mediated facilitated diffusion. Carrier proteins, such as the one that allows glucose into the cell, change shape upon solute binding. Facilitated diffusion is a type of passive transport and does not require energy (ATP).

Channel Proteins

Channel proteins that are involved in the transport of ions are called ion channels. These ion channel proteins can act as gated channels that will open or close in response to a stimulus. The stimulus may be electrical. The nerve cell contains a potassium ion channel that opens in response to an electrical stimulus. Potassium ions can flow through the channel protein, thereby leaving the cell. Similarly, sodium ions may move outside a resting nerve cell base on an electrochemical gradient. When the cell is stimulated, a gated channel protein opens, thereby facilitating the diffusion of sodium ions. Driven by the concentration gradient of the sodium ions, the cations move down the electrochemical gradient.

Polarization of Membranes

Cells have specific voltages across the plasma membrane. This voltage is called a membrane potential, and it ranges from -50 to -200 millivolts (mV). A voltage is defined as electric potential energy that results from the separation of charges. The cytoplasmic side of the cell membrane (inside the cell) is typically negative with respect to the extracellular side. The polarization is the result of the unequal distribution of cations and anions on both sides of the cell membrane. The membrane potential favors the passive transport of anions out of the cell and the passive transport of cations into the cell. The combination of the two forces, a chemical force (concentration gradient) and an electrical force (membrane potential), that drive the ion diffusion across the cell membrane is a chemical force called the electrochemical gradient.

Membrane Proteins

Facilitated diffusion is a type of passive transport in which a solute moves down its concentration gradient. No energy is needed for the passive transport of ions, and the direction of transport is not altered. Specific transport proteins can move solutes against a concentration gradient through the cell membrane, where the solute is less concentrated. Active transport is a process in which a cell must expend energy to pump a solute against its concentration gradient. Transport proteins that move a solute against its gradient are called carrier proteins. The sodium-potassium pump is an example of an active transport system.

Metabolic Energy

Active transport allows a cell to regulate the internal concentrations of small solutes. An animal cell may contain higher concentrations of potassium ions and a lower concentration of sodium ions. For an active transport process, the cell expends energy, and sodium ions are pumped out of the cell while potassium ions are pumped into the cell. Adenosine triphosphate (ATP) hydrolysis supplies the energy needed for the cell membrane to pump ions into or out of the cell. When the terminal phosphate group of ATP is transferred to the transport protein, it changes the shape of the protein and translocates the bound solute across the membrane.

Membrane Potential

To maintain the membrane potential, the Na+/K+ ATPase oscillates between two shapes that pump three sodium ions out of the cell for every two potassium ions that are pumped into the cell. First, the cytoplasmic sodium ion binds to the pump. Once three sodium ions are attached to the pump, phosphorylation by ATP follows and leads to a change in protein shape. Affinity for the sodium ion is reduced, and the proteins release the ions to the outside. The new protein shape has an affinity for the potassium ions, and the ions begin to bind on the extracellular side. The binding triggers the release of the phosphate group and restores the protein's original shape. Lastly, potassium ions are released toward the inside of the cell, and the affinity for sodium ions increases.

Tonicity and Osmoregulation

Concentration Gradients

Water is a molecule that travels via facilitated diffusion through proteins called aquaporins. Water movement is determined by its environment, of which there are three types:

- Isotonic environments are achieved when there is a dynamic equilibrium between two solutions. Water will move in and out at equal rates.
- Hypotonic solutions are ones that have a lower solute concentration than the solution they are being compared to. The solution will be low in solute and high in water, so water will move out to achieve equilibrium.
- Hypertonic solutions are ones that have a higher solute concentration than the one they are being compared to. They will be high in solute and low in water, so water will move in to achieve equilibrium.

Animal cells in a hypotonic environment are subject to a net water movement into the cell, so the cell will swell and possibly burst if equilibrium is never achieved. Conversely, hypertonic solutions will cause the cell to shrink as water moves out.

Plant cells are also affected by their water concentrations. The pressure of their cell wall against the cell membrane is called turgor pressure. In hypotonic environments, the cell will swell, and the cell wall will press on the cell membrane, resulting in a turgid, or firm, cell. This is healthiest for a plant because it provides the support to hold it upright. Isotonic environments mean that water will diffuse in and out of the plants cells at equal rates. In a hypertonic environment, the plant cell will undergo a process called plasmolysis, where the cell membrane shrinks and separates from the cell wall, resulting in a wilted plant due to lack of turgor pressure.

Protists such as paramecium that live in hypotonic environments will constantly have water moving inward and will never achieve equilibrium. They have a contractile vacuole that actually pumps out extra water using energy.

Water potential (Ψ) always indicates the direction of net water flow. It is determined by the sum of the pressure potential (Ψ_p) and solute potential (Ψ_s).

$$\Psi = \Psi_s + \Psi_p$$

Pressure potential is the force a plant cell wall exerts on its cell membrane (turgor pressure).

Osmoregulatory Mechanisms

Osmoregulators must use energy to maintain osmotic gradients that result in water loss and gain. Animals use the electron transport chain to generate ATP and control the solute concentrations in their bodily fluids. The kidneys regulate the ion-salt concentration and balance the amount of water.

Salt concentrations must be maintained so that the body's cells, muscles, and neurons function normally. An animal adapts to its environment and learns to regulate its salt concentrations and conserve water. Osmolarity is the molarity or the moles of solute per one liter of solution. If two solutions have the same osmolarity, they are isoosmotic. Animals may balance water in two ways. An animal may be an osmoconformer, meaning it will be isoosmotic with its surroundings. Marine animals are osmoconformers, and their internal osmolarity is the same as the environment's; no water is gained or lost. Organisms that are osmoregulators can control their internal osmolarity and are independent of the external environment. Organisms that live in freshwater or terrestrial environments are osmoregulators.

Bony marine fish such as cod lose water through osmosis, but they balance water loss by drinking seawater. The excess salt they ingest is removed through the kidneys and gills. To prevent the denaturation of proteins and to maintain homeostasis, nitrogenous waste such as urea is excreted from the kidneys. Freshwater animals are hyperosmotic since their cells cannot handle salt concentrations that are as low as those in river or lake water. Freshwater animals have the problem of gaining water through osmosis. Therefore, water balance requires excreting mostly dilute urine and consuming little water. Freshwater fish uptake salt from their gills and through food to replenish salts lost by diffusion or urination.

Growth and Homeostasis

Maintaining the osmolarity between an animal's body and environment requires energy. Osmosis is a process in which water diffuses through a semipermeable membrane. Tonicity is the concentration of a solute between two solutions, one inside the cell and one outside. If the solution outside the cell contains a higher concentration of solute outside the cell, it is a hypertonic solution. Water will leave the cell, and the cell will shrink. If the solution is hypotonic, meaning it has a high concentration of solute inside the cell, water will enter the cell, and the cell will swell. An isotonic solution has an equal concentration of solutes and water on both sides of the membranes. A solute moves from a hypertonic to a hypotonic solution. The solvent (water) moves from hypotonic to hypertonic solutions.

Different types of cells adapt to different tonicity relationships. For example, the healthy state of most plant cells is a turgid or very firm cell (hypotonic). If the plant cells are isotonic, there is no tendency for water to move into the cell. Consequently, the plant cell becomes flaccid and will eventually wilt. In a hypertonic environment, a plant cell loses water and shrinks. The plasma membrane moves away from the cell wall, and the plant undergoes plasmolysis; the plant wilts and dies.

Osmoregulation and Water Balance

Solute potential (also called **osmotic potential**) is defined by the pressure needed to be added to a solution in order to prevent the influx of water into the other solution. It is influenced by concentration, by molarity of the solution, by ionization of the solute, and by temperature of the system. Solute potential decreases as solute is added to a solution, thus the negative sign in the equation below. Distilled water has a solute potential of zero.

$$\Psi_s = -iCRT$$

The equation above shows the relationship between the variables. R is not a variable — it is the pressure constant equal to $0.0831\ \frac{\mathrm{L \times bar}}{\mathrm{mol \times K}}$. A bar is a very large unit of pressure. The actual variables are as follows:

- First, i is a measure of the solute's ionization. If the solute disassociates, the number of individual particles in the solution increases, which decreases the solute potential. Organic and nonpolar molecules have an i value of 1. Ions have an i value dependent on their disassociation into a cation (a positive ion) and anion (a negative ion). NaCl disassociates into 2 ions (Na^+ and Cl^-) and has an i value of 2. $CaCl_2$ separates into 3 ions (Ca^{2+} and 2 Cl^-) and has an i value of 3.
- C (concentration) is the molarity (moles per liter) of the solution.
- T is the absolute temperature of the system in Kelvin ($°C + 273$).

Acid-Base Imbalance

A person requires a homeostatic balance of acidic compounds and basic compounds within their body. This balance is regulated by the lungs, which remove carbon dioxide, and by hormones that regulate the kidneys in releasing compounds that are causing an acid-base imbalance. An acid-base imbalance occurs when a patient's blood becomes too acidic or too alkaline. A number of respiratory and renal conditions can cause acid-base imbalance, as these impact the respiratory and renal organs' ability to remove compounds contributing to the imbalance. These conditions include chronic lung disease, obesity, chronic kidney disease, alcoholism, uncontrolled Type 1 diabetes, and acute infections that cause dehydration. Symptoms of acidosis include difficulty breathing or rapid breath, fatigue, dizziness, and confusion. Symptoms of alkalosis include muscle spasms, nausea, and vomiting. Treatment includes administering electrolytes and fluids to correct the imbalance, oxygen or ventilation support, or treatment of any underlying infections that may be contributing.

Describe the Relationship Between Genetic Material and the Structure of Proteins

Chromosome Structure

In an electron micrograph, chromosomes appear as short X-shaped bar-like rods composed of condensed coiled chromatin threads. A chromosome consists of two sister chromatids, which are joined by a centromere. A chromatid is a duplicated chromosome that has not separated. The chromosome is just a condensed form of deoxyribonucleic acid (DNA). Chromatids are about 700 nanometers in diameter and consist of tight helical fibers that are 30 nanometers in diameter. Chromatin is DNA wrapped around histone proteins and appears as bumpy threads under a light microscope. Chromatin comprises 30% genetic material (DNA), 60% globular histone proteins, and 10% newly forming or formed ribonucleic acid (RNA). The main units of chromatin are the nucleosomes, which contain flat disc-shaped clusters of eight histone proteins. Nucleosomes are about 10 nanometers in diameter and are connected like beads with a DNA molecule. DNA wraps around the nucleosome twice and is connected to another cluster via a DNA segment or linker. The histone proteins package very long strands of DNA in an ordered manner and have a role in gene regulation. Methyl groups found on histones can shut down DNA, and adding acetyl groups to histones exposes a variety of genes or DNA segments. Histones determine the specifications for producing various types of RNA species and proteins.

Nucleic Acids

Nucleic acids have two important duties in the body. As monomers, they are crucial for energy transfer. As polymers, they are a fundamental component of genetic material. Monomers form the building blocks of macromolecules, while polymers are formed when monomers link together in chains, forming larger macromolecules.

Nucleotides are the monomers that link together to form nucleic acids. Nucleotides have three components: a nitrogenous base and a phosphate functional group both attached to a five-carbon (pentose) sugar. There are two classes of nitrogenous bases: purines and pyrimidines. The two types of purines are guanine (G) and adenine (A), while the three types of pyrimidines are thymine (T), cytosine (C), and uracil (U). The two types of pentose sugars are deoxyribose and ribose. Nucleotides containing deoxyribose are termed deoxyribonucleic acids (DNA) and utilize guanine, adenine, cytosine, and thymine as their nitrogen bases. Nucleotides containing ribose are termed ribonucleic acids (RNA) and utilize guanine, adenine, cytosine, and uracil as their nitrogenous bases.

Chromosomes are composed of hundreds to thousands of genes. Human cells contain 23 pairs of chromosomes for a total of 46 chromosomes. As explained above, genes are inherited in pairs, one from each parent.

Proteins are made of long chains of amino acids. In total, there are 20 amino acids, 11 of which humans can synthesize on their own and the remaining 9 of which are procured through diet. DNA contains the information for the synthesis of proteins, but that information on DNA has to undergo transcription and translation by RNA in order to produce proteins.

Codons

A codon represents a sequence of three nucleotides that codes for either one specific amino acid or a stop signal during protein synthesis. Codons are found on messenger RNA (mRNA).

Twenty essential amino acids are utilized in the process of protein synthesis. The full set of codons encompasses 64 possible combinations and is termed the **genetic code**. In the genetic code, 61 codons represent amino acids and three codons are stop signals. The genetic code is redundant due to the fact that a single amino acid may be produced by multiple codons. For example, the codons AAA and AAG produce the amino acid lysine. The codons UAA, UAG, and UGA are stop signals. The codon AUG codes for both the amino acid methionine and the start signal. As a result, when found in mRNA, the codon AUG marks the initiation point of protein translation.

RNA

Ribonucleic acid (RNA) plays crucial roles in protein synthesis and gene regulation. RNA is made of nucleotides consisting of ribose (a sugar), a phosphate group, and one of four possible nitrogenous bases—adenine (A), cytosine (C), guanine (G), and uracil (U). RNA utilizes the nitrogenous base uracil in place of the base thymine found in DNA. Another difference between RNA and DNA is that RNA is typically found as a single-stranded structure, while DNA typically exists in a double-stranded structure.

RNA can be categorized into three major groups—messenger RNA (mRNA), ribosomal RNA (rRNA), and transfer RNA (tRNA). Messenger RNA (mRNA) transports instructions from DNA in the nucleus of a cell to the areas responsible for protein synthesis in the cytoplasm of a cell. This process is known as transcription. Transfer RNA (tRNA) deciphers the amino acid sequence for the construction of proteins found in mRNA. Both tRNA and ribosomal RNA (rRNA) are found in the ribosomes of cells. Ribosomes are responsible for protein synthesis. The process is also known as translation, and both tRNA and rRNA play crucial roles. Both translation and transcription are further described below.

DNA

Deoxyribonucleic acid, or DNA, contains the genetic material that is passed from parents to offspring. It contains specific instructions for the development and function of a unique eukaryotic organism. The vast majority of cells in any eukaryotic organism contains the same DNA.

The majority of DNA can be found in the cell's nucleus and is referred to as nuclear DNA. A small amount of DNA can be located in the mitochondria and is referred to as mitochondrial DNA. Mitochondria are the site of aerobic energy production for the cell. All offspring inherit mitochondrial DNA from their mother. James Watson, an American geneticist, and Frances Crick, a British molecular biologist, first outlined the structure of DNA in 1953.

The structure of DNA visually approximates a twisting ladder, and is described as a double helix. DNA is made of nucleotides consisting of deoxyribose (a sugar), a phosphate group, and one of four possible nitrogenous bases—thymine (T), adenine (A), cytosine (C), and guanine (G). It is estimated that human DNA contains three billion bases. The sequence of these bases dictates the instructions contained in the DNA, making each species singular. The bases in DNA pair in a particular manner—thymine (T) with adenine (A) and guanine (G) with cytosine (C). Weak hydrogen bonds between the nitrogenous bases ensures easy uncoiling of DNA's double helical structure in preparation for replication.

Transcription

Transcription refers to a portion of DNA being copied into RNA, specifically mRNA. It represents the first crucial step in gene expression. The process begins with the enzyme RNA polymerase binding to the promoter region of DNA, which initiates transcription of a specific gene. RNA polymerase then untwists the double helix of DNA by breaking weak hydrogen bonds between its nucleotides. Once DNA is untwisted, RNA polymerase travels down the strand reading the DNA sequence and adding complementary nitrogen bases. With the assistance of RNA polymerase, the pentose sugar and phosphate functional group are added to the nitrogen base to form a nucleotide. Lastly, the weak hydrogen bonds uniting the DNA-RNA complex are broken to free the newly formed mRNA. The mRNA travels from the nucleus of the cell out to the cytoplasm of the cell where translation occurs.

Translation

Translation refers to the process of ribosomes synthesizing proteins. It represents the second crucial step in gene expression. The instructions encoding specific proteins to be made are contained in codons on mRNA, which have previously been transcribed from DNA. Each codon represents a specific amino acid or stop signal in the genetic code.

Amino acids are the building blocks of proteins. Ribosomes contain transfer RNA (tRNA) and ribosomal RNA (rRNA). Translation occurs in ribosomes located in the cytoplasm of cells and consists of the following three phases:

Initiation: The ribosome gathers at a target point on the mRNA, and tRNA attaches at the start codon (AUG), which is also the codon for the amino acid methionine.

Elongation: A new tRNA reads the next codon on the mRNA and links the two amino acids together with a peptide bond. The process is repeated until a polypeptide, or long chain of amino acids, is formed.

Termination: The ribosome disengages from the mRNA when it encounters a stop codon (UAA, UAG, or UGA). The event releases the polypeptide molecule. Proteins are made of one or more polypeptide molecules.

DNA Replication

During DNA replication, identical copies of the cell's genome are passed to the two formed daughter cells. Replication occurs on the chromatin threads. Because of the DNA molecule's length, replications occur at several origin points along the chain. There are four sequences of events during the replication of DNA: uncoiling, separation, assembly, and restoration.

During the first phase, called uncoiling, the DNA molecule unwinds with the help of enzymes to form a replication bubble. In the separation sequence, the hydrogen bonds between the DNA base pairs (Guanine-Cytosine, Adenine-Thymine) are broken. The unzipping of the strands forms a replication fork. In the third stage or assembly, DNA polymerase places free nucleotides along the parental or template strands to create new strands. The DNA polymerases function in one direction and create leading and lagging strands. Both strands are produced in opposite directions. The leading strand is made in the 5' to 3' direction, and the lagging strand is produced in the 3' to 5' direction. The Okazaki fragments are not produced simultaneously but are later connected together with DNA ligase to produce a lagging strand. In the last stage, restoration, the ligase enzymes splice Okazaki fragments, the short sequences of DNA nucleotides, to rebuild the double-helix structure.

Genetic Mutations

Mutations occur when single DNA base-pairs are altered or when an improper codon is added to the chain. The change in the DNA sequence may incorporate improper amino acids in specific positions within a protein. Consequently, the modified protein may not function or it may function abnormally, which can lead to disease. Any change, insertion, or deletion of a different single base-pair, called a point change, can range from synonymous to frameshift mutations. Synonymous, or silent, mutations produce the same codons owing to the redundancy in genetic code. Frameshift mutations are genetic mutations caused by insertions or deletions (indels) of many nucleotides in a sequence of DNA that is not divisible by three; for example, the insertion of two different base-pairs is not divisible by three. Frameshift mutations can lead to various diseases such as cancer, cystic fibrosis, and Crohn's disease.

Apply Concepts Underlying Mendel's Laws of Inheritance

Genes are the basis of heredity. The German scientist Gregor Mendel first suggested the existence of genes in 1866. A gene can be pinpointed to a **locus**, or a particular position, on DNA. It is estimated that humans have approximately 20,000 to 25,000 genes. For any particular gene, a human inherits one copy from each parent for a total of two.

Genotype refers to the genetic makeup of an individual within a species. **Phenotype** refers to the visible characteristics and observable behavior of an individual within a species.

Genotypes are written with pairs of letters that represent alleles. Alleles are different versions of the same gene, and, in simple systems, each gene has one dominant allele and one recessive allele. The letter of the dominant trait is capitalized, while the letter of the recessive trait is not capitalized. An individual can be homozygous dominant, homozygous recessive, or heterozygous for a particular gene. **Homozygous** means that the individual inherits two alleles of the same type, while **heterozygous** means inheriting one dominant allele and one recessive allele.

If an individual has homozygous dominant alleles or heterozygous alleles, the dominant allele is expressed. If an individual has homozygous recessive alleles, the recessive allele is expressed. For example, imagine a species of bird develops either white or black feathers. The white feathers are the dominant allele, or trait (*A*), while the black feathers are the recessive allele (*a*). Homozygous dominant (*AA*) and heterozygous (*Aa*) birds will develop white feathers. Homozygous recessive (*aa*) birds will develop black feathers.

Genotype (genetic makeup)	Phenotype (observable traits)
AA	white feathers
Aa	white feathers
aa	black feathers

Influence of Phenotype on Genotype

The genetic material (DNA) inherited from an individual's parents determines the genotype. Natural selection leads to adaptations within a species, which affects the phenotype. Over time, individuals within a species with the most advantageous phenotypes will survive and reproduce. As result of reproduction, the subsequent generation of phenotypes receives the fittest genotype. Eventually, the individuals within a species with genetic fitness flourish and those without it are erased from the environment, which describes the concept of "survival of the fittest". When this process is duplicated over numerous generations, the outcome is offspring with a level of genetic fitness that meets or exceeds that of their parents.

Mendel's Laws of Genetics and Punnett Squares

Mendel's first law of genetics is the principle of **segregation** and states that alleles will segregate into different cells during the formation of gametes in meiosis. Mendel's second law of genetics is the principle of **independent assortment** and states that genes for different traits will be assigned to different gametes independent of the others. Together, these two laws state the assumptions upon which genetic probabilities are based.

Punnett squares are simple graphic representations of all the possible genotypes of offspring, given the genotypes of the parent organisms. For instance, in the above example with the species of bird with black or white feathers, *A* represents a dominant allele and determines white colored feathers on a bird. The recessive allele *a* determines black colored feathers on a bird. If both parents are heterozygous (*Aa*, the *x* and *y*-axis of the square), the offspring will have the possible genotypes *AA, Aa, Aa*, and *aa*. Phenotypically, three offspring would have white feathers and one would have black feathers, as shown in the following Punnett square:

	A	a
A	White	White
a	White	Black

Monohybrid and Dihybrid Genetic Crosses

Genetic crosses represent all possible permutations of gene combinations, or alleles. A **monohybrid cross** investigates the inheritance pattern of a single gene such as in the above example of the birds with black or white feathers. Both parents must have heterozygous gene pairs in a monohybrid cross.

The phenotypic ratio for a monohybrid cross is 3:1 (AA, Aa, Aa, aa), in favor of the dominant gene. A dihybrid cross investigates the inheritance patterns of two genes that are related, for example A and B. A dihybrid cross has a phenotypic ratio of 9:3:3:1, with nine offspring inheriting both dominant genes, six offspring inheriting a single dominant and a single recessive gene, and one offspring inheriting both recessive genes.

Describe Structure and Function of the Basic Macromolecules in A Biological System

There are four classes of macromolecules that allow organisms to exist: carbohydrates, lipids, proteins, and nucleic acids. Carbon is the backbone of these organic molecules because of its ability to form up to four covalent bonds. Carbon (C), hydrogen (H), oxygen (O), nitrogen (N), sulfur (S), and phosphorus (P) are the most prevalent elements in these biological molecules. The following chart gives an overview of each organic molecule.

Organic Molecule	Example	Monomer (smallest repeating unit)	Structure	Function
Carbohydrate	• Sugar • Cellulose	Monosaccharide	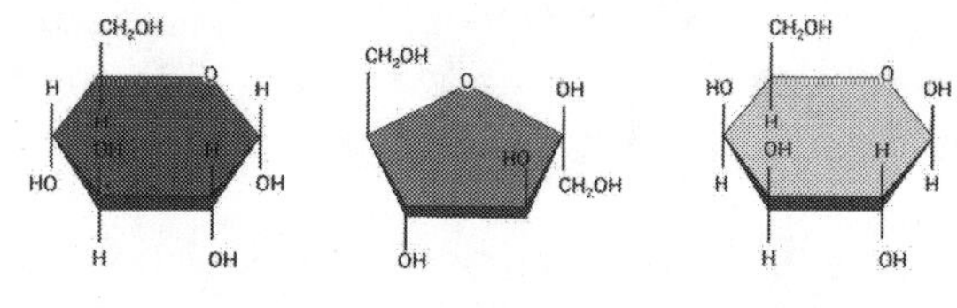 Glucose Fructose Galactose	• Energy • Structure
Protein	• Actin • Insulin	Amino Acid	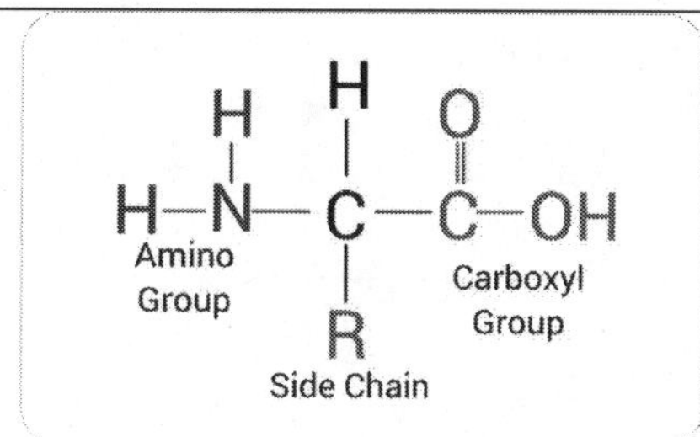	• Structure • Support • Some hormones
Lipid	• Fat • Oil	Technically none because the glycerol and fatty acids are not repeating.	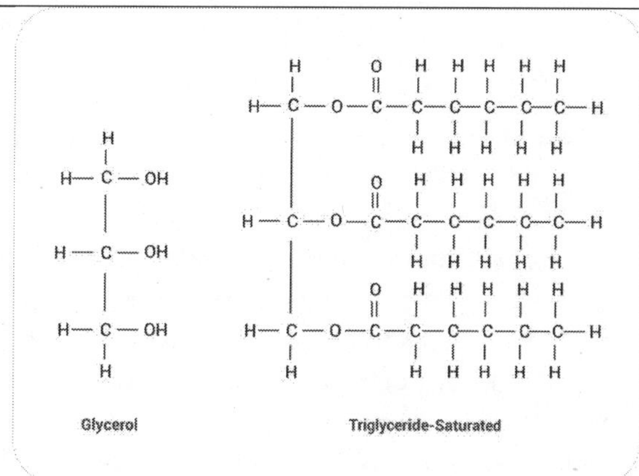	• Long-term energy • Steroid Hormones • Cell membranes
Nucleic Acid	• DNA • RNA	Nucleotide	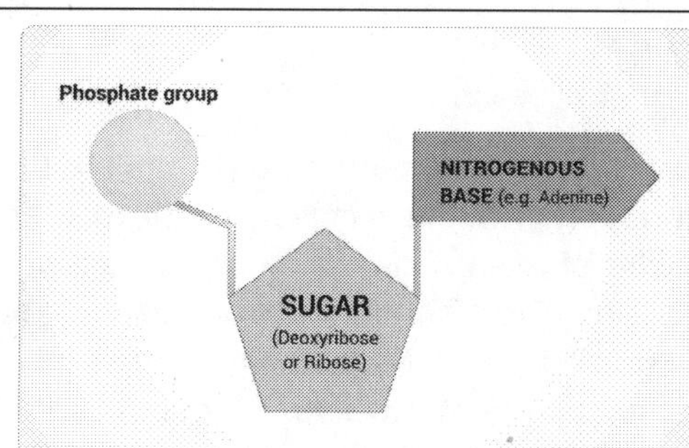	• Genetic code • Makes Protein

Carbohydrates

Carbohydrates are usually sweet, ring-like sugar molecules that are built from carbon (carbo-), oxygen, and hydrogen (-hydrates, meaning water). They can exist as one-ring monosaccharides, like glucose, fructose, and galactose, or as two-ring disaccharides, like lactose, maltose, and sucrose. These simple sugars can be easily broken down and used via glycolysis to provide a source of quick energy. Polysaccharides are repeating chains of monosaccharide rings. They are more complex carbohydrates, and there are several types. For example:

- Plants store energy in the form of starch.
- Animals store energy in the form of glycogen. Vertebrates store glycogen in the liver and in muscle cells.
- Cellulose is the chief structural component of plant cell walls.
- Chitin is the chief structural component of fungi cell walls and the exoskeletons of arthropods.

Through gluconeogenesis, the body can produce carbohydrates such as glucose from glycogen, galactose, fructose, or non-carbohydrate substrates such as pyruvate, lactate, glycerol, and some gluconeogenic amino acids. Some enzymes in gluconeogenesis include fructose 1,6-bisphosphatase and glucose 6-phosphatase. Simple carbohydrates such as glucose can combine with another monomer of glucose to form a glycosidic bond. Carbohydrates can be broken down by hydrolysis, which results in the formation of one water molecule and a smaller polysaccharide or simple carbohydrate. Starch is a polysaccharide of glucose that can be broken down into maltose by the enzyme amylase. Maltase can break down maltose by hydrolyzing the glycosidic bond into two glucose molecules. During glycolysis, simple carbohydrates such as glucose are broken down into two molecules of pyruvate. The glycolysis pathway goes from glucose to glucose-6-phosphate to fructose-6-phosphate and finally to pyruvate.

Proteins

Proteins are composed of chains of amino acids. There are several different kinds.

- Enzymes catalyze chemical reactions in the body.
- Storage proteins like albumin in eggs are important for development.
- Hormonal proteins are responsible for initiating signal transduction cascades that regulate gene expression.
- Motor proteins like actin and myosin are responsible for movement.
- Immune proteins like antibodies and antigens are important for fighting disease.
- Transport proteins like channel proteins and protein pumps move molecules.
- Receptor proteins receive chemical messages like neurotransmitters.
- Marker proteins serve as a cell's identification or fingerprint that distinguishes between cells of different types and sources.
- Structural proteins like keratin are important for things like spider webs, hair, and feathers.

All proteins are made from a combination of some of all of the same 20 amino acids. The varying amino acids are linked by peptide bonds and form the primary structure of the polypeptide, or chain of amino acids. The primary structure is just the string of amino acids. It is the secondary, tertiary, and quaternary structure that determines protein shape and function. The secondary structure can be beta sheets or alpha helices formed by hydrogen bonding between the polar regions of the polypeptide backbone. Tertiary structure results from the interactions between the side chains. Quaternary structure is the overall protein structure that occurs when subunits merge, take the correct shape, and become functional.

Proteins are synthesized through translation, whereby a sequence of messenger RNA (mRNA) is translated into a specific amino acid sequence. An amino acid bonded to translation RNA (tRNA), containing a codon, docks on a ribosome that is attached to mRNA. An amino acid chain grows on the end of the tRNA chain containing the amino acid. A condensation reaction between an amino acid containing a carboxyl group and another amino acid with an amino group produces a peptide bond and a molecule of water. Peptidyl transferase catalyzes peptide bond formation during the formation of the polypeptide chain during translation. Proteins can be broken down by a catabolic process. During degradation, transcription factors help break down proteins. The primary change of a protein consists of a sequence of amino acids held together by peptide bonds. A peptide or amide bond (-CO-NH-) is a covalent bond that can be broken with the addition of water, a process called hydrolysis. Proteases break peptide bonds by hydrolysis.

Lipids

Lipids are mostly nonpolar, hydrophobic molecules that are not soluble in water. Triglycerides are a type of lipid with a glycerol backbone attached to three long fatty acid chains. These energy-storage molecules can exist as any of the following types.

- Saturated fats have no double bonds within their fatty acid tails. These are solid at room temperature and are mostly animal fats like bacon fat.
- Unsaturated fats have double bonds within any of their fatty acid tails. Due to the kinks caused by the double bonds, these fats are liquid at room temperature and are mostly plant fats like olive oil.

Phospholipids are also composed of glycerol except they have two fatty acid tails. The third tail is replaced with a hydrophilic phosphate group. The amphipathic nature of this molecule results in a lipid bilayer where the "water-loving" hydrophilic heads face the extracellular matrix and cytoplasm and the "water-hating" hydrophobic tails face each other on the inside.

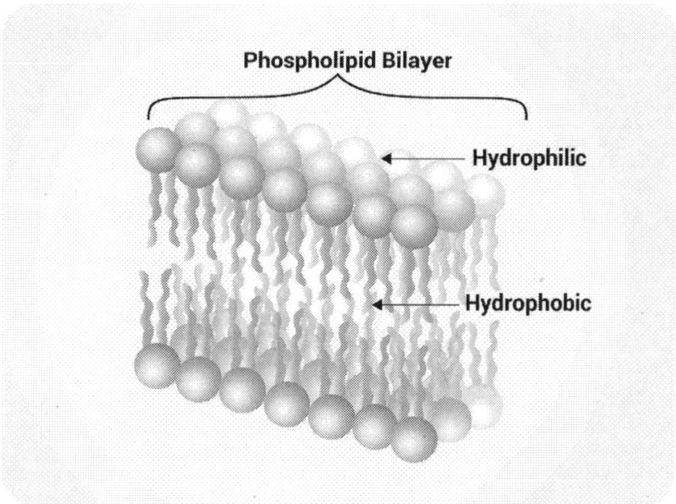

Steroids are another type of lipid. Cholesterol is a steroid that is embedded in animal cell membranes and acts as a fluidity buffer. Steroid hormones such as testosterone and estrogen are responsible for transcriptional regulation in certain cells.

Lipids consist of triglycerides, phospholipids, and steroids. Triglycerides consist of fats (solids) or oils (liquid) that are produced by the addition of a single glycerol molecule to three fatty acid chains. The addition is carried out by a dehydration synthesis which creates an E-shaped molecule. The body constantly requires energy and can break down triglycerides into their smaller building blocks which include glycerol and fatty acids. The degradation reaction is called a hydrolysis reaction, or lipolysis, which takes place in the cell's cytoplasm. In a lab setting, triglycerides can be broken down by boiling in a strong base; a process called saponification.

Nucleic acids

Nucleic acids are made of nucleotides. Nucleotides consist of a five-carbon sugar, a nitrogen-containing base, and a phosphate group. Deoxyribonucleic acid (DNA) exists as two nucleotide chains arranged in a double helix. Each deoxyribose sugar is connected to a nitrogenous base and an electrically-negative phosphate group. The nitrogenous bases are adenine and guanine, the two-ringed purines, and cytosine and thymine, the one-ringed pyrimidines. The double helix is held together by weak hydrogen bonds that connect adenine to thymine and cytosine to guanine. Ribonucleic acid (RNA) has a slightly different structure. It is usually single-stranded, has a ribose sugar as opposed to deoxyribose, and contains uracil instead of thymine.

Take a look at this chart:

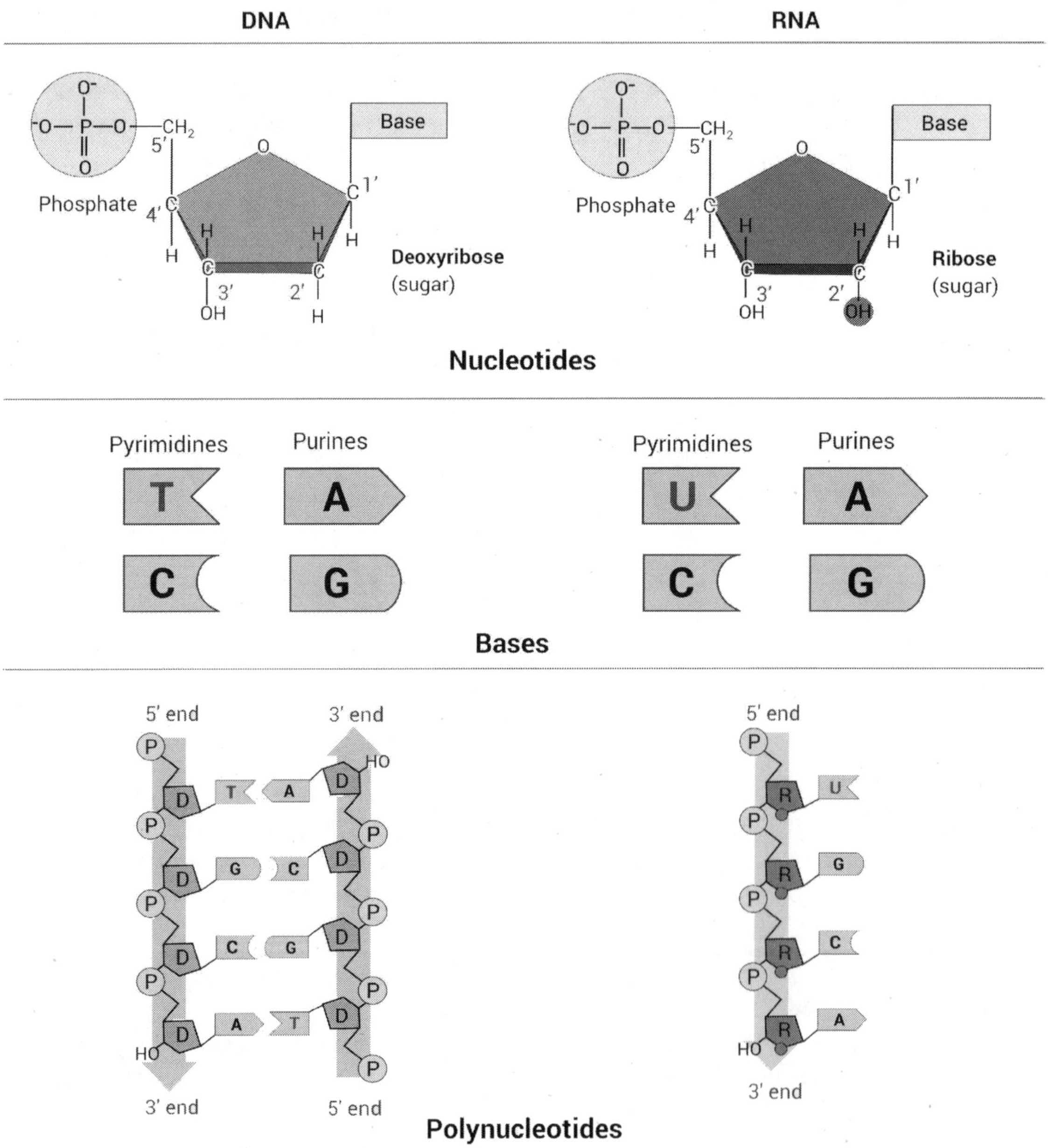

DNA forms the genetic code in the nucleus of eukaryotes, and RNA is the interpreter of that code. RNA exists in the following subtypes:

- Messenger RNA (mRNA) copies the DNA into a complementary transcript. This process is called transcription.
- Ribosomal RNA (rRNA) makes up the protein-making structure called the ribosome, which reads the transcript in a process called translation.
- Transfer RNA (tRNA) carries amino acids and delivers them to the ribosome. Each three letters of the mRNA transcript, or codon, recruits the anti-codon of a tRNA molecule that carries the corresponding amino acid.

A variety of enzymes participate in the synthesis of nucleic acids, which include dihydrofolate reductase and dihydroorotate dehydrogenase. The building blocks of RNA are nucleosides, and for DNA, they are nucleotides. The synthesis of nucleic acids begins with the production of pyrimidine and purine ribonucleotides. DNA and RNA contain bases that can be synthesized through de novo synthesis, which is energetically more expensive. Each ribonucleotide may be produced from small molecules such as amino acids, ribose sugars, and carbon dioxide. In a less energetic route, the pyrimidine nucleosides and purine bases can be salvaged from the breakdown of nucleotide cofactors and nucleic cells. The breakdown process will then produce nucleotides that can be added to nucleic acids. The breakdown of nucleic acids may also occur by DNA unwinding, where helicases and topoisomerases can cut one or both DNA strands to facilitate uncoiling.

Describe the Role of Micro-Organisms in Disease

Microorganisms

Microorganisms are tiny single-celled or multicellular organisms that can only be seen through a microscope. They include all bacteria and archaea (prokaryotes that live in extreme environmental conditions), and almost all protozoa, fungi, algae, and some rotifers (round microorganisms that reside in freshwater and have three-layered body cavities). Microorganisms have an important role in the environment, as they're found all over and help to recycle nutrients and energy.

Biodiversity

Biodiversity refers to the variety of life and species on Earth. There are many types of microorganisms on our planet. Four main classes of microorganisms are viruses, bacteria, protozoa, and fungi. Although *viruses* are acellular, they use a host species to replicate themselves, allowing for the cycling of nutrients, bacteria, and algae. They can also be pathogens and spread diseases. *Bacteria* are unicellular and obtain energy through photosynthesis, chemosynthesis (the synthesis of organic material from inorganic material for use as energy particularly in the absence of sunlight), and heterotropism (the ability to only produce organic material from carbon derived from animal or plant biosynthesis). *Protozoa* are a diverse group of unicellular organisms that carry out complex metabolic activities. They're also non-photosynthetic, so they cannot use light as an energy source. Amoebae, flagellates, and ciliates are all protozoa. *Fungi* can be unicellular or multicellular and they convert organic matter into nutrients. They are the primary decomposers of an ecological system.

Microbial Systematics

Microbial systematics is the scientific study of the types of microorganisms and the relationships between them. It can be divided into three areas: classification, nomenclature, and identification. This area of discipline allows microbiologists to further study genomic similarities between different species or microorganisms.

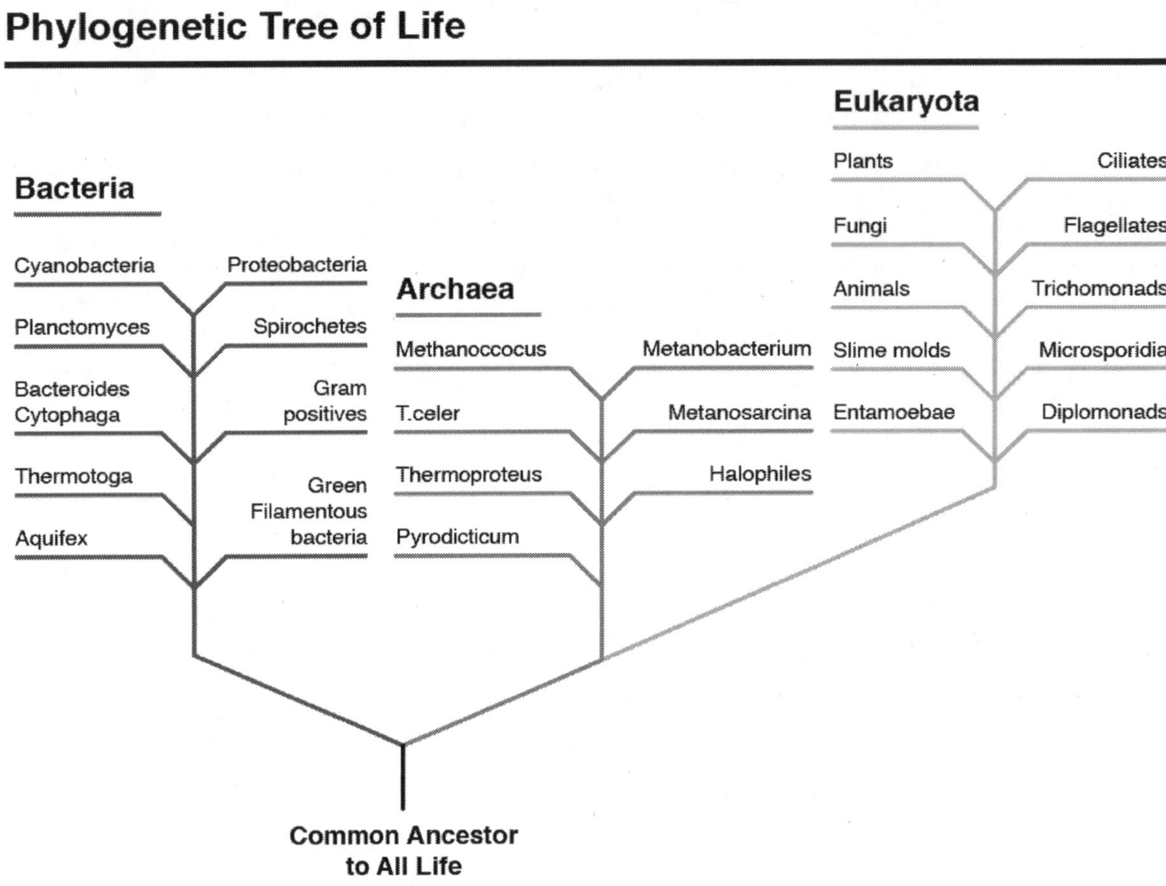

Domain Bacteria

The domain *Bacteria* includes many of the prokaryotic species that people encounter daily. Most are *heterotrophic*, which means they acquire their food from organic matter. Some are *parasitic*, which means they live within a host and cause disease. Some are *autotrophic* and synthesize their own food, such as by photosynthesis or chemosynthesis. They can be aerobic or anaerobic. Bacteria can also be beneficial to the environment by turning nitrogen from the air into organic compounds available to plants. They also help with the decay of landfill materials and other environmental debris. Bacteria swap genetic material through horizontal gene transfer, which can happen by transformation, transduction, or conjugation. *Transformation* involves the naturally-transforming bacteria taking up short fragments of naked DNA. *Transduction* involves the uptake of DNA by bacteriophages. *Conjugation* requires cell-to-cell contact and DNA is transferred by sexual pilus.

Domain Archaea

The domain *Archaea* is comprised of single-cell *prokaryotes*, which means that they don't have a cell nucleus or any membrane-bound organelles within them. Although they are similar in size and shape to bacteria, they contain genes on a single circular chromosome and have several metabolic pathways including transcription and translation.

There are three types of archaeal species that use different sources of energy: *Phototrophs* use sunlight for energy, *lithotrophs* use inorganic compounds for energy, and *organotrophs* use organic compounds for energy.

Protists

Protists are a diverse group of unicellular eukaryotic organisms. They are often grouped by convenience and because they are not an animal, plant, or fungus. As eukaryotes, they have a nucleus and organelles. Photosynthetic protists contain plastids, which are organelles responsible for converting light to energy. Protists that use oxygen for energy contain mitochondria. Those that live in hypoxic environments, which lack oxygen, have hydrogenosomes, which appear to be like modified mitochondria. Protists can gain nutrition in many ways, such as photosynthesis or heterotrophism. A few common protists are euglena, amoeba, paramecium, and volvox.

Fungi

Fungi are a group of microorganisms that includes yeasts, molds, and mushrooms. They have the distinct characteristic of having chitin in their cell walls. *Chitin* is a long carbohydrate chain that adds rigidity to the walls of the fungi cells. Fungi are also solely heterotrophic; they break down dead organic material and use the released nutrients. They play an important role in cycling nutrients throughout an ecosystem. Many vascular plants only grow because of the symbiotic fungi that inhabit their roots and supply them with essential nutrition. Some fungi are responsible for the production of antibiotics, such as penicillin. Contrastingly, fungi can also cause many diseases in plants and animals, such as rusts and stem rot in plants and ringworm and athlete's foot in humans.

Helminths

Helminths are large multicellular organisms generally known as parasitic worms. Many worms classified as helminths are the cause of intestinal infections. They live in and feed off their living hosts. They disrupt their host's nutrient absorption, causing them to feel weak and be ridden with disease. Although they share a similar form, many species classified as helminths are not actually evolutionarily related.

Viruses and Virus-Like Agents

Viruses are acellular units comprised of a nucleic acid core surrounded by a layer of protein. As they are acellular and therefore non-living, they cannot reproduce or metabolize on their own—they must use a host organism to do both. Viruses can have a variety of effects on their host. Many viruses disable their hosts and cause cell death. Other viruses are latent and don't show signs of infection within their host.

Microbial Growth, Nutrition, and Metabolism

Most microorganisms reproduce by binary fission, a process where a cell grows to twice its normal size and then divides in half to produce two equally-sized daughter cells. These two cells can eventually divide again and become four cells, and the four cells can grow and divide to become eight total cells, and so on, to make the microorganism population larger. The growth of the microorganisms depends on intake and metabolism of appropriate nutrients. The most important nutrients are carbon, oxygen, nitrogen, and hydrogen. Different microorganisms can metabolize these elements for use as both food and energy. The flagella of protozoa are like those of human sperm and can aid in the study of human reproduction.

Microbial Genetics

Microbial genetics looks at the genotype and phenotypic expression of microorganisms. Because microorganisms have a rapid growth rate and a short generation time, they have been used for centuries to study different processes and pathways. The distinct traits of microorganisms allow for a variety of things to be studied. Bacteria have been used to study gene transfer systems. Archaea can withstand harsh environments and are used to study extreme environmental conditions *in vitro*. Fungi are used to study cell cycle regulation, chromatin structure, and gene regulation. Although their gene function isn't well understood, it is thought that both archaea and fungi have horizontal gene transfer functions like bacteria. Viruses are important for the study of genetics, as well as the study of viral pathogenic properties. Molecular biologists often use viral vectors to insert genetic material into cells.

Physical and Chemical Methods of Controlling Microorganisms

It is important to be able to control microorganisms to prevent the transmission and spread of diseases, and to stop decomposition of organisms and food spoilage. They can be controlled by both physical and chemical methods. Physical control can occur through changes in temperature, humidity, osmotic pressure, and by filtration. These changes can inhibit microorganism growth and make the environment less ideal for their survival. Filtration includes the physical removal of microorganisms by preventing their passage through a porous material. Chemical control occurs using disinfectants, antibiotics, antiseptics, and antimicrobial chemicals, which all work by selective toxicity. These agents seek out and kill the microorganisms without harming anything else.

Tools for Studying Microorganisms

Microorganisms cannot be seen by the naked eye and can only be visualized using a microscope. Certain types of microscopy, such as bright field, phase-contrast, and dark field, allow the cells to be seen without staining. Cells can also be stained and then viewed under a microscope so that different characteristics of the cell can be illuminated. Electron microscopy uses a beam of electrons to magnify specimens so that their details can be seen more clearly.

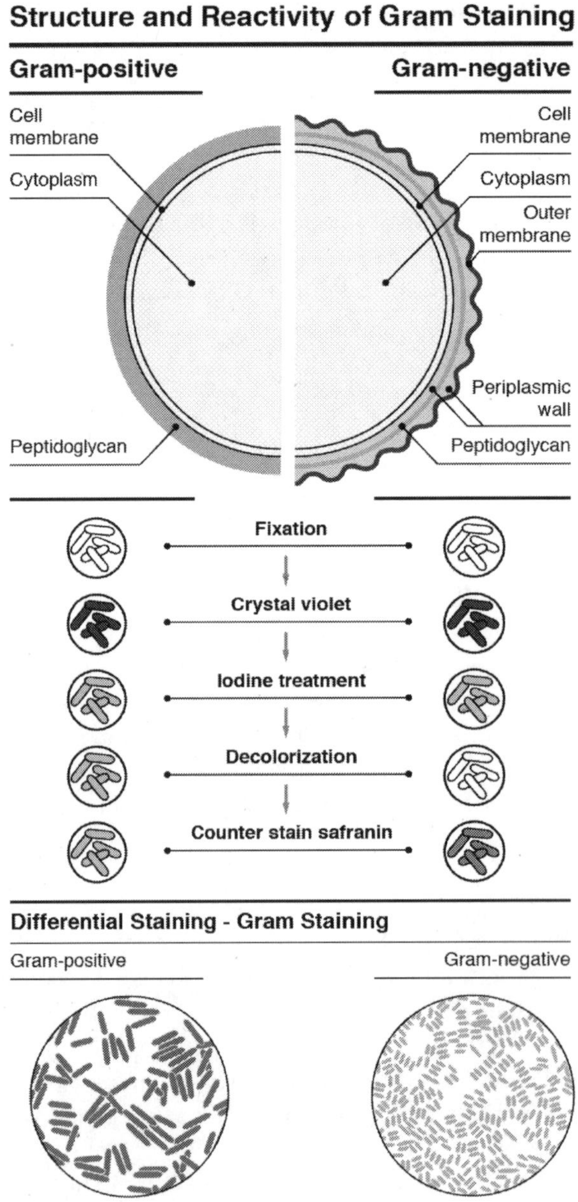

Infectious Diseases & Prevention

Infectious diseases are caused by the spread of microorganisms from one person to another, either directly or indirectly. *Direct contact* involves that exchange of bodily fluids or droplets between an infected person and another person. *Indirect contact* involves airborne spread or touching a contaminated object. Individuals with compromised immune systems are often more susceptible hosts than healthy individuals. The spread of infectious diseases can be prevented by thorough sanitization and disinfection, such as hand washing, vaccination, and the use of disinfectants while cleaning surfaces.

Immunity and Serology

Serology is the study of *blood serum*, the clear fluid that separates when blood clots, and how it relates to the immune system. The body's immune system is the network of cells, tissues, and organs that helps fight off infections. *Immunity* is the ability of an organism to use specific antibodies to fight an infection or toxin. Serology includes identifying these antibodies present in blood serum and investigating problems with the immune system. Three important serology tests include those for immunoglobulins (proteins responsible for antibody activity), rheumatoid factor (involved in certain types of arthritis), and human leukocyte antigen (HLA) typing (which determines organ, tissue, and bone marrow transplant compatibility).

AIDS and Immune Disorders

Immunodeficiency disorders occur when the body's immune system is unable to defend itself against foreign cells that can cause infection. This can cause unusual, prolonged, and/or frequent infections or cancers. Primary and secondary disorders are the two kinds of immunodeficiency disorders. Primary disorders are generally hereditary and present at birth. Secondary disorders develop later in life and result from the use of certain drugs or from another disorder. Acquired immune deficiency syndrome (AIDS) is a secondary disorder that develops from the human immunodeficiency virus (HIV). AIDS develops from HIV when a specific set of T cells, CD4+, from the immune system are depleted. The absence of these cells prevents the body from effectively fighting infections or killing cancerous cells. Immunodeficiency disorders can also include autoimmune disorders, which occur when the body's immune system attacks itself as if it were a foreign pathogen.

Antimicrobial Medications and Drugs

An antimicrobial medication or drug is used to treat a microbial infection. It can be antibiotic, antifungal, antiprotozoal, or antiviral. These drugs work by penetrating the cell wall of the microorganism and then disrupting the inside of the cell. They work to inhibit microbial growth and reproduction. The *therapeutic index* of a drug is a measure of its relative toxicity to a patient. It is calculated by taking the lowest dose that is toxic to a patient and dividing it by the dose typically used for therapy. Drugs that have antimicrobial selective toxicity are more harmful to microorganisms than patients. Some strains of microorganisms can change and become antimicrobial-resistant. When this happens, the microorganisms are no longer harmed by the medications, so they continue to survive, multiply, and harm the patient.

Systemic Infectious Diseases

Systemic infections are infections that occur in the bloodstream and therefore affect the whole body. As the infection is carried in the blood, it can affect multiple organs and tissues and cause multiple systemic infectious disease syndrome (MSIDS). Patients affected by MSIDS can have a variety of concurrent symptoms, making it hard to identify the source of the infection and thus also making it hard to treat the infection. The flu is an example of a systemic infection, and hypertension is an example of a systemic disease.

Infectious Diseases Affecting the Cardiovascular, Respiratory, Lymphatic and Nervous Systems

Infections of the cardiovascular system affect the blood, blood vessels, and the heart. *Septicemia* is the general term given to a microbial infection of the blood and blood vessels. If this infection reaches the heart valves, it results in endocarditis. Generally, this can be treated with antibiotics, but if there's too much damage to the heart, surgery may be needed. Common infections of the respiratory tract are the common cold and flu. *Bacterial infections* are less common than viral infections in the respiratory system. These affect the sinuses, throat, airways, or lungs. *Pneumonia* is an example of a bacterial infection of the lower respiratory tract. When microorganisms infect the lymphatic system, the lymph, lymph vessels, lymph nodes, and lymphoid organs—such as the spleen, tonsils, and thymus—are affected. When bacteria or viruses invade the vessels of the lymphatic system through a wound, this is known as infectious lymphangitis. Infections of the central nervous system can be very serious, as they affect the brain and spinal cord. Brain abscesses and bacterial meningitis are caused by bacteria or fungi, while viral meningitis and encephalitis are caused by viruses.

Infectious Diseases Affecting the Digestive, Urinary, and Reproductive Systems

When microorganisms enter the digestive tract, they cause gastrointestinal infections, which are an inflammation of the gastrointestinal (GI) tract that involves the stomach and the small intestine. Dehydration is the largest worry with GI infections, as the patient may not be absorbing enough water while affected by the virus, bacteria, or parasite. Infections of the urinary tract (UTIs) are most often caused by bacteria. They are often the result of bacteria from the large intestine entering the urethra and traveling up to the bladder. If they are not treated in a timely manner, the infection can also continue up to the kidneys and cause a serious infection. Symptoms of a kidney infection can include chills, fever, back pain, and nausea. There are three types of reproductive tract infections: sexually-transmitted diseases, endogenous infections, and iatrogenic infections. Sexually-transmitted diseases (STDs), such as chlamydia, gonorrhea, and HIV, are transmitted from one person to another by bodily fluids that are part of the reproductive system. Endogenous infections are caused by the abnormal growth of organisms that are normally present, such as bacterial vaginosis. Iatrogenic infection of the reproductive system occurs when microorganisms are introduced during an unsterile medical procedure. Serious reproductive infections may result in infertility.

Infectious Diseases Affecting the Skin and Eyes

Although the skin provides a barrier from infection, it sometimes gets infected. Bacterial infections include cellulitis and impetigo. Viral infections include shingles, warts, and herpes simplex virus. These infections can start with a rash, itching, pain, and tenderness. Most can be treated with antibiotics. Fungal infections include yeast infections, athlete's foot, and ringworm. They often occur when there is a cut on the skin's surface and the body's immune system is weakened. Microorganisms can also affect the surface or interior of the eyes. The most common eye infection is *conjunctivitis*, or pink eye, which is caused by the viruses and bacteria that cause the common cold. *Bacterial keratitis* is an infection of the cornea. When microorganisms reach the interior of the eyes, pain is not usually felt, but vision starts to deteriorate.

Chemistry

Recognize Basic Atomic Structure

Measurable Properties of Atoms

All matter is made of atoms. An **atom** is the most basic component of an element that still retains its properties. All of the elements known to man are catalogued in the **periodic table**, a chart of elements arranged by increasing atomic number. The **atomic number** refers to the number of protons in an atom's nucleus. It can be found either in the upper left-hand corner of the box or directly above an element's chemical symbol on the periodic table. For example, the atomic number for hydrogen (H) is 1. The term "atomic mass" refers to the sum of protons and neutrons in an atom's nucleus. The atomic mass can be found beneath an element's abbreviation on the periodic table. For example, the average atomic mass of hydrogen (H) is 1.008. Because protons have a positive charge and neutrons have a neutral charge, an atom's nucleus typically has a positive electrical charge. Electrons orbiting the nucleus have a negative charge. As a result, elements with equal numbers of protons and electrons have no net charge.

Atoms that have gained or lost electrons wind up having a net electrical charge and are termed **ions**. The following are the primary ions pertinent to human health:

Bicarbonate	HCO^{3-}	A major buffer in blood. The lungs and kidneys regulate its concentration.
Chloride	Cl^-	Important in stomach acid and usually ingested as the salts sodium chloride (NaCl) and potassium chloride (KCl).
Calcium	Ca^{2+}	Important for muscle contraction and bone construction.
Copper	Cu	Specialized chemical reactions in the cell.
Iodine	I	Specialized chemical reactions in the cell.
Iron	Fe	Important in hemoglobin for transport of oxygen as well as part of the electron transport chain.
Magnesium	Mg^{2+}	Important in chlorophyll and animal energy production as well as a constituent of bone.
Phosphate	PO_4^{3-}	A minor intracellular pH buffer that is regulated by the kidneys and is an important factor in bone.
Potassium	K^+	The most plentiful mineral inside of cells and is important for nerve and muscle function.
Sodium	Na^+	The most common mineral outside of cells and is important for water and osmolarity regulation as well as nerve and muscle function.
Sulfate	SO_4^{2-}	A minor pH buffer for body fluids.

For the majority of light atoms, the number of protons is similar to the number of neutrons. An **isotope** is a variation of an element having the same number of protons, but a different number of neutrons. For example, all isotopes of carbon (C) have six protons. However, C-12 has six neutrons, C-13 has seven neutrons, and C-14 has eight neutrons.

Some isotopes are radioactive and result in nuclear decay. Not all radioactive isotopes are harmful, and some are even useful to scientists and physicians. For example, C-14 is radioactive and can be used in the process of radiocarbon dating, which can be used to determine the age of organic remains. A radioactive isotope of gold (Au-198) can be utilized to treat ovarian, prostate, and brain cancer.

Periodicity and the Periodic Table

Periodicity

Periodicity refers to the repeating patterns, or trends, in the properties of elements. The atomic number and atomic structure are the key determinants of the properties of elements. During the mid-1800s, the Russian chemist Dmitri Mendeleev utilized the principal of periodicity to arrange elements in a manner similar to the modern periodic table. Mendeleev's periodic table was arranged in rows according to increasing atomic mass and in columns according to similar chemical behavior. The modern periodic table is arranged in order of increasing **atomic**

number, which is defined as the number of protons in an atom's nucleus. Elements near each other are more similar than elements that are distant on the periodic table.

Periodic Table

The periodic table catalogues all of the elements known to man, currently 118. It is one of the most important references in the science of chemistry. Information that can be gathered from the periodic table includes the element's atomic number, atomic mass, and chemical symbol. The first periodic table was rendered by Mendeleev in the mid-1800s and was ordered according to increasing atomic mass. The modern periodic table is arranged in order of increasing atomic number. It is also arranged in horizontal rows known as **periods**, and vertical columns known as **families**, or **groups**. The periodic table contains seven periods and eighteen families. Elements in the periodic table can also be classified into three major groups: metals, metalloids, and nonmetals. Metals are concentrated on the left side of the periodic table, while nonmetals are found on the right side. Metalloids occupy the area between the metals and nonmetals.

Due to the fact the periodic table is ordered by increasing atomic number, the electron configurations of the elements show periodicity. As the atomic number increases, electrons gradually fill the shells of an atom. In general, the start of a new period corresponds to the first time an electron inhabits a new shell. Other trends in the properties of elements in the periodic table are:

- **Atomic radius**: One-half the distance between the nuclei of atoms of the same element
- Electronegativity: A measurement of the tendency of an atom to form a chemical bond
- Ionization energy: The amount of energy needed to remove an electron from a gas or ion
- Electron affinity: The ability of an atom to accept an electron

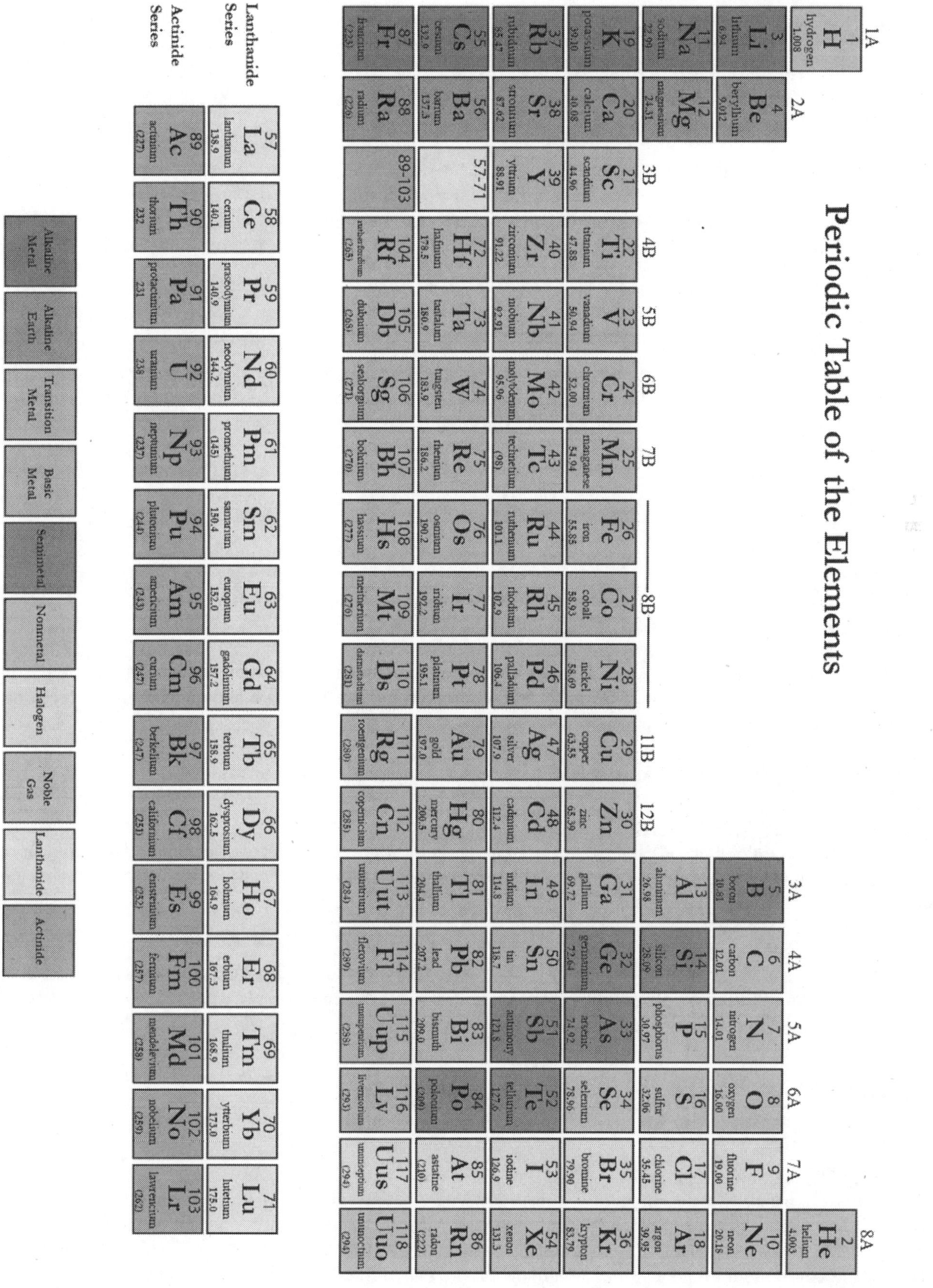
Periodic Table of the Elements
Lanthanide Series
Actinide Series
Alkaline Metal
Alkaline Earth
Transition Metal
Basic Metal
Semimetal
Nonmetal
Halogen
Noble Gas
Lanthanide
Actinide

Moving left to right in a period, trends reveal decreasing atomic radius, increasing electronegativity, increasing ionization energy, and increasing electron affinity. Moving from top to bottom in a group, trends reveal increasing atomic radius, decreasing electronegativity, and decreasing ionization energy. Helium, for example, being in Period 1 and Group 8A, has the smallest atomic radius. The trend of decreasing electron affinity is only seen in Group 1 of the periodic table.

Protons, Neutrons, and Electrons

The structure of an atom has two major components: the atomic nucleus and the atomic shells (also known as orbitals). The nucleus is found in the center of an atom. The three major subatomic particles are protons, neutrons, and electrons and are found in the atomic nucleus and shells.

Protons are found in the atomic nucleus and are positively-charged particles. The addition or removal of protons from an atom's nucleus creates an entirely different element. **Neutrons** are also found in the atomic nucleus and are neutral particles, meaning they have no net electrical charge. The addition or removal of neutrons from an atom's nucleus does not create a different element but instead creates a lighter or heavier form of that element called an isotope. **Electrons** are found orbiting in the atomic shells around the nucleus and are negatively-charged particles. A proton or a neutron has nearly 2,000 times the mass of an electron.

Electrons and Chemical Bonds

Electrons orbit the nucleus in atomic shells, or electron clouds, each of which can accommodate a certain number of electrons. For example, the first atomic shell can accommodate two electrons, the second atomic shell can hold a maximum of eight electrons, and the third atomic shell can house a maximum of eight electrons. The negatively-charged electrons orbiting the nucleus are attracted to the positively-charged protons in the nucleus via electromagnetic force. The attraction of opposite electrical charges gives rise to chemical bonds, which refers to the ways atoms are attached to each other.

Chemical bonding typically results in the formation of a new substance, called a **compound**. Only the electrons in the outermost atomic shell are able to form chemical bonds. These electrons are known as **valence electrons**, and they are what determines the chemical properties of an atom.

Physical Properties and Changes of Matter

States of Matter—Liquids, Gases, and Solids

There are three fundamental states of matter—liquid, gas, and solid. The molecules in a liquid are not in an orderly arrangement and can move past one another. Weak intermolecular forces contribute to a liquid having an indefinite shape, but definite volume. Lastly, a liquid conforms to the shape of its container, is not easily compressible, and flows quite easily.

The molecules in a gas have a large amount of space between them. A gas will diffuse indefinitely if unconfined, while it will assume the shape and volume of its container if enclosed. In other words, a gas has no definite shape or volume. Lastly, a gas is compressible and flows quite easily.

The molecules in a solid are closely packed together, which restricts their movement. Very strong intermolecular forces contribute to a solid having a definite shape and volume. Furthermore, a solid is not easily compressible and does not flow easily.

Vaporization, Evaporation, and Condensation

States of matter are able to undergo phase transitions. Vaporization refers to the transformation of a solid or liquid into a gas. There are two types of vaporization—evaporation and boiling. Evaporation is a surface phenomenon and involves the conversion of a liquid into a gas below the boiling temperature at a given pressure. Evaporation is also an important component of the water cycle. Boiling occurs below the surface and involves the conversion of liquid into a gas at or above the boiling temperature. Condensation represents the conversion of a gas into a liquid. It is the reverse of evaporation. Condensation is also most often synonymous with the water cycle. It is a crucial component of distillation.

The physical properties of matter do not change the chemical composition of a substance. The mass of an object or substance refers to the amount of matter found in that substance. Matter takes up space and is perceived by the human senses. The units of mass are reported in grams or kilograms. A laboratory balance is used to measure the mass. Based on the law of conservation of mass, chemical change will not change the total mass. Mass is not synonymous with weight, which is the force of gravity exerted on an object or substance. The mass of a specific object does not change, but the weight can. The astronaut's mass remains the same on earth and the moon, but the weight does not.

The volume of a substance refers to the length cubed and has units based on the metric or SI system (e.g., cm^3, m^3). Cubic centimeters (cm^3 or cc) is a standard laboratory unit. Chemists often use the unit of volume called the liter (L), which is equal to a cubic decimeter ($1 \text{ L} = \text{dm}^3$). Laboratory glassware is calibrated in milliliters or liters ($1{,}000 \text{ mL} = 1 \text{ L}$). A cubic centimeter is equivalent to one milliliter ($1 \text{ cm}^3 = 1{,}000 \text{ cm}^3$). Some examples of laboratory glassware that measure the volume are the beaker, volumetric flask, Erlenmeyer flask, graduated cylinder, and pipet.

An object's density is the object mass per volume unit and is given by the equation:

$$d = \frac{m}{V}$$

The density(d) can be determined by knowing the object's mass (m) and volume (V). For example, if the mass of an object is 10.0 g and the volume is 20.0 cm^3, then the density is:

$$d = \frac{10.0 \text{ g}}{20.0 \text{ cm}^3}$$

The density is very helpful for identifying a substance and can determine its purity. For instance, the density of pure gold is greater than silver mixed with gold.

Phase Transitions

Matter exists in phases and is mostly in the solid, liquid, or gas form. Solid matter has particles packed closely together. Solids are not compressible because they are already so compact that they are actually vibrating due to the significant attractive and repulsive intermolecular forces. Solids have no flow and do not take the shape of their container. Liquids, on the other hand, have flow because particles are not as tightly packed. They take the shape of their container but are not easily compressible because the particles are still fairly close together. Gas particles are different from solids and liquids in that they are very easily compressible. They are so far apart that intermolecular forces are negligible.

Below is an image that illustrates the stages of phase change:

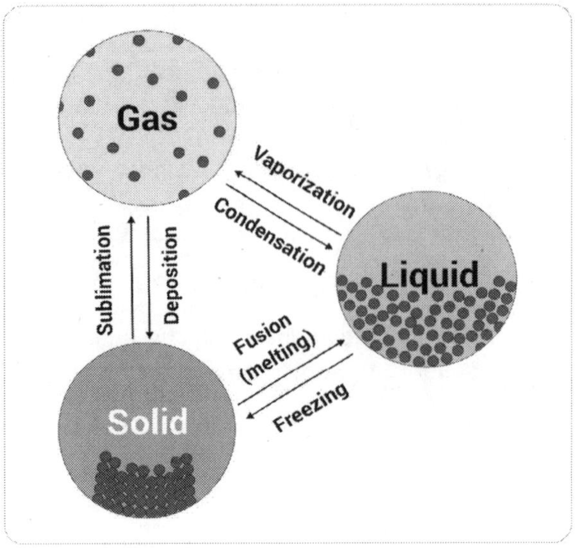

Phase changes are best described in terms of temperature and kinetic energy. Consider a tightly packed solid that has particles very close together. If heat is added, kinetic energy of the molecules increase. If enough heat is added, the particles will move quickly enough that they will begin to slide past each other and form a liquid. Moving from a solid to a liquid is called **melting**. The opposite change is **freezing**. Freezing occurs when liquid particles move slower and pack closely together into a solid.

Think of liquid water heating on a stove. When the boiling point is reached, some of the particles will turn into gas because they have so much kinetic energy. Moving from a liquid into a gas is called **vaporization**. The opposite reaction is **condensation**, which occurs when gas particles slow down and form a liquid. This is seen on the exterior of a cold drink when water vapor in the air cools on the glass and forms water beads.

Less common are direct changes from either solid to gas, or **sublimation**, or from a gas to a solid, or **deposition**. Sublimation appears as a solid emitting a cloud, like dry ice. Deposition can happen with water in extremely cold temperatures. Frost is water that has gone directly from a gas to a solid.

Describe Chemical Reactions

Valence Electrons

Valence electrons are found on the outermost shell of an atom. These electrons are found on atoms without a pseudo-noble gas or noble gas core. Atoms containing valence electrons are involved in chemical reactions. Elements with similar valence-shell configurations have similar chemical properties within a group in the periodic table. The nitrogen atom belongs to group 5A. Five valence electrons in nitrogen are represented by the following valence shell electron configuration ($2s^2 2p^3$).

Three valence electrons are needed to fill the p orbital, which means nitrogen will form three bonds. In ammonia (NH_3), nitrogen is bonded to three hydrogen atoms and has a neutral electrical charge. In ammonium (NH_4^+), the nitrogen atom shares an extra valence electron to form four N-H bonds; it has a positive electrical charge. Compounds with a positive electrical charge are cations. When the nitrogen atom in amide (NH_2^-) shares two valence electrons, it forms an anion since it bears a negative electrical charge.

The formation of molecules or compounds tends to follow the octet rule, which is the trend where atoms within a molecule/compound contain eight valence electrons within the valence shell. The nitrogen in ammonia, ammonium, and amide has an octet, but the hydrogen atom has a duet. A duet is an atom that has only two electrons in its valence shell. Electronegativity (EN) is the ability of an atom to pull electrons towards the atom's nucleus. Moving across or down the periodic table increases the EN for an atom. Consequently, the bonding of two atoms will have different polarities. A C-C covalent bond is nonpolar since the electronegativity value is the same for each carbon atom. A C-H bond is polar covalent since carbon has a greater EN value than hydrogen. Bonds with the greatest polarity are ionic and consist of a metal and nonmetal, such as sodium chloride (NaCl).

Chemical Bonds Between Atoms

Chemical bonds refer to the manner in which atoms are attached to one another. Atoms may be held together with three fundamental types of chemical bonds—ionic, covalent, or hydrogen.

Ionic Bonding

Ionic bonds are formed from the electrostatic attractions between oppositely charged atoms. They result from the transfer of electrons from a metal on the left side of the periodic table to a nonmetal on the right side. In an ionic bond, an atom loses one or more electrons to another atom which gains them. The atoms do this so that they can achieve a full outermost shell of electrons, which is the configuration that is most stable, and these are typically the strongest types of bonds. The metallic substance often has a low ionization energy and will transfer an electron easily to the nonmetal, which has a high electron affinity.

An example of this is the compound NaCl, which is sodium chloride or table salt, where the Na atom transfers an electron to the Cl atom. Due to their very strong bonding, ionic compounds have several distinct characteristics. They have high melting points and high boiling points, and are brittle and crystalline. They are arranged in rigid, well-defined structures, which allows them to break apart along smooth, flat planes. The formation of ionic bonds is a reaction that is very exothermic. In the opposite scenario, the energy it takes to break up a one mole quantity of an ionic compound is referred to as **lattice energy**, which is generally very endothermic. The Lewis structure for NaCl is written as follows:

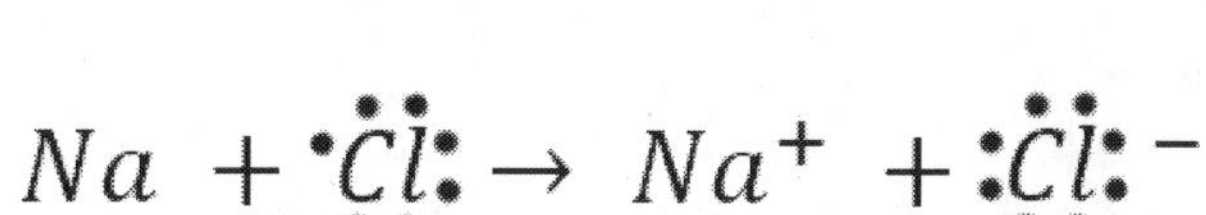

When an atom has a different number of electrons than its number of protons, it is termed an **ion**. A positively charged ion is referred to as a **cation**, while a negatively charged ion is referred to as an **anion**. For example, a sodium cation (Na^{+1}) can form an ionic bond with a chlorine anion (Cl^{-1}), which forms sodium chloride (NaCl), which is also known as table salt. The majority of the molecules formed with ionic bonds such as this have a crystalline structure.

Covalent Bonding

Covalent bonds are formed when two atoms share electrons, instead of transferring them like in ionic compounds. The atoms in covalent compounds have a balance of attraction and repulsion between their protons and electrons, which keeps them bonded together. Two atoms can be joined by single, double, or even triple covalent bonds. As the number of electrons that are shared increases, the length of the bond decreases. Covalent substances have low melting and boiling points and are also poor conductors of heat and electricity. The Lewis structure for Cl_2 is written as follows:

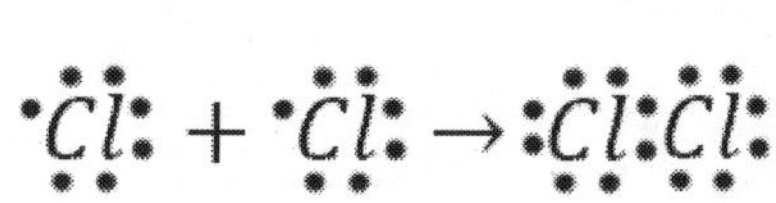

Covalent bonds are the most common type of bond in the human body. They are typically found in molecules containing carbon. Only six elements typically form covalent bonds: carbon (C), nitrogen (N), phosphorus (P), oxygen (O), sulfur (S), and hydrogen (H). Covalent bonds are a crucial source of energy for living organisms. Covalent bonds are comparable in strength to ionic bonds, but stronger than hydrogen bonds, and are typically used to bind the basic macromolecules—carbohydrates, lipids, nucleic acids, and proteins—together.

Hydrogen Bonding

Hydrogen bonds are temporary and weak. They typically occur between two partial, opposite electrical charges. For example, hydrogen bonds form when a hydrogen (H) atom is in the vicinity of nitrogen (N), fluorine (F), or oxygen (O) atoms. These partial electrical charges are called **dipoles** and are caused by the unequal sharing of electrons between covalent bonds. Water is the most prevalent molecule that forms hydrogen bonds.

Hydrogen bonds contribute to the adhesiveness and cohesiveness properties of molecules like water. Adhesiveness confers glue-like properties to molecules, which ensure they stick or connect more easily with other molecules—much like wetting a suction cup before sticking it to a surface. Cohesiveness refers to a molecule's ability to form hydrogen bonds with itself. For example, the cohesiveness of water is the reason why it has a high boiling point, which is a physical property.

Metallic Bonds

Metallic bonds are formed by electrons that move freely through the metal. They are the product of the force of attraction between electrons and metal ions. The electrons are shared by many metal ions and act like a glue holding the metallic substance together, similar to the attraction between oppositely charged atoms in ionic substances except the electrons are more fluid and float around the bonded metals and form a "sea of electrons". Metallic compounds have characteristic properties including strength, conduction of heat and electricity, and malleability. They can conduct electricity by passing energy through the freely moving electrons, creating a current. These compounds also have high melting and boiling points. Lewis structures are not common for metallic structures because of the free-roaming ability of the electrons.

Types of Chemical Reactions

Chemical reactions are characterized by a chemical change in which the starting substances, or **reactants**, differ from the substances formed, or **products**. Chemical reactions may involve a change in color, the production of gas, the formation of a precipitate, or changes in heat content. The following are the basic types of chemical reactions:

Reaction Type	Definition	Example
Decomposition	A compound is broken down into two or more smaller elements or compounds.	$2H_2O \rightarrow 2H_2 + O_2$
Synthesis	Two or more elements or compounds are joined together.	$2H_2 + O_2 \rightarrow 2H_2O$
Single Displacement	A single element or ion takes the place of another in a compound. (**substitution reaction**)	$Zn + 2HCl \rightarrow ZnCl_2 + H_2$
Reaction Type	**Definition**	**Example**
Double Displacement	Two elements or ions exchange a single atom each to form two different compounds, resulting in different	$H_2SO_4 + 2NaOH \rightarrow Na_2So_4 + 2H_2O$

Reaction Type	Definition	Example
	combinations of cations and anions in the final compounds. (**metathesis reaction**)	
Oxidation-Reduction	Elements undergo a change in oxidation number. Also known as a **redox reaction**.	$2S_2O_3{}^{2-}(aq) + I_2(aq) \rightarrow S_4O_6{}^{2-}(aq) + 2I^-(aq)$
Acid-Base	Involves a reaction between an acid and a base, usually producing a salt and water	$HBr + NaOH \rightarrow NaBr + H_2O$
Combustion	A hydrocarbon (a compound composed of only hydrogen and carbon) reacts with oxygen to form carbon dioxide and water.	$CH_4 + 2O_2 \rightarrow CO_2 + 2H_2O$

Balancing Chemical Reactions

Chemical reactions are expressed using chemical equations. Chemical equations must be balanced with equivalent numbers of atoms for each type of element on each side of the equation. Antoine Lavoisier, a French chemist, was the first to propose the **Law of Conservation of Mass** for the purpose of balancing a chemical equation. The law states, "Matter is neither created nor destroyed during a chemical reaction."

The reactants are located on the left side of the arrow, while the products are located on the right side of the arrow. Coefficients are the numbers in front of the chemical formulas. Subscripts are the numbers to the lower right of chemical symbols in a formula. To tally atoms, one should multiply the formula's coefficient by the subscript of each chemical symbol. For example, the chemical equation $2H_2 + O_2 \rightarrow 2H_2O$ is balanced.

For H, the coefficient of 2 multiplied by the subscript 2 equals 4 hydrogen atoms. For O, the coefficient of 1 multiplied by the subscript 2 equals 2 oxygen atoms. Coefficients and subscripts of 1 are understood and never written. When known, the form of the substance is noted with (g) meaning gas, (s) meaning solid, (l) meaning liquid, or (aq) meaning aqueous.

Demonstrate How Conditions Affect Chemical Reactions

Factors that Affect the Rate of a Reaction

There are a variety of factors that affect the rate of a reaction, such as temperature, surface area of the reactants, and a variety of environmental factors. Reaction concentration is another major factor, except in zero-order processes. In a **zero-order process**, the reaction rate does not depend on the concentration of the reactants and is equal to the rate constant: reaction *rate* = *k*. In **nonzero order processes**, the rate will depend on many factors. Steel wool does not burn in air; however, when the oxygen or reactant concentration is increased from 20 percent to 100 percent, the material burns and forms a white flame, thereby increasing the rate of reaction. As the temperature increases, the rate of reaction also increases because more reactant molecules contain enough kinetic energy to surmount the activation energy barrier and form reaction products. Adding a strip of zinc into a solution of hydrochloric acid will take longer to decompose compared to adding the same strip but chopped into pieces. This observation is due to the surface area of zinc, which increases when it's cut into pieces, allowing the rate of reaction to increase. A **catalyst** is a chemical substance or enzyme that allows the rate of reaction to increase without it being consumed and lowers the activation energy needed to form a product. If the surface area of the catalyst increases, so does the rate of the reaction.

Introduction to Equilibrium

Reversible Reactions in the Lab and Real World

Many chemical reactions are **reversible**, which means that the reactants can form the products, or the products can react to form the reactants. Depending on the environmental and experimental conditions, the reaction can be driven in either direction. Substances can move between different states of matter by changing the conditions of the reaction. When heat is added to water, it will become gaseous water vapor. If the temperature is lowered, i.e., heat is removed from the environment, the water vapor will condense into liquid water. Heat can also be used to dissolve a salt in water to make an aqueous solution. The conditions can be changed to then precipitate the salt out of the aqueous solution. The transfers of protons and electrons in acid-base and redox reactions, respectively, are also reversible reactions. The conditions of the solutions can cause acid and base ions to either disassociate or reattach to each other. Similarly, electrons can be transferred back and forth in chemical equations that involve both reduction and oxidation reactions.

There are many relevant, biological examples of reversible reactions that we experience every day. Hemoglobin is a protein that is used to transport oxygen in the blood throughout the human body. Oxygen molecules bind to the hemoglobin and when hemoglobin reaches the cells and tissues that need oxygen, the reaction is reversed, and the oxygen molecules are released from the hemoglobin molecule. As another example, olfactory molecules bind to the receptors in the nose to trigger a reaction from the brain. Once the reaction is triggered, the molecules are released.

The environment also has many reversible reactions that occur every day. Carbon is constantly transferred between the biosphere and the atmosphere. When living organisms exhale, they release carbon dioxide from their bodies into the atmosphere. Plants and other anaerobic elements of the biosphere then reabsorb carbon dioxide from the atmosphere and use it to produce energy. The **hydrosphere** is the system of the Earth that contains all of its water, such as oceans, seas, and lakes. Many substances—such as carbon dioxide, sulfur, and nitrogen—dissolve easily in water. When the water heats up, such substances can enter the atmosphere as a gas. The cycle continues when the substances condense again with drops in temperature and reenter the hydrosphere.

Equilibrium Conditions

Chemical reactions reach a state of equilibrium when the rate of the forward reaction is equivalent to the rate of the reverse reaction. The concentrations of the reactants and products are proportional to each other with regard to the stoichiometry of the equation and are no longer changing at equilibrium. The reaction quotient, Q, represents the proportional concentrations of reactants and products in the equation and at equilibrium, it is equal to the equilibrium constant, K. The equilibrium constant can be calculated from the equilibrium concentrations of the products and reactants of a chemical reaction. In the reaction $2H_2 + S_2 \rightarrow 2H_2S$, the equilibrium concentrations of the components are 0.25 moles $2H_2$, 0.625 moles S_2, and 0.75 moles $2H_2S$. K can be calculated using the following generic equation for the chemical reaction $aA + bB \rightarrow cC + dD$, using the equilibrium concentrations of the reactants and products:

$$K = \frac{[C]^c[D]^d}{[A]^a[B]^b}$$

For hydrogen and sulfur reacting, K can be calculated as:

$$K = \frac{[H_2S]^2}{[H_2]^2[S_2]}$$

Given the equilibrium concentrations:

$$K = \frac{(0.75)^2}{(0.25)^2(0.625)} = 14.4$$

Using Concentration Over Time Graphs to Understand the Establishment of Chemical Equilibrium

Simple graphs can be used to see the changes in the rate of a reaction and in the concentrations of the reactants and products as a reaction progresses and reaches equilibrium. The rates of the forward and reverse reactions equalize at equilibrium. Depending on the dynamics of the reaction, there may be more products or more reactants at the equilibrium, but both concentrations should change and then become steady as equilibrium is reached.

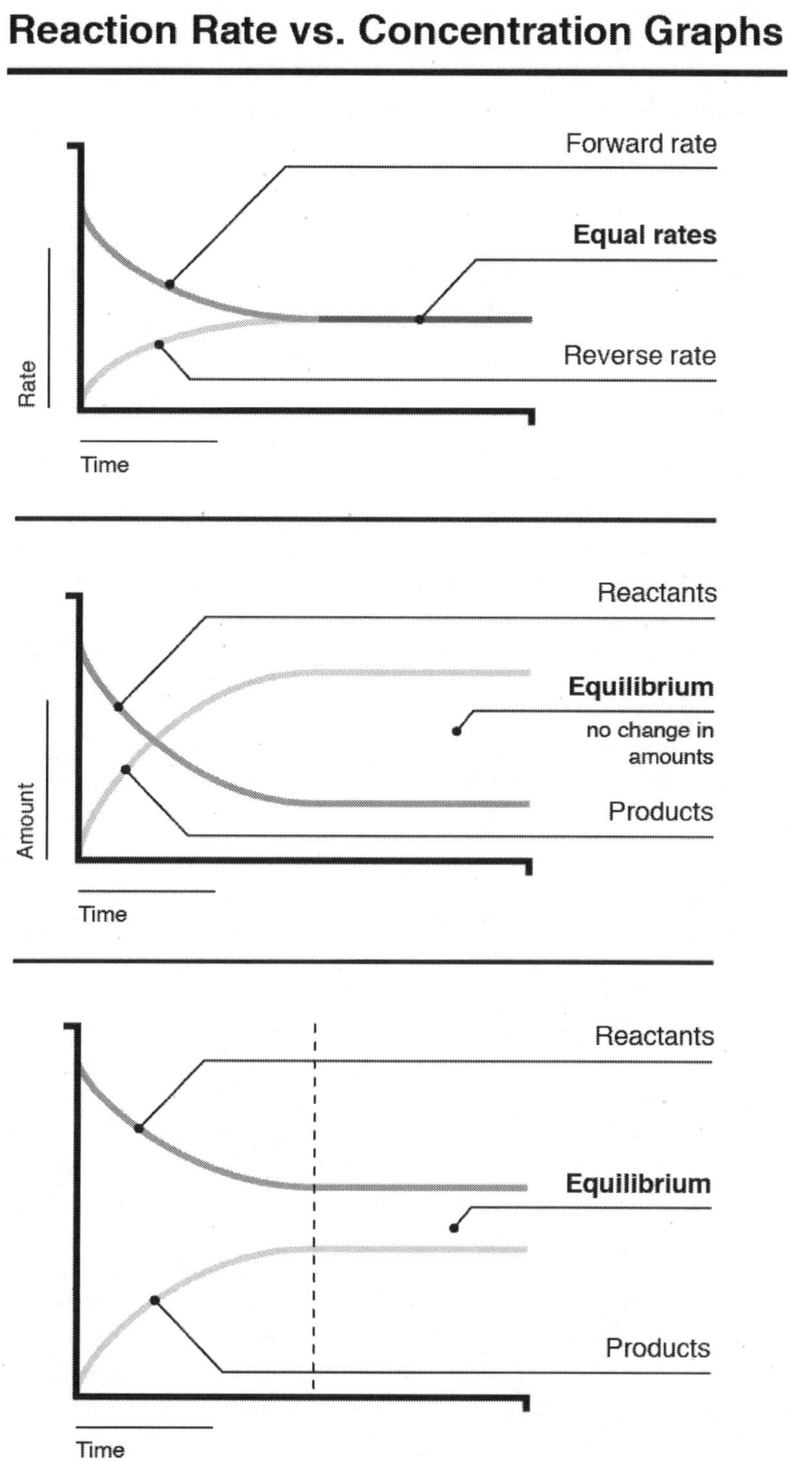

Direction of Reversible Reactions

Net Conversion Between Reactions and Products Based on Rate vs. Equilibrium State

In reversible reactions, if the forward reaction proceeds at a faster rate than the reverse reaction, there is a net conversion of the reaction's reactants to the products. On the other hand, if the reverse reaction proceeds at a faster rate than the forward reaction, there is a net conversion of the reaction's products to the reactants.

Reaction Quotient and Equilibrium Constant

The Reaction Quotient, Q

The reactant quotient, Q, measures the proportions of the reactants and products at any given point in the reaction, not just at equilibrium. In the equation aA + bB → cC + dD, the reaction quotient can be calculated as:

$$Q = \frac{[C]^c[D]^d}{[A]^a[B]^b}$$

The value of Q gives a picture of the progression of the reaction. As its value approaches that of the equilibrium constant K, the reaction gets closer to an equilibrium state. When Q = K, equilibrium is reached.

Q, and K in Reversible Reactions

When Q < K, product formation is favored, and if the reaction is reversible and Q > K, reactant formation is favored. At the start of a reaction that has only reactants, the concentrations of A and B are high, and C and D are zero, so Q would be zero. As the reaction progresses to produce more products, the value of Q can become infinitely high. The measure of Q is only dependent on concentrations of reactants and products that change as the reaction progresses. It is not affected by substances whose concentrations are independent of the reaction, such as with solids that are in contact with an aqueous solution or gas or pure solids or liquids that are in contact with a gas. When two reactions occur consecutively due to the formation of an intermediary substance, the Q and K values of the resulting reaction are calculated by multiplying the individual Q values and individual K values for each equation.

Important Reversible Reactions

Examples of common and important reversible reactions include the transfer of electrons between species in oxidation-reduction reactions, the transfer of protons in acid-base reactions, and the dissolution of a solid in a solution.

Introduction to Le Châtelier's Principle

Using Le Chatelier's Principle to Predict the Response of a System to Different Stresses

Le Chatelier's principle is a law of equilibrium that states that if a system at equilibrium is subjected to a change in the environment, the system will react accordingly to counter the change and restore its state of equilibrium. Disruptions to the system can include changes to the temperature, volume, or pressure of a gas, or the concentration of any of the reactants or products. The equilibrium constant, K, only changes with changes to the temperature of the system. With all other changes, the value of K remains the same. For exothermic reactions, energy, or heat, is released from the system. If the temperature is decreased, or energy is taken out of the system, formation of the products would be favored because more energy, or heat, would need to be produced to restore equilibrium and vice versa for energy being added to an exothermic reaction. For an endothermic reaction, in the same situation of energy being taken away from the system, the formation of the reactants would be favored because energy is needed to form the products. If energy was added, the reactants would use the energy to react and form more products. When the volume of a gas increases, the pressure decreases and vice versa. If volume increases and pressure decreases in a system, the reaction will run toward the side of the equation that has the largest number of gas moles to increase the pressure of the system and restore equilibrium. With a decrease in volume and an increase in pressure, the reaction would run toward the direction of the fewest number of gas moles.

If the concentration of the reactants was increased or that of the products was decreased, the reaction would run in the forward direction to form more product/s. If the concentration of the reactants was decreased or that of the products was increased, the reaction would run in the reverse direction to form more reactants. Diluting the reactants with water is one way in which the concentration of the reactants could be decreased.

Some reactants and products have different colors. Looking at the mix of colors of the solution at equilibrium can elucidate the proportion of reactants and products in the solution. For example, if the reactant is blue, the product is yellow, and at equilibrium the solution is perfectly green, a green color is evidence that the reactant and product may be present in equal amounts. The pH of a solution can also be checked to monitor the dissociation of acids and bases in a solution at equilibrium.

Qualitative Reasoning with Le Chatelier's Principle

Le Chatelier's principle states that when a property of a chemical reaction changes and the reaction becomes unbalanced, the system will compensate for the property that changed to restore equilibrium to the system. Equilibrium concentrations can be calculated quantitatively using ICE tables that show the initial concentration of the substances in a reaction and the change that takes place. The value of K—the equilibrium constant—indicates the proportion of reactants and products that are present at equilibrium. At equilibrium, both reactants and products are present; most reactions do not completely favor one side of the reaction. The rates of the forward and reverse reactions are equal at equilibrium so that the concentrations of the reactants and products are constant and do not change. Q—the reaction quotient—becomes equal to K at equilibrium. If a change in the system created more products, the reaction would run in the reverse direction to create more reactants in order to restore equilibrium and bring the products and reactants back to their equilibrium proportions. If the change created more reactants, the reaction would run in the forward direction to create more products until the equilibrium proportions were reached again.

Reaction Quotient and Le Chatelier's Principle

Stresses that Shift Q or K

The reaction quotient, Q, can be measured at any given point of the chemical reaction. Once the reaction has reached equilibrium, Q becomes equal to K, the equilibrium constant. K describes the state of the reactants and products when the reaction has reached equilibrium and the concentrations are no longer changing with time. The forward and reverse reactions occur at equal rates to keep the reactant and product concentrations steady. In reality, stresses can occur to change the equilibrium status of the chemical reaction. When a stress occurs, the value of Q changes immediately and is no longer equivalent to the value of K. Changes in volume, pressure, concentration, and temperature all cause the value of Q to change. The reaction then shifts to counteract the stressor and bring the values of Q and K back to equivalency. If there was an increase in any of these properties, the reaction would run in the opposite direction to decrease the increases. As mentioned, temperature is the only stressor that also changes the value of K. The value of K is dependent on steady state conditions, which includes a certain temperature. If the temperature changes, the value of K changes, and the concentrations of the reactants and products at equilibrium changes.

Introduction to Solubility Equilibria

Solubility Products and the Solubility of Salts

When a salt substance is dissolved in a solvent, it is considered a **reversible reaction** because the substance can be precipitated out of the solvent again. The reaction quotient, Q, of the reaction describes the concentration of the reactants and products at any time of the reaction. The equilibrium constant for solubility reactions is K_{sp}. The value of K_{sp} is dependent on the solubility of the salt in the solvent. Large Ksp values indicate greater dissociation of the salt molecule and greater solubility.

Catalysts

Catalysts are substances that accelerate the speed of a chemical reaction. A catalyst remains unchanged throughout the course of a chemical reaction. In most cases, only small amounts of a catalyst are needed. Catalysts increase the rate of a chemical reaction by providing an alternate path requiring less activation energy. Activation energy refers to the amount of energy required for the initiation of a chemical reaction.

Catalysts can be homogeneous or heterogeneous. Catalysts in the same phase of matter as its reactants are homogeneous, while catalysts in a different phase than reactants are heterogeneous. It is important to remember catalysts are selective. They don't accelerate the speed of all chemical reactions, but catalysts do accelerate specific chemical reactions.

Enzymes

Enzymes are a class of catalysts instrumental in biochemical reactions, and are almost always proteins. Like all catalysts, enzymes increase the rate of a chemical reaction by providing an alternate path for the reaction to proceed, lowering the activation energy of the reaction. Enzymes catalyze thousands of chemical reactions in the human body. Enzymes possess an active site, which is the part of the molecule that binds the reacting molecule, or substrate. The "lock and key" analogy is used to describe the substrate key fitting precisely into the active site of the enzyme lock to form an enzyme-substrate complex.

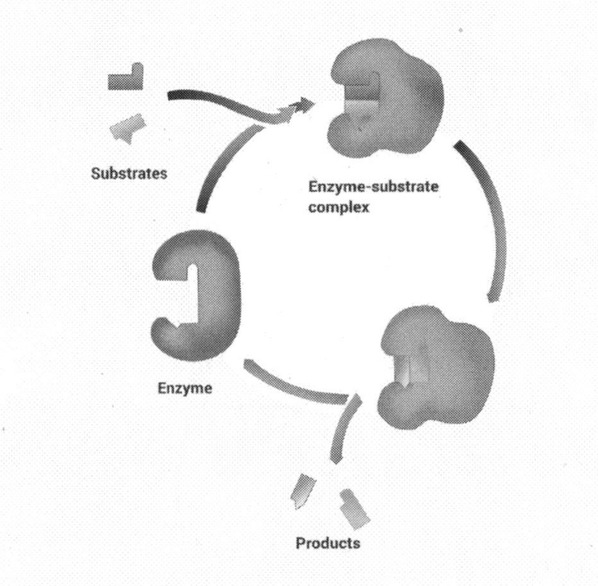

Many enzymes work in tandem with cofactors or coenzymes to catalyze chemical reactions. **Cofactors** can be either inorganic (not containing carbon) or organic (containing carbon). Organic cofactors can be either coenzymes or prosthetic groups tightly bound to an enzyme. **Coenzymes** transport chemical groups from one enzyme to another. Within a cell, coenzymes are continuously regenerating and their concentrations are held at a steady state.

Several factors including temperature, pH, and concentrations of the enzyme and substrate can affect the catalytic activity of an enzyme. For humans, the optimal temperature for peak enzyme activity is approximately body temperature at 98.6 °F, while the optimal pH for peak enzyme activity is approximately 7 to 8. Increasing the concentrations of either the enzyme or substrate will also increase the rate of reaction, up to a certain point.

The activity of enzymes can be regulated. A common form of metabolic control is **feedback inhibition**, where the pathway is controlled by inhibitory binding of the product to an enzyme earlier in the pathway.

Understand Properties of Solutions

Explaining Characteristic Properties of Substances

Properties of Water

Water is the most abundant molecule on Earth. It is a compound composed of hydrogen and oxygen, and has the chemical formula H_2O. Water is also **polar**, which means it is negatively charged at one end and positively charged at the other end. The oxygen is more **electronegative** than the hydrogens, meaning that its protons pull in more of the electrons than the hydrogens. This leaves the oxygen with a partial negative charge and the hydrogens with a partial positive charge.

Water is **amphoteric** and **self-ionizable** in that it tends to dissociate, or split, into hydrogen ions (H^+) and hydroxyl ions (OH^-) randomly. No other substance on Earth may be found naturally in all three states of matter—liquid, solid, and gas. Water is also unique due to its liquid state being more dense than its solid state (ice), which is why ice floats in liquid water. Water is colorless, odorless, and tasteless. It freezes at 32 °F and boils at 212 °F. Pure water has a pH of 7, which makes it neutral. Water is considered the universal solvent because it can dissolve many substances. Many of the properties of water are due to its polarity and hydrogen bonding. Water has the following properties:

- **Cohesiveness**: Refers to the force of attraction between molecules of identical substances. Cohesiveness is mainly the result of hydrogen bonding in water.
- **Adhesiveness**: Refers to the force of attraction between molecules of different substances, like water and glass. Adhesiveness is mainly the result of hydrogen bonding in water.
- **High specific heat**: Refers to the amount of heat required to raise the temperature of water by one degree Celsius. Water's high specific heat is a consequence of hydrogen bonding. As a result, water can store a great deal of heat energy.
- **High surface tension**: The cohesiveness of water molecules is responsible for its high surface tension. The strong cohesion of its molecules makes water sticky and elastic.
- **High heat of vaporization**: Refers to the energy needed to change an amount of water from a liquid to a gas at a particular pressure. Water's high heat of vaporization is due to hydrogen bonding.

Characteristic Properties of Molecules

Molecules have both physical and chemical properties. Physical properties describe a substance in isolation, while chemical properties describe how a substance reacts with others. There are two types of physical properties: **extensive** and **intensive**. Extensive physical properties depend on the amount of a substance. Volume, length, and mass are all examples of extensive properties. Intensive physical properties are static and unchanging properties of a substance that identify it.

Examples of intensive physical properties include the following:

- Color
- Smell
- Taste
- Odor
- Luster: Ability to reflect light, also known as "shininess"
- Hardness: Ability to scratch
- Brittleness: Response to pressure. The more brittle, the easier it is to break.
- Malleability: Ability to bend
- Ductility: Ability to form wire

- Conductivity: Ability to conduct heat and electricity
- Polarity: Extent to which a covalent molecule has a partial charge due to the unequal sharing of electrons
- Melting Point
- Boiling Point
- Density (mass/volume)

Extensive properties are important for measurement and recording data but do not identify a substance. Intensive properties are critical for identification, as indicated by the following examples.

You find a brittle, yellow, dull rock that smells like rotten eggs. *What is it?* All signs point to sulfur; however, pure sulfur has no smell so it has to be some sort of sulfur mixture.

You buy a beautiful ring and are unsure if it is silver, white gold, or platinum. They all have the same color, are shiny, and conduct heat. *So which metal is it?* To determine which specific metal the ring is made out of, more information would be needed. Platinum is much harder than gold and not easily scratched. Silver is significantly less dense than the other two. By examining the physical properties and comparing them to the physical properties of silver, white gold, and platinum, determining the composition of the ring should be no problem.

Physical changes do not change the intensive physical properties of a substance. For example, cutting paper into pieces will not change its density, hardness, or luster. Shattering glass does not change the physical properties either; it is still clear and not malleable or ductile. Pouring water into a differently shaped container won't change its melting or boiling points.

Chemical changes, on the other hand, transform substances so that they have new physical properties. For example, upon exposing iron to air, it will form a completely different substance. The product of iron and oxygen is rust, a reddish substance.

While physical properties describe the characteristics of a substance, chemical like properties describe how it **behaves** in chemical reactions.

- If substances are flammable, they burn easily in chemical reactions.
- If substances are radioactive, they emit radiation in nuclear reactions.
- If substances are corrosive, they are capable of degrading or eating away other substances.
- If substances are easily oxidized, they will react quickly with air.

Solutions and Mixtures

Types of Solutions

A **solution** is a homogenous mixture of more than one substance. A **solute** is another substance that can be dissolved into a substance called a **solvent.** If only a small amount of solute is dissolved in a solvent, the solution formed is said to be **diluted**. A solution is considered **concentrated** if a large amount of solute is dissolved into the solvent. For example, water from a typical, unfiltered household tap is diluted because it contains other minerals in very small amounts.

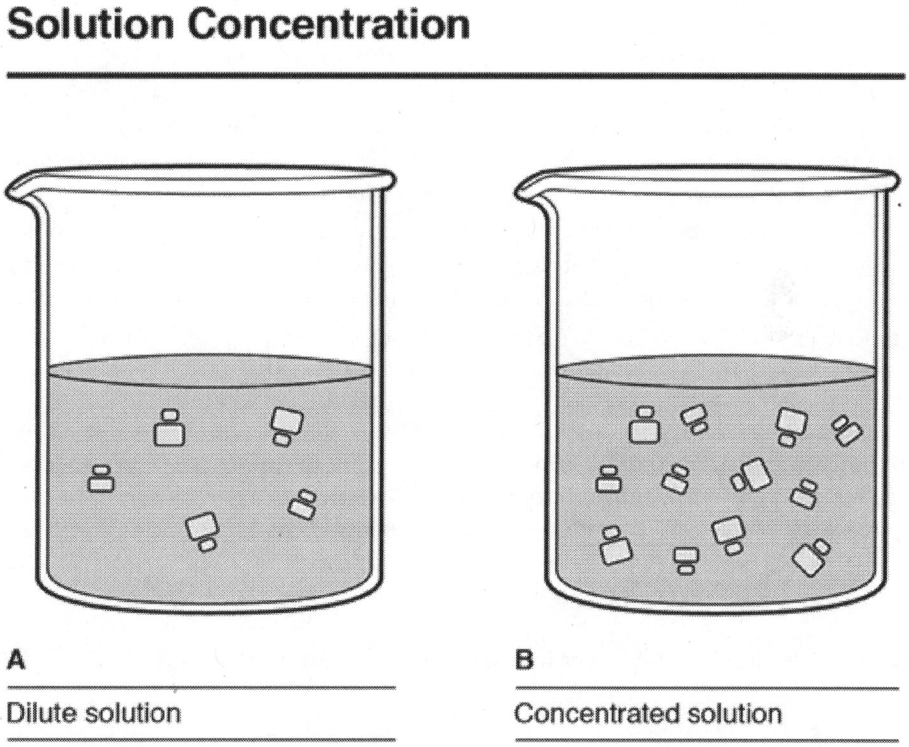

If more solute is being added to a solvent, but not dissolving, the solution is called **saturated.** For example, when hummingbirds eat sugar-water from feeders, they prefer it as sweet as possible. When trying to dissolve enough sugar (solute) into the water (solvent), there will be a point where the sugar crystals will no longer dissolve into the solution and will remain as whole pieces floating in the water. At this point, the solution is considered saturated and cannot accept more sugar. This level, at which a solvent cannot accept and dissolve any more solute, is called its **saturation point**. In some cases, it is possible to force more solute to be dissolved into a solvent, but this will result in crystallization. The state of a solution on the verge of crystallization, or in the process of crystallization, is called a **supersaturated** solution. This can also occur in a solution that seems stable, but if it is disturbed, the change can begin the crystallization process.

Again, **solutions** are homogeneous mixtures of different components. They are made up of a **solute** and a **solvent** component, where the solute is dissolved in the solvent. All parts of a solution are identical. Solutions can be solids, liquids, or gases. In a liquid solution, the solute that is dissolved into the solvent can be a solid, liquid, or gas. Because of their homogeneous composition, solutions cannot be separated by filtration. They also cannot scatter visible light.

Examples of solutions include gaseous, liquid, and solid solutions. An example of a gaseous solution is air, which contains miscible gases such as nitrogen (N_2), argon (Ar), oxygen (O_2), and trace gases. An example of a solid solution is dental fillings, which may consist of silver (Ag) or different metal alloys. Liquid solutions include soda, which contains carbon dioxide (CO_2) gas dissolved in liquid water, and alcohol, which contains ethanol mixed with liquid water. Remember that the terms *solute* and *solvent* describe the types of components in a solution. The solute is the component in the lesser amount, and the solvent is the component in the greater amount. Ethanol is often mixed with octane to form a miscible gasoline solution with a ratio of 1:9 ethanol to octane. Ethanol is the solute, while octane is the solvent. In contrast, oil and water are not miscible. It's important to understand the factors that explain solubility, as they explain why solutions are either miscible or immiscible.

Preparing Solutions with Specified Molarity

The strength of a solution can be described in several ways. Although the terms *dilute*, *concentrated*, *saturated*, and *supersaturated* give qualitative descriptions of solutions, a more precise quantitative description needs to be established for the use of chemicals. This holds true especially for mixing strong acids or bases. The method for calculating the concentration of a solution is done through finding its **molarity**. The **molality** of a solution, abbreviated as m, is defined as the moles of solute dissolved in one kilogram of solvent. More commonly, solutions are described in terms of molarity, abbreviated as M, which describes the number of moles of solute dissolved per liter of solution. In the laboratory, use of accurately graduated glassware, including graduated cylinders and volumetric flasks, is imperative for making solutions. In some instances, such as environmental reporting, molarity is measured in **parts per million** (ppm). Parts per million, is the number of milligrams of a substance dissolved in one liter of water.

Concentrated solutions are often diluted with additional solvent to make a solution of the desired strength. First, take a known volume of concentrated solution and calculate the number of moles of solute in it. Next, dilute that amount of concentrated solution to the appropriate volume with solvent to give the desired molarity of the new solution. For example, say you have a 10 M NaCl solution, which has 10 moles NaCl per liter of solution, and need a 1 M NaCl solution, which has 1 mole NaCl per liter of solution. You can take 0.1 L 10 M NaCl, which contains 1 mole NaCl, and dilute it to 1 L total volume by adding 0.9 mL solvent to achieve a 1 M NaCl solution.

To find the molarity, or the amount of solute per unit volume of solution, for a solution, the following formula is used:

$$c = \frac{n}{V}$$

In this formula, *c* is the molarity (or unit moles of solute per volume of solution), *n* is the amount of solute measured in moles, and *V* is the volume of the solution, measured in liters.

Example:

What is the molarity of a solution made by dissolving 2.0 grams of NaCl into enough water to make 100 mL of solution?

To solve this, the number of moles of NaCl needs to be calculated:

First, to find the mass of NaCl, the mass of each of the molecule's atoms is added together as follows:

23.0g (Na) + 35.5g (Cl) = 58.8g NaCl

Next, the given mass of the substance is multiplied by one mole per total mass of the substance:

2.0g NaCl × (1 mol NaCl/58.5g NaCl) = 0.034 mol NaCl

Finally, the moles are divided by the number of liters of the solution to find the molarity:

(0.034 mol NaCl)/(0.100L) = 0.34 M NaCl

To prepare a solution of a different concentration, the **mass solute** must be calculated from the molarity of the solution. This is done via the following process:

Example:

How would you prepare 600.0 mL of 1.20 M solution of sodium chloride?

To solve this, the given information needs to be set up:

1.20 M NaCl = 1.20 mol NaCl/1.00 L of solution

0.600 L solution × (1.20 mol NaCl/1.00 L of solution) = 0.72 moles NaCl

0.72 moles NaCl × (58.5g NaCl/1 mol NaCl) = 42.12 g NaCl

This means that one must dissolve 42.12 g NaCl in enough water to make 600.0 L of solution.

Passive Transport Mechanisms

Passive transport refers to the migration of molecules across a cell membrane that does not require energy. The three types of passive transport include simple diffusion, facilitated diffusion, and osmosis.

Simple diffusion relies on a concentration gradient, or differing quantities of molecules inside or outside of a cell. During simple diffusion, molecules move from an area of high concentration to an area of low concentration. Facilitated diffusion utilizes carrier proteins to transport molecules across a cell membrane. Osmosis refers to the transport of water across a selectively permeable membrane. During osmosis, water moves from a region of low solute concentration to a region of high solute concentration.

Describe Concepts of Acids and Bases

pH, Acids, and Bases

pH refers to the power or potential of hydrogen atoms and is used as a scale for a substance's acidity. In chemistry, pH represents the hydrogen ion concentration (written as $[H^+]$) in an aqueous, or watery, solution. The hydrogen ion concentration, $[H^+]$, is measured in moles of H^+ per liter of solution.

The pH scale is a logarithmic scale used to quantify how acidic or basic a substance is. pH is the negative logarithm of the hydrogen ion concentration: $\mathrm{pH} = -\log{[H^+]}$. A one-unit change in pH correlates with a ten-fold change in hydrogen ion concentration. The pH scale typically ranges from zero to 14, although it is possible to have pHs outside of this range. Pure water has a pH of 7, which is considered neutral.

pH values less than 7 are considered acidic, while pH values greater than 7 are considered basic, or alkaline:

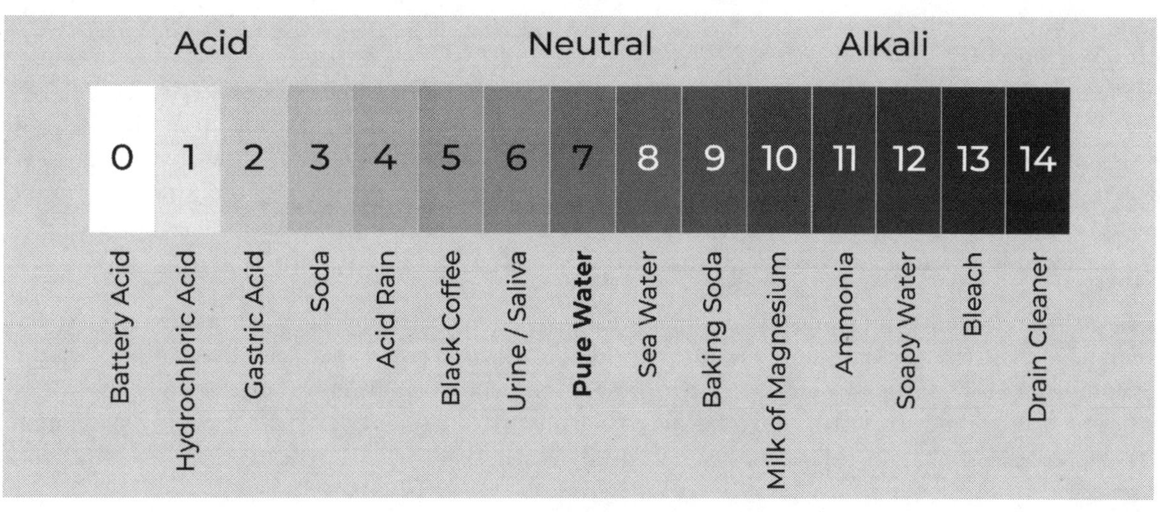

Generally speaking, an acid is a substance capable of donating hydrogen ions, while a base is a substance capable of accepting hydrogen ions. A buffer is a molecule that can act as either a hydrogen ion donor or acceptor. Buffers are crucial in the blood and body fluids, and prevent the body's pH from fluctuating into dangerous territory. pH can be measured using a pH meter, test paper, or indicator sticks.

The combination of an acid with a base produces water and an ionic compound in a process referred to as a neutralization reaction. The general form of this reaction is as follows, where A is an acid and B is a base, and H is the dissociable hydrogen from the acid:

$$AH + B \rightarrow A + BH$$

One well-known example is the reaction of hydrochloric acid (HCl) with sodium hydroxide (NaOH) to produce water and sodium chloride:

$$HCl + NaOH \rightarrow H_2O + NaCl$$

The product of a neutralization reaction most often forms water and a salt (an ionic chemical compound), though whether the salt is soluble or insoluble in water depends on the reactants.

Scientific Reasoning

Use Basic Scientific Measurements and Measurement Tools

Technology and mathematics are crucial to the advancement of scientific investigations and communications. Individuals in specialized scientific fields need answers to problems swiftly, as they are frequently under time constraints. Accurate and prompt scientific investigation is dependent on technological and mathematical skills and their advancement. Advances in technology and mathematics can help accelerate the pace of scientific investigations and communications.

Although scientific investigations can be communicated to some degree through subjective qualitative data, objective quantitative data is preferred to establish rigorous mathematical conclusions. Connections can also be conveyed through the use of graphs, formulas, and equations. Mathematical relationships can be proven with numerical models.

Software like spreadsheets and networks like the Internet have expanded scientific communication by providing multiple avenues to distribute information. Increased computing capacity and fiber optics have also increased the speed and processing time of scientific communication.

Reasons for Including Technology and Mathematics in Science Research

There are many different reasons for including technology and mathematics in science research. Technology is always advancing and its application is playing an increasingly larger role in science research. Technology enhances the gathering and manipulation of scientific data. Technology also increases the accuracy and precision of scientific data, which in many ways is becoming more dependent on the type of technology adopted. Graphs or models can be produced to highlight emerging patterns or trends in scientific data which can be used to improve the interpretation and understanding of specific scientific data from the past or present.

Mathematics has been around for centuries and has constantly been called upon in scientific research to help understand and explain the workings of the natural world. It is a crucial part of the scientific method. Mathematics can help improve and refine the asking of questions or hypotheses in a scientific argument. Advances in mathematics have led to improvements in gathering data, constructing scientific explanations, and communicating results of scientific investigations. Lastly, mathematics has improved the efficiency of processing and manipulating often complicated scientific data.

When recording data, it is of the utmost importance to also record units. Acceptable customary units in the U.S. include feet, gallons, and pounds, which measure length, volume, and mass, respectively. Laboratory data is typically recorded with SI units which are universally used. Standard SI units include the following:

- Second (s) for time
- Meter (m) for length
- Gram (g) for mass
- Liter (L) for volume
- Celsius (oC) or Kelvin (K) for temperature ($°C + 273 = K$)

Prefixes also indicate the scale, as seen in the chart below.

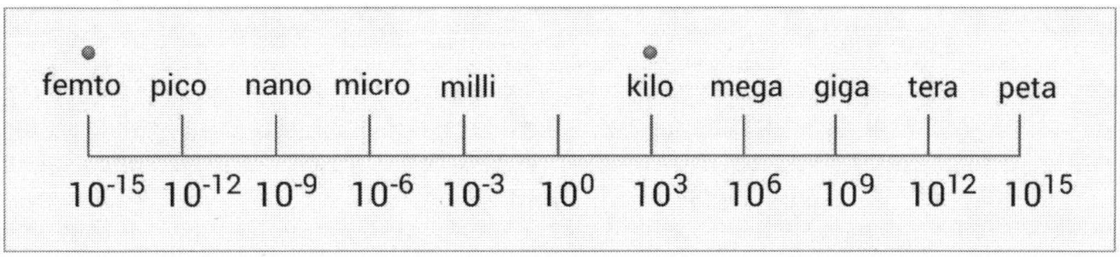

Other important concepts regarding collecting data are scientific notation, rounding, and significant figures.

Scientific notation should be used when appropriate. The correct form is to have the ones unit followed by the decimal point with the appropriate number of significant figures followed by an indication of the power of ten.

$$1{,}320{,}000 = 1.32 \times 10^{6}$$

$$0.000867 = 8.67 \times 10^{-4}$$

Rounding should be used to the correct number of significant figures. 0-4 always keeps the preceding number as is while 5-9 raises it.

1.325 rounds to 1.33
4.289 rounds to 4.29
5.998 rounds to 6.00

Significant figures should be used, meaning that measurements too precise to be recorded should not be included. This concept is illustrated in the following scenarios.

A balance that goes to the hundredths place measures a rock as 1.92. It would be incorrect to record the value as 2 or 1.9 (remember rounding rules) because that is not precise enough. It would also be incorrect to record the value as 1.920 because that implies a level of precision that does not exist with that measuring device.

Examine the three rulers below and the line being measured.

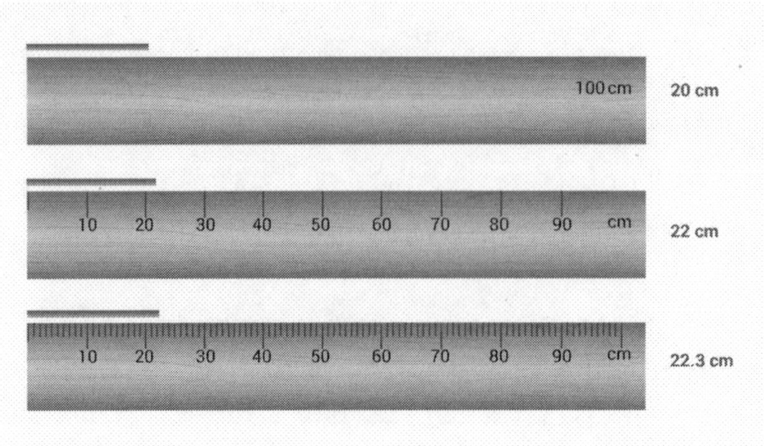

While the length of the line remains the same, the different calibrations of the rulers result in answers with different numbers of significant figures. The top ruler cannot even give a level of certainty to the ones place, so the appropriate number of significant figures is 1. The middle ruler does have a calibration that allows a measurement to the ones place, so there are two significant figures. The bottom ruler can record a reading with 3 significant figures.

Measuring volume with a graduated cylinder is tricky because the liquid will look curved. The curve, or **meniscus**, is due to the adhesion of the water to the sides of the device. The bottom of the meniscus indicates the actual volume of the liquid. In this case, recording the value as 35 would be incorrect. The calibration of the graduated cylinder calls for a greater level of precision in any data taken, and the data recorded needs to reflect that. The correct value is 35.0.

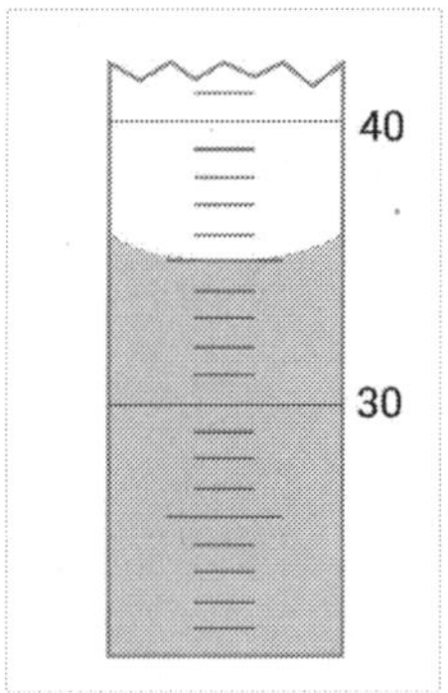

Significant figures have a few rules. Any non-zero number preceding a decimal point is significant and any trailing zeros are not significant. Zeroes between numbers are always significant. After the decimal point, any preceding zeroes are not significant while any trailing zeroes are.

- 3,570,000 has 3 significant figures.
- 4,000,560 has 6 significant figures.
- 0.000008320 has 4 significant figures.
- 0.00903 has 3 significant figures.

Scale

Different situations call for different units of measurement, or different scales. It is important to be mindful of scale, especially when working in medicine. Anesthesia administration is weight-dependent, so it is critical to make sure that the weight is correctly labeled as either kilograms or pounds.

Kilograms or pounds, on the other hand, are inappropriate units for very small objects. Chemists and physicists do calculations with atoms and molecules, which require a completely different unit. They use a unit called the mole, which contains 6.02×10^{23} particles of a substance.

Temperature has three different scales: Kelvin, Celsius, and Fahrenheit. Kelvin is required for gas calculations, and should engineers use the wrong conversion, gas tanks could explode or be completely non-functional.

Apply Logic and Evidence to A Scientific Explanation

A scientific explanation has three crucial components—a claim, evidence, and logical reasoning. A **claim** makes an assertion or conclusion focusing on the original question or problem. The **evidence** provides backing for the claim and is usually in the form of scientific data. The scientific data must be appropriate and sufficient. The scientific **reasoning** connects the claim and evidence and explains why the evidence supports the claim.

Scientific explanations must fit certain criteria and be supported by logic and evidence. The following represent scientific explanation criteria. The proposed explanation:

- Must be logically consistent
- Must abide by the rules of evidence
- Must report procedures and methods
- Must be open to questions and possible modification
- Must be based on historical and current scientific knowledge

The scientific method encourages the growth and communication of new information and procedures among scientists. Explanations of how the natural changes and works based on fiction, personal convictions, religious morals, mystical influences, superstitions, or authorities are not scientific; therefore, these explanations are irrelevant to the scientific community.

Cause and effect relationships seek to provide explanations to an experiment and to provide solutions. These relationships may be simple or complex. Through well-designed experiments, a scientist can uncover or understand these relationships. To identify a cause-and-effect relationship, a scientist must ask the following:

1. How does it work, or what is the mechanism of the relationship?

2. Why does that phenomenon occur?

One example to consider is the effects of salinity on relative density when a bag containing fresh water is placed in a container with saltwater. 1. A freshwater bag floats in a container of saltwater. 2. The phenomenon occurs because the density of saltwater ($d = \frac{m}{v}$) is greater than freshwater.

Scientific explanations have two fundamental characteristics. First, they should explain all scientific data and observations gleaned from experiments. Second, they should allow for predictions that can be verified with future experiments.

It's important to focus on the **empirical**, or observable/tangible evidence, in an experiment. After all, an experiment is about testing something, not theorizing about it in the abstract. Doing so helps remove a researcher's personal **bias** towards what they think or hope to be true.

Predict Relationships Among Events, Objects, and Processes

Cause and Effect

A cause is like a stimulus in the nervous system in that it results in a response. An effect is what happens because of the stimulus.

Cause	Effect
I forgot to wear shoes.	I stubbed my toe.
I forgot to practice piano.	I messed up at the recital and was embarrassed.
I studied for my math exam.	I got a 100.

The cause is *why* something happens, and the effect is what actually happens.

While it is typical for there to be a single cause and a single effect as noted above, there are many situations that call for a cause to have many effects, such as exploring the effects of a certain event. In exploring the effects of exercise, for example, the cause is exercise. Effects are stress relief, increased energy, and weight loss, among others.

There is the possibility that one effect can have many causes. For example, type 2 diabetes is not a one-cause disease, but rather a combination of exercise habits, diet, and genetics.

A cause-and-effect chain is when an effect then causes another effect. For example, the initial cause could be when a young gentleman played video games instead of studying for a biology test, which sets off a chain reaction of effects.

- 1st effect: He failed the test.
- 2nd effect: He got in trouble with his parents.
- 3rd effect: He couldn't hang out with his friends on Friday night.
- 4th effect: He had a boring night.

Unit Size

In understanding relationships between objects encountered in science (such as parts of the human body), it's important to roughly understand the scale of them. This is accomplished by understanding the size of different units of measurement and knowing which unit makes the most sense for measuring something.

For example, you could record the distances between cities in centimeters, but miles or kilometers makes the most sense. Be sure to memorize the metric prefixes discussed in the math section. That will give you an indication of how big or small a unit is.

Apply the Scientific Method to Interpret a Scientific Investigation

The scientific method provides the framework for studying and learning about the world in a scientific fashion. The scientific method has been around since at least the 17th century and is a codified way to answer natural science questions. Due to objectivity, the scientific method is impartial and its results are highly repeatable; these are its greatest advantages.

There is no consensus as to the number of steps involved in executing the scientific method, but the following six steps are needed to fulfill the criteria for correct usage of the scientific method:

- *Ask a* question: Most scientific investigations begin with a question about a specific problem.
- Make observations: Observations will help pinpoint research objectives on the quest to answer the question.
- Create or propose a hypothesis: The hypothesis represents a possible solution to the problem. It is a simple statement predicting the outcome of an experiment designed to investigate the research question.
- Formulate an experiment: The experiment tests the proposed hypothesis.
- Test the hypothesis: The outcome of the experiment to test the hypothesis is the most crucial step in the scientific method.
- Accept or reject the hypothesis: Using results from the experiment, a scientist can conclude to accept or reject the hypothesis.

Several key nuances of the scientific method include:

- The hypothesis must be verifiable and falsifiable. Falsifiable refers to the possibility of a negative solution to the hypothesis. The hypothesis should also have relevance, compatibility, testability, simplicity, and predictive power.
- Investigation must utilize both deductive and inductive reasoning. Deductive reasoning employs a logical process to arrive at a conclusion using premises considered true, while inductive reasoning employs an opposite approach. Inductive reasoning allows scientists to propose hypotheses in the scientific method, while deductive reasoning allows scientists to apply hypotheses to particular situations.

An experiment should incorporate an independent, or changing, variable and a dependent, or non-changing, variable. It should also utilize both a control group and an experimental group. The experimental group will ultimately be compared against the control group.

Science Practice Quiz

1. What is an adaptation?
    a. The original traits found in a common ancestor
    b. Changes that occur in the environment
    c. When one species begins behaving like another species
    d. An inherited characteristic that enhances survival and reproduction

2. If a person with AB blood and a person with O blood have children, what is the probability that their children will have the same phenotype as either parent?
    a. 0%
    b. 25%
    c. 50%
    d. 75%

3. What does the scientific method describe?
    a. How to review a scientific paper
    b. How to organize a science laboratory
    c. The steps utilized to conduct an inquiry into a scientific question
    d. How to use science to earn money in society

4. When de-oxygenated blood first enters the heart, which of the following choices is in the correct order for its journey to the aorta?

    I. Tricuspid valve → Lungs → Mitral valve
    II. Mitral valve → Lungs → Tricuspid valve
    III. Right ventricle → Lungs → Left atrium
    IV. Left ventricle → Lungs → Right atrium

    a. I and III only
    b. I and IV only
    c. II and III only
    d. II and IV only

5. Which element's atoms have the greatest number of electrons?
    a. Hydrogen
    b. Iron
    c. Copper
    d. Iodine

See answers on the next page.

Answer Explanations

1. D: Charles Darwin based the idea of adaptation around his original concept of natural selection. He believed that evolution occurred based on three observations: the unity of life, the diversity of life, and the suitability of organisms to their environments. There was unity in life based on the idea that all organisms descended from a common ancestor. Then, as the descendants of common ancestors faced changes in their environments or moved to new environments, they began adapting new features to help them. This concept explained the diversity of life and how organisms were matched to their environments. Natural selection helps to improve the fit between organisms and their environments by increasing the frequency of features that enhance survival and reproduction.

2. A: There is no chance that an offspring will have O blood or AB blood (see Punnett square).

	I^A	I^B
i	I^Ai	I^Bi
i	I^Ai	I^Bi

3. C: The scientific method refers to how to conduct a proper scientific inquiry, including recognizing a question/problem, formulating a hypothesis, making a prediction of what will happen based on research, experimenting, and deciding whether the outcome confirmed or denied the hypothesis.

4. A: Carbon dioxide-rich blood is delivered from systemic circulation to the right atrium. It is pumped into the right ventricle. The tricuspid valve prevents backflow between the two chambers. From there, the pulmonary artery takes blood to the lungs where diffusion causes gas exchange. Then, oxygenated blood returns to the left atrium before getting pumped into the left ventricle. The mitral valve prevents the backflow of blood from the left ventricle to the atrium. Finally, blood is ejected from the left ventricle through the aorta to enter systemic circulation.

5. D: Iodine has the greatest number of electrons at 53 electrons. The number of electrons increases in elements going from left to right across the periodic table. Hydrogen, Choice *A*, is at the top left corner of the periodic table, so it has the fewest electrons (one electron). Iron has 26 electrons, copper has 29 electrons, Choices *B* and *C*, respectively.

Conventions of Standard English

Conventions of Standard English Spelling

Spelling might or might not be important to some, or maybe it just doesn't come naturally, but those who are willing to discover some new ideas and consider their benefits can learn to spell better and improve their writing. Misspellings reduce a writer's credibility and can create misunderstandings. Spell checkers built into word processors are not a substitute for accuracy. They are neither foolproof nor without error. In addition, a writer's misspelling of one word may also be a word. For example, a writer intending to spell *herd* might accidentally type *s* instead of *d* and unintentionally spell *hers*. Since *hers* is a word, it would not be marked as a misspelling by a spell checker. In short, use spell check, but don't rely on it.

Guidelines for Spelling

Saying and listening to a word serves as the beginning of knowing how to spell it. Keep these subsequent guidelines in mind, remembering there are often exceptions because the English language is replete with them.

Guideline #1: Syllables must have at least one vowel. In fact, every syllable in every English word has a vowel.

- dog
- haystack
- answering
- abstentious
- simple

Guideline #2: The long and short of it. When the vowel has a short vowel sound as in *mad* or *bed,* only the single vowel is needed. If the word has a long vowel sound, add another vowel, either alongside it or separated by a consonant: bed/*bead*; mad/*made.* When the second vowel is separated by two consonants— *madder*—it does not affect the first vowel's sound.

Guideline #3: Suffixes. Refer to the examples listed above.

Guideline #4: Which comes first; the *i* or the *e*? Remember the saying, "*I* before *e* except after *c* or when sounding as *a* as in *neighbor* or *weigh*." Keep in mind that these are only guidelines and that there are always exceptions to every rule.

Guideline #5: Vowels in the right order. Another helpful rhyme is, "When two vowels go walking, the first one does the talking." When two vowels are in a row, the first one often has a long vowel sound and the other is silent. An example is *team*. This is true for about half of the occurrences of two vowels next to each other.

If you have difficulty spelling words, determine a strategy to help. Work on spelling by playing word games like Scrabble or Words with Friends. Consider using phonics, which is sounding words out by slowly and surely stating each syllable. Try repeating and memorizing spellings as well as picturing words in your head. Try making up silly memory aids. See what works best.

Homophones

Homophones are two or more words that have no particular relationship to one another except their identical pronunciations. Homophones make spelling English words fun and challenging like these:

Common Homophones		
affect, effect	cell, sell	it's, its
allot, a lot	do, due, dew	knew, new
barbecue, barbeque	dual, duel	libel, liable
bite, byte	eminent, imminent	principal, principle
brake, break	flew, flu, flue	their, there, they're
capital, capitol	gauge, gage	to, too, two
cash, cache	holy, wholly	yoke, yolk

Irregular Plurals

Irregular plurals are words that aren't made plural the usual way.

- Most nouns are made plural by adding –s (books, televisions, skyscrapers).
- Most nouns ending in ch, sh, s, x, or z are made plural by adding –es (churches, marshes).
- Most nouns ending in a vowel + y are made plural by adding –s (days, toys).
- Most nouns ending in a consonant + y, are made plural by the -y becoming -ies (baby becomes babies).
- Most nouns ending in an o are made plural by adding –s (pianos, photos).
- Some nouns ending in an o, though, may be made plural by adding –es (example: potatoes, volcanoes), and, of note, there is no known rhyme or reason for this!
- Most nouns ending in an f or fe are made plural by the -f or -fe becoming -ves! (example: wolf becomes wolves).
- Some words function as both the singular and plural form of the word (fish, deer).
- Other exceptions include man becomes men, mouse becomes mice, goose becomes geese, and foot becomes feet.

Contractions

The basic rule for making **contractions** is one area of spelling that is pretty straightforward: combine the two words by inserting an apostrophe (') in the space where a letter is omitted. For example, to combine *you* and *are*, drop the *a* and put the apostrophe in its place: *you're*.

he + is = he's
you + all = y'all (informal but often misspelled)

Note that *it's*, when spelled with an apostrophe, is always the contraction for *it is*. The possessive form of the word is written without an apostrophe as *its*.

Correcting Misspelled Words

A good place to start looking at commonly misspelled words here is with the word **misspelled**. While it looks peculiar, look at it this way: **mis** (the prefix meaning *wrongly*) + *spelled* = *misspelled*.

Let's look at some commonly misspelled words.

Commonly Misspelled Words					
accept	benign	existence	jewelry	parallel	separate
acceptable	bicycle	experience	judgment	pastime	sergeant
accidentally	brief	extraordinary	library	permissible	similar
accommodate	business	familiar	license	perseverance	supersede
accompany	calendar	February	maintenance	personnel	surprise
acknowledgement	campaign	fiery	maneuver	persuade	symmetry
acquaintance	candidate	finally	mathematics	possess	temperature
acquire	category	forehead	mattress	precede	tragedy
address	cemetery	foreign	millennium	prevalent	transferred
aesthetic	changeable	foremost	miniature	privilege	truly
aisle	committee	forfeit	mischievous	pronunciation	usage
altogether	conceive	glamorous	misspell	protein	valuable
amateur	congratulations	government	mortgage	publicly	vengeance
apparent	courtesy	grateful	necessary	questionnaire	villain
appropriate	deceive	handkerchief	neither	recede	Wednesday
arctic	desperate	harass	nickel	receive	weird
asphalt	discipline	hygiene	niece	recommend	
associate	disappoint	hypocrisy	ninety	referral	
attendance	dissatisfied	ignorance	noticeable	relevant	
auxiliary	eligible	incredible	obedience	restaurant	
available	embarrass	intelligence	occasion	rhetoric	
balloon	especially	intercede	occurrence	rhythm	
believe	exaggerate	interest	omitted	schedule	
beneficial	exceed	irresistible	operate	sentence	

Capitalization

Here's a non-exhaustive list of things that should be capitalized:

- The first word of every sentence
- The first word of every line of poetry
- The first letter of proper nouns (World War II)
- Holidays (Valentine's Day)
- The days of the week and months of the year (Tuesday, March)
- The first word, last word, and all major words in the titles of books, movies, songs, and other creative works (In the novel, *To Kill a Mockingbird,* note that *a* is lowercase since it's not a major word, but *to* is capitalized since it's the first word of the title.)
- Titles when preceding a proper noun (President Roberto Gonzales, Aunt Judy)

When simply using a word such as *president* or *secretary*, though, the word is not capitalized.

Officers of the new business must include a *president* and *treasurer*.

Seasons—spring, fall, etc.—are not capitalized.

North, *south*, *east*, and *west* are capitalized when referring to regions but are not when being used for directions. In general, if it's preceded by *the* it should be capitalized.

> I'm from the South.
> I drove south.

Conventions of Standard English Punctuation

Ellipses

An **ellipsis** (...) is used to show that there is more to the quoted text than is necessary for the current discussion. Writers use them in place of words, lines, phrases, list content, or paragraphs that might just as easily have been omitted from a passage of writing. This can be done to save space or to focus only on the specifically relevant material.

> Exercise is good for some unexpected reasons. Watkins writes, "Exercise has many benefits such as...reducing cancer risk."

In the example above, the ellipsis takes the place of the other benefits of exercise that are more expected.

The ellipsis may also be used to show a pause in sentence flow.

> "I'm wondering...how this could happen," Dylan said in a soft voice.

Commas

A **comma** (,) is the punctuation mark that signifies a pause—breath—between parts of a sentence. It denotes a break of flow. As with so many aspects of writing structure, authors will benefit by memorizing all of the different ways in which commas can be used so as not to abuse them.

In a **complex sentence**—one that contains a subordinate (dependent) clause or clauses— the use of a comma is dictated by where the subordinate clause is located. If the subordinate clause is before the main clause, a comma is needed between the two clauses.

> While the dog slept, I cleaned up the mess in the bathroom.

Generally, if the subordinate clause is placed after the main clause, no punctuation is needed.

> I did well on my exam because I studied for two hours the night before.

Notice how the last clause is dependent because it the earlier independent clauses to make sense.

Use a comma on both sides of an interrupting phrase.

> I will pay for the ice cream, *chocolate and vanilla*, and then will eat it all myself.

The words forming the phrase in italics are nonessential (extra) information. To determine if a phrase is nonessential, try reading the sentence without the phrase and see if it's still coherent.

A comma is not necessary in this next sentence because no interruption—nonessential or extra information—has occurred. Read sentences aloud when uncertain.

> I will pay for his chocolate and vanilla ice cream and then will eat it all myself.

If the nonessential phrase comes at the beginning of a sentence, a comma should only go at the end of the phrase. If the phrase comes at the end of a sentence, a comma should only go at the beginning of the phrase.

Other types of interruptions include the following:

- interjections: Oh no, I am not going.
- abbreviations: Barry Potter, M.D., specializes in heart disorders.
- direct addresses: Yes, Claudia, I am tired and going to bed.
- parenthetical phrases: His wife, lovely as she was, was not helpful.
- transitional phrases: Also, it is not possible.

The second comma in the following sentence is called an Oxford comma.

> I will pay for ice cream, syrup, and pop.

It is a comma used after the second-to-last item in a series of three or more items. It comes before the word *or* or *and*. Not everyone uses the Oxford comma; it is optional, but many believe it is needed. The comma functions as a tool to reduce confusion in writing. So, if omitting the Oxford comma would cause confusion, then it's best to include it.

Commas are used in math to mark the place of thousands in numerals, breaking them up so they are easier to read. Other uses for commas are in dates (*March 19, 2016*), letter greetings (*Dear Sally,*), and in between cities and states (*Louisville, KY*).

Semicolons

The **semicolon** (;) might be described as a heavy-handed comma. Take a look at these two examples:

> I will pay for the ice cream, but I will not pay for the steak.
> I will pay for the ice cream; I will not pay for the steak.

What's the difference? The first example has a comma and a conjunction separating the two independent clauses. The second example does not have a conjunction, but there are two independent clauses in the sentence. So something more than a comma is required. In this case, a semicolon is used.

Two independent clauses can only be joined in a sentence by either a comma and conjunction or a semicolon. If one of those tools is not used, the sentence will be a run-on. Remember that while the clauses are independent, they need to be closely related in order to be contained in one sentence.

Another use for the semicolon is to separate items in a list when the items themselves require commas.

> The family lived in Phoenix, Arizona; Oklahoma City, Oklahoma; and Raleigh, North Carolina.

Colons

Colons have many miscellaneous functions. Colons can be used to precede further information or a list. In these cases, a colon should only follow an independent clause.

> Humans take in sensory information through five basic senses: sight, hearing, smell, touch, and taste.

The meal includes the following components:

- Caesar salad
- spaghetti

- garlic bread
- cake

Colons can also be used to introduce an appositive.

- The family got what they needed: a reliable vehicle.

While a comma is more common, a colon can also precede a formal quotation.

He said to the crowd: "Let's begin!"

The colon is used after the greeting in a formal letter.

Dear Sir:
To Whom It May Concern:

In the writing of time, the colon separates the minutes from the hour (*4:45 p.m.*). The colon can also be used to indicate a ratio between two numbers (*50:1*).

Hyphens

The **hyphen** (-) is a small dash mark that can be used to join words to show that they are linked. Hyphenate two words that work together as a single adjective (a compound adjective):

honey-covered biscuits

Some words always require hyphens even if not serving as an adjective.

merry-go-round

Hyphens always go after certain prefixes like *anti-* & *all-*. Hyphens should also be used when the absence of the hyphen would cause a strange vowel combination (**semi-engineer**) or confusion. For example, *re-collect* should be used to describe something being gathered twice rather than being written as *recollect*, which means to remember.

Parentheses and Dashes

Parentheses are half-round brackets that look like this: *( )*. They set off a word, phrase, or sentence that is an afterthought, explanation, or side note relevant to the surrounding text but not essential. A pair of commas is often used to set off this sort of information, but parentheses are generally used for information that would not fit well within a sentence or that the writer deems not important enough to be structurally part of the sentence.

The picture of the heart (see above) shows the major parts you should memorize.
Mount Everest is one of three mountains in the world that are over 28,000 feet high (K2 and Kanchenjunga are the other two).

See how the sentences above are complete without the parenthetical statements? In the first example, *see above* would not have fit well within the flow of the sentence. The second parenthetical statement could have been a separate sentence, but the writer deemed the information not pertinent to the topic.

The **em-dash** (—) is a mark longer than a hyphen used as a punctuation mark in sentences and to set apart a relevant thought. Even after plucking out the line separated by the dash marks, the sentence will be intact and make sense.

Looking out the airplane window at the landmarks—Lake Clarke, Thompson Community College, and the bridge—she couldn't help but feel excited to be home.

The dashes use is similar to that of parentheses or a pair of commas. So, what's the difference? Many believe that using dashes makes the clause within them stand out while using parentheses is subtler. It's advised to not use dashes when commas could be used instead.

Quotation Marks

Quotation marks ("") are used in a number of ways. Here are some instances where quotation marks should be used: to indicate a quote that was taken from somewhere else, either from a verbal or written source...

- Dialogue for characters in narratives. When characters speak, the first word should always be capitalized, and the punctuation goes inside the quotes. For example:
    - Janie said, "The tree fell on my car during the hurricane."
- Around titles of songs, short stories, essays, and chapters in books
- To emphasize a certain word
- To refer to a word as the word itself

Apostrophes

This punctuation mark, the apostrophe ('), is a versatile little mark. It has a few different functions:

- Quotes: Apostrophes are used when a second quote is needed within a quote.
- In my letter to my friend, I wrote, "The girl had to get a new purse, and guess what Mary did? She said, 'I'd like to go with you to the store.' I knew Mary would buy it for her."
- Contractions: Another use for an apostrophe in the quote above is a contraction. I'd is used for I would.
- Possession: An apostrophe followed by the letter s shows possession (Mary's purse). If the possessive word is plural, the apostrophe generally just follows the word.
- The trees' leaves are all over the ground.

Correct Sentence Structures

Sentence Fluency

It's time to take what's been studied and put it all together in order to construct well-written sentences and paragraphs that have correct structure. Learning and utilizing the mechanics of structure will encourage effective, professional results, and adding some creativity will elevate one's writing to a higher level.

First, let's review the basic elements of sentences:

A **sentence** is a set of words that make up a grammatical unit. The words must have certain elements and be spoken or written in a specific order to constitute a complete sentence that makes sense.

1. A sentence must have a **subject** (a noun or noun phrase). The subject tells whom or what the sentence is addressing (i.e., what it is about).

2. A sentence must have an **action** or **state of being** (*a verb*). To reiterate: A verb forms the main part of the predicate of a sentence. This means that it explains what the noun is doing.

3. A sentence must convey a complete thought.

When examining writing, be mindful of grammar, structure, spelling, and patterns. Sentences can come in varying sizes and shapes; so, the point of grammatical correctness is not to stamp out creativity or diversity in writing.

Rather, grammatical correctness ensures that writing will be enjoyable and clear. One of the most common methods for catching errors is to mouth the words as you read them. Many typos are fixed automatically by our brain, but mouthing the words often circumvents this instinct and helps one read what's actually on the page. Often, grammar errors are caught not by memorization of grammar rules but by the training of one's mind to know whether something *sounds* right or not.

Types of Sentences

There isn't an overabundance of absolutes in grammar, but here is one: every sentence in the English language falls into one of four categories.

- Declarative: a simple statement that ends with a period
    - The price of milk per gallon is the same as the price of gasoline.
- Imperative: a command, instruction, or request that ends with a period
    - Buy milk when you stop to fill up your car with gas.
- Interrogative: a question that ends with a question mark
    - Will you buy the milk?
- Exclamatory: a statement or command that expresses emotions like anger, urgency, or surprise and ends with an exclamation mark
    - Buy the milk now!

Declarative sentences are the most common type, probably because they are comprised of the most general content, without any of the bells and whistles that the other three types contain. They are, simply, declarations or statements of any degree of seriousness, importance, or information.

Imperative sentences often seem to be missing a subject. The subject is there, though; it is just not visible or audible because it is **implied**. Look at the imperative example sentence.

Buy the milk when you fill up your car with gas.

You is the implied subject, the one to whom the command is issued. This is sometimes called *the understood you* because it is understood that *you* is the subject of the sentence.

Interrogative sentences—those that ask questions—are defined as such from the idea of the word **interrogation**, the action of questions being asked of suspects by investigators. Although that is serious business, interrogative sentences apply to all kinds of questions.

To exclaim is at the root of **exclamatory** sentences. These are made with strong emotions behind them. The only technical difference between a declarative or imperative sentence and an exclamatory one is the exclamation mark at the end. The example declarative and imperative sentences can both become an exclamatory one simply by putting an exclamation mark at the end of the sentences.

The price of milk per gallon is the same as the price of gasoline!
Buy milk when you stop to fill up your car with gas!

After all, someone might be really excited by the price of gas or milk, or they could be mad at the person that will be buying the milk! However, as stated before, exclamation marks in abundance defeat their own purpose! After a while, they begin to cause fatigue! When used only for their intended purpose, they can have their expected and desired effect.

Sentence Structures

A **simple sentence** has one independent clause.

> I am going to win.

A **compound sentence** has two independent clauses. A conjunction—*for, and, nor, but, or, yet, so*—links them together. Note that each of the independent clauses has a subject and a verb.

> I am going to win, but the odds are against me.

A **complex sentence** has one independent clause and one or more dependent clauses.

> I am going to win, even though I don't deserve it.

Even though I don't deserve it is a dependent clause. It does not stand on its own. Some conjunctions that link an independent and a dependent clause are *although*, *because*, *before*, *after*, *that*, *when*, *which*, and *while*.

A **compound-complex sentence** has at least three clauses, two of which are independent and at least one that is a dependent clause.

> While trying to dance, I tripped over my partner's feet, but I regained my balance quickly.

The dependent clause is *While trying to dance*.

Parallel Structure in a Sentence

Parallel structure, also known as parallelism, refers to using the same grammatical form within a sentence. This is important in lists and for other components of sentences.

> Incorrect: At the recital, the boys and girls were dancing, singing, and played musical instruments.
> Correct: At the recital, the boys and girls were dancing, singing, and playing musical instruments.

Notice that in the second example, *played* is not in the same verb tense as the other verbs, nor is it compatible with the helping verb *were*. To test for parallel structure in lists, try reading each item as if it were the only item in the list.

> The boys and girls were dancing.
> The boys and girls were singing.
> The boys and girls were played musical instruments.

Suddenly, the error in the sentence becomes very clear.

Here's another example:

> Incorrect: After the accident, I informed the police *that Mrs. Holmes backed* into my car, *that Mrs. Holmes got out* of her car to look at the damage, and *she was driving* off without leaving a note.
> Correct: After the accident, I informed the police *that Mrs. Holmes backed* into my car, *that Mrs. Holmes got out* of her car to look at the damage, and *that Mrs. Holmes drove off* without leaving a note.
> Correct: After the accident, I informed the police that Mrs. Holmes *backed* into my car, *got out* of her car to look at the damage, and *drove off* without leaving a note.

Note that there are two ways to fix the nonparallel structure of the first sentence. The key to parallelism is consistent structure.

Parts of Speech

Nouns

A **noun** is a person, place, thing, or idea. All nouns fit into one of two types, common or proper.

A **common noun** is a word that identifies any of a class of people, places, or things. Examples include numbers, objects, animals, feelings, concepts, qualities, and actions. *A, an,* or *the* usually precedes the common noun. These parts of speech are called **articles**.

Here are some examples of sentences using nouns preceded by articles.

> *A* building is under construction.
> *The* girl would like to move to *the* city.

A **proper noun** (also called a **proper name**) is used for the specific name of an individual person, place, or organization. The first letter in a proper noun is capitalized. "My name is *Mary*." "I work for *Walmart*."

Nouns sometimes serve as adjectives (which themselves describe nouns), such as "hockey player" and "state government."

Pronouns

A word used in place of a noun is known as a **pronoun**. Pronouns are words like *I, mine, hers,* and *us*.

Pronouns can be split into different classifications (see below) which make them easier to learn; however, it's not important to memorize the classifications.

- **Personal pronouns**: refer to people
  1. First person: we, I, our, mine
  2. Second person: you, yours
  3. Third person: he, them
- Possessive pronouns: demonstrate ownership (mine, my, his, yours)
- Interrogative pronouns: ask questions (what, which, who, whom, whose)
- Relative pronouns: include the five interrogative pronouns and others that are relative (whoever, whomever, that, when, where)
- Demonstrative pronouns: replace something specific (this, that, those, these)
- Reciprocal pronouns: indicate something was done or given in return (each other, one another)
- Indefinite pronouns: have a nonspecific status (anybody, whoever, someone, everybody, somebody)

Indefinite pronouns such as *anybody, whoever, someone, everybody,* and *somebody* command a singular verb form, but others such as *all, none,* and *some* could require a singular or plural verb form.

Antecedents

An **antecedent** is the noun to which a pronoun refers; it needs to be written or spoken before the pronoun is used. For many pronouns, antecedents are imperative for clarity. In particular, a lot of the personal, possessive, and demonstrative pronouns need antecedents. Otherwise, it would be unclear who or what someone is referring to when they use a pronoun like *he* or *this*.

Pronoun reference means that the pronoun should refer clearly to one, clear, unmistakable noun (the antecedent).

Pronoun-antecedent agreement refers to the need for the antecedent and the corresponding pronoun to agree in gender, person, and number. Here are some examples:

> The *kidneys* (plural antecedent) are part of the urinary system. *They* (plural pronoun) serve several roles.

> The kidneys are part of the *urinary system* (singular antecedent). *It* (singular pronoun) is also known as the renal system.

Pronoun Cases

The subjective pronouns —*I, you, he/she/it, we, they,* and *who*—are the subjects of the sentence.

> Example: *They* have a new house.

The objective pronouns—*me, you* (*singular*), *him/her, us, them,* and *whom*—are used when something is being done for or given to someone; they are objects of the action.

> Example: The teacher has an apple for *us*.

The possessive pronouns—*mine, my, your, yours, his, hers, its, their, theirs, our,* and *ours*—are used to denote that something (or someone) belongs to someone (or something).

> Example: It's *their* chocolate cake.
> Even Better Example: It's *my* chocolate cake!

One of the greatest challenges and worst abuses of pronouns concerns *who* and *whom*. Just knowing the following rule can eliminate confusion. *Who* is a subjective-case pronoun used only as a subject or subject complement. *Whom* is only objective-case and, therefore, the object of the verb or preposition.

> *Who* is going to the concert?
> You are going to the concert with *whom*?

Hint: When using *who* or *whom*, think of whether someone would say *he* or *him*. If the answer is *he*, use *who*. If the answer is *him*, use *whom*. This trick is easy to remember because *he* and *who* both end in vowels, and *him* and *whom* both end in the letter *M*.

Adjectives

"The *extraordinary* brain is the *main* organ of the central nervous system." The adjective *extraordinary* describes the brain in a way that causes one to realize it is more exceptional than some of the other organs while the adjective *main* defines the brain's importance in its system.

An **adjective** is a word or phrase that names an attribute that describes or clarifies a noun or pronoun. This helps the reader visualize and understand the characteristics—size, shape, age, color, origin, etc.—of a person, place, or thing that otherwise might not be known. Adjectives breathe life, color, and depth into the subjects they define. Life would be *drab* and *colorless* without adjectives!

Adjectives often precede the nouns they describe.

> *She drove her <u>new</u> car.*

However, adjectives can also come later in the sentence.

> *Her car is new.*

Adjectives using the prefix *a*– can only be used after a verb.

> Correct: The dog was alive until the car ran up on the curb and hit him.
> Incorrect: The alive dog was hit by a car that ran up on the curb.

Other examples of this rule include *awake, ablaze, ajar, alike,* and *asleep*.

Other adjectives used after verbs concern states of health.

> The girl was finally *well* after a long bout of pneumonia.
> The boy was *fine* after the accident.

An adjective phrase is not a bunch of adjectives strung together, but a group of words that describes a noun or pronoun and, thus, functions as an adjective. Very happy is an adjective phrase; so are way too hungry and passionate about traveling.

Possessives

In grammar, **possessive nouns** and **possessive pronouns** show ownership.

Singular nouns are generally made possessive with an apostrophe and an *s* (*'s*).

> My *uncle's* new car is silver.
> The *dog's* bowl is empty.
> *James's* ties are becoming outdated.

Plural nouns ending in *s* are generally made possessive by just adding an apostrophe (*'*):

> The pistachio nuts' saltiness is added during roasting. (The saltiness of pistachio nuts is added during roasting.)
> The students' achievement tests are difficult. (The achievement tests of the students are difficult.)

If the plural noun does not end in an *s* such as *women,* then it is made possessive by adding an *apostrophe s* (*'s*)—*women's.*

Possessive pronouns can be first person (*mine*), second person (*yours*), or third person (*theirs*).

Indefinite possessive pronouns such as *nobody* or *someone* become possessive by adding an *apostrophe s* to become *nobody's* or *someone's.*

Verbs

A **verb** is the part of speech that describes an action, state of being, or occurrence.

A **verb** forms the main part of a predicate of a sentence. This means that the verb explains what the noun (which will be discussed shortly) is doing. A simple example is *time flies*. The verb *flies* explains what the action of the noun, *time*, is doing. This example is a **main** verb.

Helping (auxiliary) verbs are words like *have, do, be, can, may, should, must,* and *will.* "I *should* go to the store." Helping verbs assist main verbs in expressing tense, ability, possibility, permission, or obligation.

Particles are minor function words like *not, in, out, up,* or *down* that become part of the verb itself. "I might *not.*"

Participles are words formed from verbs that are often used to modify a noun, noun phrase, verb, or verb phrase.

The *running* teenager collided with the cyclist.

Participles can also create compound verb forms.

He is *speaking*.

Verbs have five basic forms: the **base** form, the *-s* form, the *-ing* form, the *past* form, and the **past participle** form.

The **past** forms are either *regular* (*love/loved; hate/hated*) or *irregular* because they don't end by adding the common past tense suffix "-ed" (*go/went; fall/fell; set/set*).

Adverbs

Adverbs have more functions than adjectives because they modify or qualify verbs, adjectives, or other adverbs as well as word groups that express a relation of place, time, circumstance, or cause. Therefore, adverbs answer any of the following questions: *How, when, where, why, in what way, how often, how much, in what condition,* and/or *to what degree. How good looking is he? He is <u>very</u> handsome.*

Here are some examples of adverbs for different situations:

- how: quickly
- when: daily
- where: there
- in what way: easily
- how often: often
- how much: much
- in what condition: badly
- what degree: hardly

As one can see, for some reason, many adverbs end in *-ly*.

Adverbs do things like emphasize (*really, simply,* and *so*), amplify (*heartily, completely,* and *positively*), and tone down (*almost, somewhat,* and *mildly*).

Adverbs also come in phrases.

The dog ran as <u>though his life depended on it.</u>

Prepositions

Prepositions are connecting words and, while there are only about 150 of them, they are used more often than any other individual groups of words. They describe relationships between other words. They are placed before a noun or pronoun, forming a phrase that modifies another word in the sentence. **Prepositional phrases** begin with a preposition and end with a noun or pronoun, the *object of the preposition. A pristine lake is <u>near the store</u> and <u>behind the bank</u>.*

Some commonly used prepositions are *about, after, anti, around, as, at, behind, beside, by, for, from, in, into, of, off, on, to,* and *with.*

Complex prepositions, which also come before a noun or pronoun, consist of two or three words such as *according to, in regards to,* and *because of.*

Interjections

Interjections are words used to express emotion. Examples include *wow*, *ouch*, and *hooray*. Interjections are often separate from sentences; in those cases, the interjection is directly followed by an exclamation point. In other cases, the interjection is included in a sentence and followed by a comma. The punctuation plays a big role in the intensity of the emotion that the interjection is expressing. Using a comma or semicolon indicates less excitement than using an exclamation mark.

Conjunctions

Conjunctions are vital words that connect words, phrases, thoughts, and ideas. Conjunctions show relationships between components. There are two types:

Coordinating conjunctions are the primary class of conjunctions placed between words, phrases, clauses, and sentences that are of equal grammatical rank; the coordinating conjunctions are *for*, *and*, *nor*, *but*, *or*, *yet*, and *so*. A useful memorization trick is to remember that the first letter of these conjunctions collectively spell the word *fanboys*.

> I need to go shopping, *but* I must be careful to leave enough money in the bank.
> She wore a black, red, *and* white shirt.

Subordinating conjunctions are the secondary class of conjunctions. They connect two unequal parts, one **main** (or **independent**) and the other **subordinate** (or **dependent**). I must go to the store *even though* I do not have enough money in the bank.

> *Because* I read the review, I do not want to go to the movie.

Notice that the presence of subordinating conjunctions makes clauses dependent. *I read the review* is an independent clause, but *because* makes the clause dependent. Thus, it needs an independent clause to complete the sentence.

Creating Coherent Sentences

Subject and Predicate

Every complete sentence can be divided into two parts: the subject and the predicate.

Subjects: Subjects are needed in sentences to tell the reader who or what the sentence describes. Subjects can be simple or complete, and they can be direct or indirect. There can also be compound subjects.

Simple subjects are the nouns or pronouns the sentence describes, without modifiers. The simple subject can come before or after the verb in the sentence:

> The big brown dog is the calmest one.

Complete subjects are the subject together with all of its describing words or modifiers.

> The big brown dog is the calmest one. (The complete subject is big brown dog.)

Direct subjects are subjects that appear in the text of the sentence, as in the example above. **Indirect subjects** are implied. The subject is "you," but the word *you* does not appear.

Indirect subjects are usually in imperative sentences that issue a command or order:

Feed the short skinny dog first. (The understood you is the subject.)

Watch out—he's really hungry! (The sentence warns you to watch out.)

Compound subjects occur when two or more nouns join together to form a plural subject.

Carson and Emily make a great couple.

Predicates: Once we have identified the subject of the sentence, the rest of the sentence becomes the predicate. Predicates are formed by the verb, the direct object, and all words related to it.

We went to see the Cirque du' Soleil performance.

The gigantic green character was funnier than all the rest.

A **predicate nominative** renames the subject:

John is a carpenter.

A **predicate adjective** describes the subject:

Margaret is beautiful.

Direct objects are the nouns in the sentence that are receiving the action. Sentences don't necessarily need objects. Sentences only need a subject and a verb.

The clown brought the acrobat the hula-hoop. (What is being brought? the hula-hoop)

Then he gave the trick pony a soapy bath. (What is being given? a soapy bath)

Indirect objects are words that tell us to or for whom or what the action is being done. For there to be an indirect object, there first must always be a direct object.

The clown brought the acrobat the hula-hoop. (Who is getting the direct object? the acrobat)

Then he gave the trick pony a soapy bath. (What is getting the bath? the trick pony)

Phrases

A **phrase** is a group of words that go together but do not include both a subject and a verb. They are used to add information, explain something, or make the sentence easier for the reader to understand. Unlike clauses, phrases can never stand alone as their own sentence. They do not form complete thoughts. There are noun phrases, prepositional phrases, verbal phrases, appositive phrases, and absolute phrases. Here are some examples of phrases:

I know all the shortest routes.

Before the sequel, we wanted to watch the first movie. (introductory phrase)

The jumpers have hot cocoa to drink right away.

Simple and Complete Subjects

A **complete subject** includes the simple subject and all the words modifying it, including articles and adjectives. A **simple subject** is the single noun without its modifiers.

> A warm, chocolate-chip cookie sat on the kitchen table.
>
> Complete subject: *a warm, chocolate-chip cookie*
>
> Simple subject: *cookie*

The words *a, warm, chocolate,* and *chip* all modify the simple subject *cookie*.

There might also be a **compound subject**, which would be two or more nouns without the modifiers.

> A little girl and her mother walked into the shop.
>
> Complete subject: *A little girl and her mother*
>
> Compound subject: *girl, mother*

In this case, *the girl and her mother* are both completing the action of walking into the shop, so this is a compound subject.

Subject-Verb Agreement

The subject of a sentence and its verb must agree. The cornerstone rule of subject-verb agreement is that subject and verb must agree in number. Whether the subject is singular or plural, the verb must follow suit.

> Incorrect: The houses is new.
> Correct: The houses are new.
> Also Correct: The house is new.

In other words, a singular subject requires a singular verb; a plural subject requires a plural verb.

The words or phrases that come between the subject and verb do not alter this rule.

> Incorrect: The houses built of brick is new.
> Correct: The houses built of brick are new.
> Incorrect: The houses with the sturdy porches is new.
> Correct: The houses with the sturdy porches are new.

The subject will always follow the verb when a sentence begins with *here* or *there.* Identify these with care.

> Incorrect: Here *is* the *houses* with sturdy porches.
> Correct: Here *are* the *houses* with sturdy porches.

The subject in the sentences above is not *here*, it is *houses*. Remember, *here* and *there* are never subjects. Be careful that contractions such as *here's* or *there're* do not cause confusion!

Two subjects joined by *and* require a plural verb form, except when the two combine to make one thing:

> Incorrect: Garrett and Jonathan is over there.
> Correct: Garrett and Jonathan are over there.
> Incorrect: Spaghetti and meatballs are a delicious meal!
> Correct: Spaghetti and meatballs is a delicious meal!

In the example above, *spaghetti and meatballs* is a compound noun. However, *Garrett and Jonathan* is not a compound noun.

Two singular subjects joined by *or, either/or,* or *neither/nor* call for a singular verb form.

> Incorrect: Butter or syrup are acceptable.
> Correct: Butter or syrup is acceptable.

Plural subjects joined by *or, either/or,* or *neither/nor* are, indeed, plural.

> The chairs or the boxes are being moved next.

If one subject is singular and the other is plural, the verb should agree with the closest noun.

> Correct: The chair or the boxes are being moved next.
> Correct: The chairs or the box is being moved next.

Some plurals of money, distance, and time call for a singular verb.

> Incorrect: Three dollars are enough to buy that.
> Correct: Three dollars is enough to buy that.

For words declaring degrees of quantity such as *many of, some of,* or *most of,* let the noun that follows *of* be the guide:

> Incorrect: Many of the books is in the shelf.
> Correct: Many of the books are in the shelf.
> Incorrect: Most of the pie *are* on the table.
> Correct: Most of the pie *is* on the table.

For indefinite pronouns like anybody or everybody, use singular verbs.

> Everybody *is* going to the store.

However, the pronouns *few, many, several, all, some,* and *both* have their own rules and use plural forms.

> Some *are* ready.

Some nouns like *crowd* and *congress* are called *collective nouns* and they require a singular verb form.

> Congress *is* in session.
> The news *is* over.

Books and movie titles, though, including plural nouns such as *Great Expectations*, also require a singular verb. Remember that only the subject affects the verb. While writing tricky subject-verb arrangements, say them aloud. Listen to them. Once the rules have been learned, one's ear will become sensitive to them, making it easier to pick out what's right and what's wrong.

Knowledge of Language

Using Grammar to Enhance Clarity in Writing

Forming Complete Sentences

Independent and dependent clauses are strings of words that contain both a subject and a verb. An **independent clause** *can* stand alone as complete thought, but a **dependent clause** *cannot*. A dependent clause relies on other words to be a complete sentence.

> Independent clause: The keys are on the counter.
> Dependent clause: If the keys are on the counter

Notice that both clauses have a subject (*keys*) and a verb (*are*). The independent clause expresses a complete thought, but the word *if* at the beginning of the dependent clause makes it *dependent* on other words to be a complete thought.

> Independent clause: If the keys are on the counter, please give them to me.

This example constitutes a complete sentence since it includes at least one verb and one subject and is a complete thought. In this case, the independent clause has two subjects (*keys* & an implied *you*) and two verbs (*are* & *give*).

> Independent clause: I went to the store.
> Dependent clause: Because we are out of milk,
> Complete Sentence: Because we are out of milk, I went to the store.
> Complete Sentence: I went to the store because we are out of milk.

Transitions

Transitions are the glue used to make organized thoughts adhere to one another. Transitions are the glue that helps put ideas together seamlessly, within sentences and paragraphs, between them, and (in longer documents) even between sections. Transitions may be single words, sentences, or whole paragraphs (as in the prior example). Transitions help readers to digest and understand what to feel about what has gone on and clue readers in on what is going on, what will be, and how they might react to all of these factors. Transitions are like good clues left at a crime scene.

Examples of Transitional Words and Phrases

Transitions have many purposes, as can be seen below.

- to show emphasis: truly, in fact
- to show examples: for example, namely, specifically
- to show similarities: also, likewise
- to show dissimilarities: on the other hand, even if, in contrast
- to show progression of time: later, previously, subsequently
- to show sequence or order: next, finally
- to show cause and effect: therefore, so
- to show place or position: above, nearby, there
- to provide evidence: furthermore, then
- to summarize: finally, summarizing

Verb Tense

Verb tense is used to show when the action in the sentence took place. There are several different verb tenses, and it is important to know how and when to use them. Some verb tenses can be achieved by changing the form of the verb, while others require the use of helping verbs (e.g., *is, was,* or *has*).

Present tense shows the action is happening currently or is ongoing:

I walk to work every morning.

She is stressed about the deadline.

Past tense shows that the action happened in the past or that the state of being is in the past:

I walked to work yesterday morning.

She was stressed about the deadline.

Future tense shows that the action will happen in the future or is a future state of being:

I will walk to work tomorrow morning.

She will be stressed about the deadline.

Present perfect tense shows action that began in the past, but continues into the present:

I have walked to work all week.

She has been stressed about the deadline.

Past perfect tense shows an action was finished before another took place:

I had walked all week until I sprained my ankle.

She had been stressed about the deadline until we talked about it.

Future perfect tense shows an action that will be completed at some point in the future:

By the time the bus arrives, I will have walked to work already.

Mood

Mood is used to show the speaker's feelings about the subject matter. In English, there is indicative mood, imperative mood, and subjunctive mood.

Indicative mood is used to state facts, ask questions, or state opinions:

Bob will make the trip next week.

When can Bob make the trip?

Imperative mood is used to state a command or make a request:

Wait in the lobby.

Please call me next week.

Subjunctive mood is used to express a wish, an opinion, or a hope that is contrary to fact:

> If I were in charge, none of this would have happened.
>
> Allison wished she could take the exam over again when she saw her score.

Revisions

Writers should always revise and proofread to polish things up. Putting oneself in the reader's shoes helps writers identify problems—it's a movement from the mindset of the writer to the mindset of the editor. The goal is to have clean, clear writing. Make sure to get rid of any extraneous language that does not meaningfully contribute to the text's message. The following areas should be considered when proofreading:

- Sentence fragments
- Awkward sentence structure
- Run-on sentences
- Incorrect word choice
- Grammatical agreement errors
- Spelling errors
- Punctuation errors
- Capitalization errors

Meeting the Needs of an Audience

Using language effectively is important when communicating, verbally and in writing. Style, tone, and clarity of one's writing can greatly affect a writer's audience. There are some different characteristics of effective language to keep in mind when writing.

Specific Language pertains to detailed descriptions which portray more tangible visualizations for the reader. Using specific language in writing eliminates the potential for miscommunication or misunderstanding.

Concise Language involves conveying complex ideas in as few words as possible.

Familiar Language is language which readers easily recognize, understand, and relate to because it is similar to that which they use regularly. When a writer uses unfamiliar language, the meaning, or message, they are trying to convey is easily lost. An effective writer will understand their audience and use language that is familiar to said audience.

Clear Language is similar to specific and familiar language in that it is audience based as well. Language can become unclear based on the reader's background knowledge and exposure to the written work. For this reason, it is important for a writer to use as clear of language as possible when writing their content. Using clear language will eliminate any misunderstandings.

Constructive Language refers to using more positive language in writing. Rather than using words or phrases that could potentially make the reader defensive, the writer should try to incorporate language that promotes positivity and understanding toward the reader.

Appropriate Tone is crucial for creating effective writing. Knowing what kind of tone to use in one's writing involves having an understanding of the audience they are writing for. There are a couple of types of tones a writer may use: formal (professional) and informal (more conversational). Understanding one's audience is crucial to determining which tone is best for certain writing assignments.

Formal and Informal Language

It can be helpful to distinguish whether a writer or speaker is using formal or informal language because It can be helpful to distinguish whether a writer or speaker is using formal or informal language because it can give the reader or listener clues to whether the text is informative, nonfiction, or argumentative, as well as the intended tone and audience. Formal and informal language in written or verbal communication serve different purposes and are often intended for different audiences. Consequently, their tone, word choices, and grammatical structures vary. These differences can be used to identify which form of language is used in a given piece and to determine which type of language should be used for a certain context. Understanding the differences between formal and informal language will also allow a writer or speaker to implement the most appropriate and effective style for a given situation.

Formal language is less personal and more informative and pragmatic than informal language. It is more "buttoned-up" and business-like, adhering to proper grammatical rules. It is used in professional or academic contexts, to convey respect or authority. For example, one would use formal language to write an informative or argumentative essay for school and to address a superior or esteemed professional like a potential employer, a professor, or a manager. Formal language avoids contractions, slang, colloquialisms, and first person pronouns. **Slang** refers to non-standard expressions that are not used in elevated speech and writing. Slang creates linguistic in-groups and out-groups of people, those who can understand the slang terms and those who can't. Slang is often tied to a specific time period.

For example, "groovy" and "far out" are connected to the 1970s, and "as if!" and "4-1-1-" are connected to the 1990s. **Colloquial** language is language that is used conversationally or familiarly—e.g., "What's up?"—in contrast to formal, professional, or academic language—"How are you this evening?" Formal language uses sentences that are usually more complex and often in passive voice. Punctuation can differ as well. For example, exclamations point (!) are used to show strong emotion or can be used as an interjection but should be used sparingly in formal writing situations.

Informal language is often used when communicating with family members, friends, peers, and those known more personally. It is more casual, spontaneous, and forgiving in its conformity to grammatical rules and conventions. Informal language is used for personal emails, some light fiction stories, and some correspondence between coworkers or other familial relationships. The tone is more relaxed and slang, contractions, clichés, and the first and second person may be used in writing. The imperative voice may be used as well.

As a review, the perspectives from which something may be written or conveyed are detailed below:

- First-person point of view: The story is told from the writer's perspective. In fiction, this would mean that the main character is also the narrator. First-person point of view is easily recognized by the use of personal pronouns such as I, me, we, us, our, my, and myself.
- Second-person point of view: This point of view isn't commonly used in fiction or nonfiction writing because it directly addresses the reader using the pronouns you, your, and yourself. Second-person perspective is more appropriate in direct communication, such as business letters or emails.
- Third-person point of view: In a more formal essay, this would be an appropriate perspective because the focus should be on the subject matter, not the writer or the reader. Third-person point of view is recognized by the use of the pronouns he, she, they, and it. In fiction writing, third-person point of view has a few variations.
- Third-person limited point of view refers to a story told by a narrator who has access to the thoughts and feelings of just one character.

- In third-person omniscient point of view, the narrator has access to the thoughts and feelings of all the characters.
- In third-person objective point of view, the narrator is like a fly on the wall and can see and hear what the characters do and say but does not have access to their thoughts and feelings.

Sensitivity

In speech and writing, it's important to be cognizant as to how your words are perceived by others depending on your audience. You will want to write from a perspective and use diction that is appropriate for the context and audience for your content.

Developing a Well-Organized Paragraph

Forming Paragraphs

A good **paragraph** should have the following characteristics:

- Be logical with organized sentences
- Have a unified purpose within itself
- Use sentences as building blocks
- Be a distinct section of a piece of writing
- Present a single theme introduced by a topic sentence
- Maintain a consistent flow through subsequent, relevant, well-placed sentences
- Tell a story of its own or have its own purpose, yet connect with what is written before and after
- Enlighten, entertain, and/or inform

Though certainly not set in stone, the length should be a consideration for the reader's sake, not merely for the sake of the topic. When paragraphs are especially short, the reader might experience an irregular, uneven effect; when they're much longer than 250 words, the reader's attention span, and probably their retention, is challenged. While a paragraph can technically be a sentence long, a good rule of thumb is for paragraphs to be at least three sentences long and no more than ten sentence long. An optimal word length is 100 to 250 words.

Coherent Paragraphs

Coherence is simply defined as the quality of being logical and consistent. In order to have coherent paragraphs, therefore, authors must be logical and consistent in their writing, whatever the document might be. Two words are helpful to understanding coherence: flow and relationship. Earlier, transitions were referred to as being the "glue" to put organized thoughts together. Now, let's look at the topic sentence from which flow and relationship originate.

The topic sentence, usually the first in a paragraph, holds the essential features that will be brought forth in the paragraph. It is also here that authors either grab or lose readers. It may be the only writing that a reader encounters from that writer, so it is a good idea to summarize and represent ideas accurately.

The coherent paragraph has a logical order; depending on the purpose of the paragraph, that order may be chronological, based on cause and effect, or something else. It utilizes transitional words and phrases, parallel sentence structure, clear pronoun references, and reasonable repetition of key words and phrases. Use common sense for repetition. Consider synonyms for variety. Be consistent in verb tense whenever possible.

When writers have accomplished their paragraph's purpose, they prepare it to receive the next paragraph. While writing, read the paragraph over, edit, examine, evaluate, and make changes accordingly. Possibly, a paragraph has gone on too long. If that occurs, it needs to be broken up into other paragraphs, or the length should be reduced. If a paragraph didn't fully accomplish its purpose, consider revising it.

Main Point of a Paragraph

What is the main point of a paragraph? It is *the* point all of the other important and lesser important points should lead up to, and it should be summed up in the topic sentence.

Sometimes there is a fine line between a paragraph's topic sentence and its main point. In fact, they actually might be one and the same. Often, though, they are two separate, but closely related, aspects of the same paragraph.

Depending upon the writer's purpose, the topic sentence or the paragraph's main point might not be fully revealed until the paragraph's conclusion.

Sometimes, while developing paragraphs, authors deviate from the main point, which means they have to delete and rework their materials to stay on point. Only relevant information should be included within the paragraph; irrelevant content should be removed.

Examining Paragraphs

Throughout this text, composing and combining sentences, using basic grammar skills, employing rules and guidelines, identifying differing points of view, using appropriate context, constructing accurate word usage, and discerning correct punctuation have all been discussed. Whew! The types of sentences, patterns, transitions, and overall structure have been covered as well.

While authors write, thoughts coalesce to form words on "paper" (aka a computer screen). Authors strategically place those thoughts in sentences to give them "voice" in an orderly manner, and then they manipulate them into cohesive sentences for cohesion to express ideas. Like a hunk of modeling clay (thanks to computers, people are no longer bound to erasers and whiteout), sentences can be worked and reworked until they cooperate and say what was originally intended.

Before calling a paragraph complete, identify its main point, making sure that related sentences stay on point. Pose questions such as, "Did I sufficiently develop the main point? Did I say it succinctly enough? Did I give it time to develop? *Is* it developed?" Be sure to add information where the message could be unclear or confusing.

Let's examine the following two paragraphs, each an example of a movie review. Read them and form a critique.

> Example 1: *Eddie the Eagle* is a movie about a struggling athlete. Eddie was crippled at birth. He had a lot of therapy and he had a dream. Eddie trained himself for the Olympics. He went far away to learn how to ski jump. It was hard for him, but he persevered. He got a coach and kept trying. He qualified for the Olympics. He was the only one from Britain who could jump. When he succeeded, they named him, "Eddie the Eagle."

> Example 2: The last movie I saw in the theater was *Eddie the Eagle,* a story of extraordinary perseverance inspired by real life events. Eddie was born in England with a birth defect that he slowly but surely overcame, but not without trial and error (not the least of which was his father's perpetual *dis*couragement). In fact, the old man did everything to get him to give up, but Eddie was dogged beyond anyone in the neighborhood; in fact, maybe beyond anyone in the whole town or even the whole world! Eddie, simply, did not know to quit. As he grew up, so did his dream; a strange one, indeed, for someone so unaccomplished: to compete in the Winter Olympics as a ski jumper (which he knew absolutely nothing about). Eddie didn't just keep on dreaming about it. He actually went to Germany and *worked* at it, facing unbelievable odds, defeats, and put-downs by Dad and the other Men in Charge, aka the Olympic decision-makers. Did that stop him? No way! Eddie got a coach and persevered. Then, when he failed, he persevered some more, again and again. You should be able to open up a dictionary, look at the word "persevere," and see a picture of Eddie the Eagle because, when everybody told him he couldn't, he did. The result? He is forever dubbed, "Eddie the Eagle."

Both reviews tell something about the movie *Eddie the Eagle*. Does one motivate the reader to want to see the movie more than the other? Does one just provide a few facts while the other paints a virtual picture of the movie? Does one give a carrot and the other a rib eye steak, mashed potatoes, and chocolate silk pie?

Paragraphs sometimes only give facts. Sometimes that's appropriate and all that is needed. Sometimes, though, writers want to use the blank documents on their computer screens to paint a picture. Writers must "see" the painting come to life. To do so, pick a familiar topic, write a simple sentence, and add to it. Pretend, for instance, there's a lovely view. What does one see? Is it a lake? Try again—picture it as though it were the sea! Visualize a big ship sailing out there. Is it sailing away or approaching? Who is on it? Is it dangerous? Is it night and are there crazy pirates on board? Uh-oh! Did one just jump ship and start swimming toward shore?

Expressing Ideas in Writing

Elements of the Writing Process

Practice Makes Prepared Writers

Like any other useful skill, writing only improves with practice. While writing may come more easily to some than others, it is still a skill to be honed and improved. Regardless of a person's natural abilities, there is always room for growth in writing. Practicing the basic skills of writing can aid in preparations for the TEAS.

One way to build vocabulary and enhance exposure to the written word is through reading. This can be through reading books, but reading of any materials such as newspapers, magazines, and even social media count towards practice with the written word. This also helps to enhance critical reading and thinking skills, through analysis of the ideas and concepts read. Think of each new reading experience as a chance to sharpen these skills.

Planning

Brainstorming

One of the most important steps in writing an essay is prewriting. Before drafting an essay, it's helpful to think about the topic for a moment or two, in order to gain a more solid understanding of what the task is. Then, spending about five minutes jotting down the immediate ideas that could work for the essay is recommended. **Brainstorming** is a way to get some words on the page and offer a reference for ideas when drafting. Scratch paper is provided for writers to use any prewriting techniques such as webbing, free writing, or listing. The goal is to get ideas out of the mind and onto the page.

Once the ideas are on the page, it's time to turn them into a solid plan for the essay. The best ideas from the brainstorming results can then be developed into a more formal outline.

Outlining

An **outline** is a system used to organize writing. When reading texts, outlining is important because it helps readers organize important information in a logical pattern using Roman numerals. Usually, outlines start out with the main idea(s) and then branch out into subgroups or subsidiary thoughts or subjects. The outline should be methodical, with at least two main points follow each by at least two subpoints. Not only do outlines provide a visual tool for readers to reflect on how events, characters, settings, or other key parts of the text or passage relate to one another, but they can also lead readers to a stronger conclusion.

The sample below demonstrates what a general outline looks like.

I. Main Topic 1
  a. Subtopic 1
  b. Subtopic 2
    1. Detail 1
    2. Detail 2
II. Main Topic 2
  a. Subtopic 1
  b. Subtopic 2
    1. Detail 1
    2. Detail 2

Free Writing

Like brainstorming, free writing is another prewriting activity to help the writer generate ideas. This method involves setting a timer for 2 or 3 minutes and writing down all ideas that come to mind about the topic using complete sentences. Once time is up, review the sentences to see what observations have been made and how these ideas might translate into a more coherent direction for the topic. Even if sentences lack sense as a whole, this is an excellent way to get ideas onto the page in the very beginning stages of writing. Using complete sentences can make this a bit more challenging than brainstorming, but overall it is a worthwhile exercise, as it may force the writer to come up with more complete thoughts about the topic.

Writing

Now it comes time to actually write your essay. Follow the outline you developed in the brainstorming process and try to incorporate the sentences you wrote in the free writing exercise.

Remember that your work here does not have to be perfect. This process is often referred to as **drafting** because you're just creating a rough draft of your work.

Don't get bogged down on the small details. For instance, if you're not sure whether or not a word should be capitalized, mark it somehow and look up the capitalization rule while in the revision process. The same goes for referencing sources. That should not be focused on until after the writing process.

Referencing Sources

Anytime you quote or paraphrase another piece of writing you will need to include a citation. A citation is a short description of the work that your quote or information came from. The manual of style your teacher wants you to follow will dictate exactly how to format that citation. For example, this is how you would cite a book according to the APA manual of style:

- **Format**: Last name, First initial, Middle initial. (Year Published) Book Title. City, State: Publisher.
- **Example**: Sampson, M. R. (1989). *Diaries from an Alien Invasion. Springfield, IL*: Campbell Press.

Revising

Revising and proofreading offers an opportunity for writers to polish things up. Putting one's self in the reader's shoes and focusing on what the essay actually says helps writers identify problems—it's a movement from the mindset of writer to the mindset of editor. The goal is to have a clean, clear copy of the essay. The following areas should be considered when proofreading:

- Sentence fragments
- Awkward sentence structure
- Run-on sentences
- Incorrect word choice
- Grammatical agreement errors
- Spelling errors
- Punctuation errors
- Capitalization errors

Recursive Writing Process

While the writing process may have specific steps, the good news is that the process is recursive, meaning the steps need not be completed in a particular order. Many writers find that they complete steps at the same time such as drafting and revising, where the writing and rearranging of ideas occur simultaneously or in very close order. Similarly, a writer may find that a particular section of a draft needs more development, and will go back to the prewriting stage to generate new ideas. The steps can be repeated at any time, and the more these steps of the recursive writing process are employed, the better the final product will be.

Analyzing Word Parts

By analyzing and understanding Latin, Greek, and Anglo-Saxon word roots, prefixes, and suffixes one can better understand word meanings. Of course, people can always look words up if a dictionary or thesaurus, if available, but meaning can often be gleaned on the spot if the writer learns to dissect and examine words.

A word can consist of the following:

- root
- root + suffix
- prefix + root
- prefix + root + suffix

For example, if someone was unfamiliar with the word *submarine,* they could break the word into its parts.

prefix + root
sub + marine

It can be determined that *sub* means *below* as in *subway* and *subpar*. Additionally, one can determine that *marine* refers to *the sea* as in *marine life*. Thus, it can be figured that *submarine* refers to something below the water.

Roots

Roots are the basic components of words. Many roots can stand alone as individual words, but others must be combined with a prefix or suffix to be a word. For example, *calc* is a root but it needs a suffix to be an actual word (*calcium*).

Prefixes

A **prefix** is a word, letter, or number that is placed before another. It adjusts or qualifies the root word's meaning. When written alone, prefixes are followed by a dash to indicate that the root word follows.

Some of the most common prefixes are the following:

Prefix	Meaning	Example
dis-	not or opposite of	disabled
in-, im-, il-, ir-	not	illiterate
re-	again	return
un-	not	unpredictable
anti-	against	antibacterial
fore-	before	forefront
mis-	wrongly	misunderstand
non-	not	nonsense
over-	more than normal	overabundance
pre-	before	preheat
super-	above	superman

Suffixes

A suffix is a letter or group of letters added at the end of a word to form another word. The word created from the root and suffix is either a different tense of the same root (*help + ed = helped*) or a new word (*help + ful = helpful*). When written alone, suffixes are preceded by a dash to indicate that the root word comes before.

Some of the most common suffixes are the following:

Suffix	Meaning	Example
ed	makes a verb past tense	wash*ed*
ing	makes a verb a present participle verb	washing
ly	to make characteristic of	love*ly*
s/es	to make more than one	chairs, boxes
able	can be done	deplor*able*
al	having characteristics of	comic*al*
est	comparative	great*est*
ful	full of	wonder*ful*
ism	belief in	commun*ism*
less	without	faithless
ment	action or process	accomplish*ment*
ness	state of	happi*ness*
ize, ise	to render, to make	steril*ize*, advert*ise*
cede/ceed/sede	go	concede, proceed, supersede

Prefixes and suffixes can both be used as *affixes* (linguistic elements attached to a root to form another word). When different affixes are attached appropriately to the same root, they form cognates, which are words that derive from the same linguistic origin. Here are some helpful tips when utilizing affixes:

- When adding a suffix that starts with a vowel (for example, *-ed*) to a one-syllable root whose vowel has a short sound and ends in a consonant (for example, *stun*), double the final consonant of the root (*n*).

    stun + ed = stun*n*ed

    Exception: If the past tense verb ends in *x* such as *box*, do not double the *x*.

    box + ed = boxed

- If adding a suffix that starts with a vowel (*-er*) to a multi-syllable word ending in a consonant (*begin*), double the consonant (*n*).

    begin + er = begin*n*er

- If a short vowel is followed by two or more consonants in a word such as *i+t+c+h = itch*, do not double the last consonant.

    itch + ed = itched

- If adding a suffix that starts with a vowel (*-ing*) to a word ending in *e* (for example, *name*), that word's final *e* is generally (but not always) dropped.

    name + ing = naming
    exception: manage + able = manag*e*able

- If adding a suffix that starts with a consonant (*-ness*) to a word ending in *e* (*complete*), the *e* generally (but not always) remains.

    complete + ness = completeness
    exception: judge + ment = judgment

- There is great diversity on handling words that end in y. For words ending in a vowel + y, nothing changes in the original word.

    play + ed = played

- For words ending in a consonant + *y*, change the *y* to *i* when adding any suffix except for *–ing*.

    marry + ed = married
    marry + ing = marrying

English & Language Usage Practice Quiz

1. Which sentence contains an error in punctuation or capitalization?
    a. "The show is on," Jackson said.
    b. The Grand Canyon is a national park.
    c. Lets celebrate tomorrow.
    d. Oliver, a social worker, got a new job this month.

2. Which of the following sentences contains an error in usage?
    a. Their words was followed by a signing document.
    b. No one came to the theater that evening.
    c. Several cats were living in the abandoned house down the road.
    d. It rained that morning; they had to cancel the kayaking trip.

3. A rough plan for the structure of your paper is known as what?
    a. Character development
    b. A rough draft
    c. A blueprint
    d. An outline

4. Which of the following is a transition word used to show similarities? Select all that apply.
    a. Likewise
    b. Specifically
    c. Also
    d. Subsequently

5. Which of the following is the most formal greeting?
    a. Hey.
    b. What's up?
    c. Hello.
    d. Howdy

See answers on the next page.

Answer Explanations

1. C: The correct answer choice is *Lets celebrate tomorrow*. *Lets* is supposed to be short for *let us*, and therefore needs an apostrophe between the *t* and the *s*: *Let's*.

2. A: This error is marked by a subject/verb disagreement. *Words* is plural, so the verb must be plural as well. The correct usage would be: *Their words were followed by a signing document.*

3. D: An outline is the term used to describe a system used to plan out what you are going to write. Choice *A*, *character development*, refers to the changes a character undergoes throughout a story. Choice *B*, *a rough draft*, refers to a non-final version of an essay or other work of literature. Choice *C*, *a blueprint*, has a similar meaning, but is a term generally used in construction.

4. A, C: *Likewise* and *also* are transition words used to show similarities between two things. Choice *B*, *specifically*, is a transition word used to introduce an example. Choice *D*, *subsequently*, is a transition word used to show progression of time.

5. C: *Hello* is a formal greeting and the most formal in the list of options. The other choices are informal.

TEAS 7 Practice Test #1

Reading

1. Xavier propagated his belief that dragons were real to his friends gathered around the campfire.

Which of the following words could most logically replace the underlined word without altering the intent of the sentence?

a. Whispered
b. Expressed
c. Persuaded
d. Shouted

2. Which of the following statements least supports the argument that the American economy is healthy?

a. The gross domestic product (GDP), which is the measure of all the goods and services produced in a country, increased by two percent last year.
b. Unemployment is the lowest it's been in over a decade due to a spike in job creation.
c. Average household income just hit a historical high point for the twentieth consecutive quarter.
d. Last year, the output of the manufacturing sector decreased despite repeated massive investments by both the private and public sectors.

The next three questions are based on the following table. The Dewey Decimal System is a library classification system.

The Dewey Decimal Classes
000 Computer science, information, and general works
100 Philosophy and psychology
200 Religion
300 Social sciences
400 Languages
500 Science and mathematics
600 Technical and applied science
700 Arts and recreation
800 Literature
900 History, geography, and biography

3. Teddy has been assigned to write a history paper about the United States during the Cold War. His teacher advised him to read some of the works of Noam Chomsky, an American linguist, philosopher, social scientist, cognitive scientist, historian, social critic, and political activist. Teddy was not sure where to begin, so he consulted the Dewey Decimal classes. While not all inclusive, what choice of three classes would likely be the most useful?

a. 100, 300, 700
b. 100, 300, 800
c. 100, 400, 900
d. 200, 300, 900

4. While researching Chomsky's many theories and arguments, Teddy became interested in post-World War II anarchism, a social science theory asserting the political philosophy that rejects a compulsory government. He wants to find the most appropriate works related to the subject. Which section of the library is the most likely to contain the relevant books?

a. 000
b. 200
c. 300
d. 900

5. Also during his research, Teddy discovered information about Chomsky's Jewish heritage, and he wants to research traditional Judaism as practiced in the early twentieth century. Which section of the library would most likely contain the most relevant information?

a. 100
b. 200
c. 300
d. 900

6. Samuel teaches at a high school in one of the biggest cities in the United States. His students come from diverse family backgrounds. Samuel observes that the best students in his class are from homes where parental supervision is minimal. The parents of the bottom five students are the most involved, by a large margin. There are 24 students in his class. Samuel is going to write an academic paper based on his students' family backgrounds and academic performance. The paper will argue that parental involvement is not an important factor in academic success.

Which of the following statements best describes Samuel's sample size?

a. The sample is biased because he has firsthand experience and personal knowledge of its participants.
b. The sample contains too few members to make meaningful claims applicable to a large group.
c. The sample contains too many members to understand the context and specifics of any given student's situation.
d. The sample is unbiased and appropriately sized to draw conclusions on the role of parental supervision in education.

The next question is based on the following passage.

> Annabelle Rice started having trouble sleeping. Her biological clock was suddenly amiss, and she began to lead a nocturnal schedule. She thought her insomnia was due to spending nights writing a horror story, but then she realized that even the idea of going outside into the bright world scared her to bits. She concluded she was now suffering from heliophobia.

7. Which of the following most accurately describes the meaning of the underlined word in the sentence above?

a. Fear of dreams
b. Fear of sunlight
c. Fear of strangers
d. Anxiety spectrum disorder

The next question is based on the following directions.

Follow these instructions in chronological order to transform the word into something new.

1. Start with the word LOATHING.
2. Eliminate the first and last letter in the starting word.
3. Eliminate all the vowels, except I, from the word.
4. Eliminate the letter H from the word.

8. What new word has been spelled?
    a. TON
    b. THIN
    c. TIN
    d. TAN

9. Which of these descriptions would give the most detailed and objective support for the claim that drinking and driving is unsafe?
    a. A dramatized television commercial reenacting a fatal drinking and driving accident, including heart-wrenching testimonials from loved ones
    b. The Department of Transportation's press release noting the additional drinking and driving special patrol units that will be on the road during the holiday season
    c. Congressional written testimony on the number of drinking and driving incidents across the country and their relationship to underage drinking statistics, according to experts
    d. A highway bulletin warning drivers of penalties associated with drinking and driving

The next question is based on the following passage.

> A famous children's author recently published a historical fiction novel under a pseudonym; however, it did not sell as many copies as her children's books. In her earlier years, she had majored in history and earned a graduate degree in Antebellum American History, which is the time frame of her new novel. Critics praised this newest work far more than the children's series that made her famous. In fact, her new novel was nominated for the prestigious Albert J. Beveridge Award, but it still isn't selling like her children's books, which fly off the shelves because of her name alone.

10. Which one of the following statements might be accurately inferred based on the above passage?
    a. The famous children's author produced an inferior book under her pseudonym.
    b. The famous children's author is the foremost expert on Antebellum America.
    c. The famous children's author did not receive the bump in publicity for her historical novel that it would have received if it were written under her given name.
    d. People generally prefer to read children's series over historical fiction.

The next four questions are based on the following passage.

> Smoking tobacco products is terribly destructive. A single cigarette contains over 4,000 chemicals, including 43 known carcinogens and 400 deadly toxins. Some of the most dangerous ingredients include tar, carbon monoxide, formaldehyde, ammonia, arsenic, and DDT. Smoking can cause numerous types of cancer, including throat, mouth, nasal cavity, esophageal, gastric, pancreatic, renal, bladder, and cervical cancer.
>
> Cigarettes contain a drug called nicotine, which is one of the most addictive substances known. Addiction is defined as a compulsion to seek the substance despite negative consequences. According to the National Institute on Drug Abuse, nearly 35 million smokers expressed a desire to

quit smoking in 2015; however, more than 85 percent of those who struggle with addiction will not achieve their goal. Almost all smokers regret picking up that first cigarette. You would be wise to learn from their mistake if you have not yet started smoking.

According to the US Department of Health and Human Services, 16 million people in the United States presently suffer from a smoking-related condition, and nearly nine million suffer from a serious smoking-related illness. According to the Centers for Disease Control and Prevention (CDC), tobacco products cause nearly six million deaths per year. This number is projected to rise to over eight million deaths by 2030. Smokers, on average, die ten years earlier than their nonsmoking peers.

In the United States, local, state, and federal governments typically tax tobacco products, which leads to high prices. Nicotine users who struggle with addiction sometimes pay more for a pack of cigarettes than for a few gallons of gas. Additionally, smokers tend to stink. The smell of smoke is all-consuming and creates a pervasive nastiness. Smokers also risk staining their teeth and fingers with yellow residue from the tar.

Smoking is deadly, expensive, and socially unappealing. Clearly, smoking is not worth the risks.

11. Which of the following best describes the passage?
    a. Narrative
    b. Persuasive
    c. Expository
    d. Technical

12. Which of the following statements most accurately summarizes the passage?
    a. Tobacco is less healthy than many alternatives.
    b. Tobacco is deadly, expensive, and socially unappealing, and smokers would be much better off kicking the addiction.
    c. In the United States, local, state, and federal governments typically tax tobacco products, which leads to high prices.
    d. Tobacco products shorten smokers' lives by ten years and kill more than six million people per year.

13. The author would be most likely to agree with which of the following statements?
    a. Smokers should only quit cold turkey and should avoid all nicotine cessation devices.
    b. Other substances are more addictive than tobacco.
    c. Smokers should quit for whatever reason gets them to stop smoking.
    d. People who want to continue smoking should advocate for a reduction in tobacco product taxes.

14. Which of the following represents an opinion statement on the part of the author?
    a. According to the Centers for Disease Control and Prevention (CDC), tobacco products cause nearly six million deaths per year.
    b. Nicotine patches are just as terrible as cigarettes.
    c. Smokers also risk staining their teeth and fingers with yellow residue from the tar.
    d. Additionally, smokers tend to stink. The smell of smoke is all-consuming and creates a pervasive nastiness.

The next question is based on the following passage.

In 2015, 28 countries, including Estonia, Portugal, Slovenia, and Latvia, scored significantly higher than the United States on standardized high school math tests. In the 1960s, the United States consistently ranked first in the world. Today, the United States spends more than $800 billion on education, which exceeds the next highest country by more than $600 billion. The United States also leads the world in spending per school-aged child by an enormous margin.

15. If the statements above are true, which of the following statements must be correct?
    a. Outspending other countries on education has benefits beyond standardized math tests.
    b. The United States' education system is corrupt and broken.
    c. The standardized math tests are not representative of American academic prowess.
    d. Spending more money does not guarantee success on standardized math tests.

16. At the top of an encyclopedia's page are the following two guide terms: *kingcraft* and *klieg light*. Which one of the following words will be found on this page?
    a. Kleptomania
    b. Knead
    c. Kinesthesia
    d. Kickback

17. Which of the following is a primary source? *Select all that apply.*
    a. A critic's summary and review of a new book on the life of Abraham Lincoln
    b. A peer-reviewed scientific journal's table of contents
    c. A personal journal from a commander during World War II
    d. An encyclopedia entry discussing the Industrial Revolution

The next question is based on the following passage.

Cynthia keeps to a strict vegetarian diet, which is part of her religion. She absolutely cannot have any meat or fish dishes. This is more than a preference; her body has never developed the enzymes to process meat or fish, so she becomes violently ill if she accidentally eats any of the offending foods.

Cynthia is attending a full day event at her college next week. When at an event that serves meals, she always likes to bring a platter of vegetarian food for herself and to share with other attendees who have similar dietary restrictions. She requested a menu in advance to determine when her platter might be most useful to vegetarians. Here is the menu:

Breakfast: Hazelnut coffee or English breakfast tea, French toast, eggs, and bacon strips

Lunch: Assorted sandwiches (vegetarian options available), French fries, and baked beans

Cocktail hour: Alcoholic beverages, fruit, and cheese

Dinner: Roasted pork loin, seared trout, and bacon-bit topped macaroni and cheese

18. If Cynthia wants to pick the meal where there would be the least options for her and fellow vegetarians, during what meal should she bring the platter?
   a. Breakfast
   b. Lunch
   c. Cocktail hour
   d. Dinner

The next three questions are based on the following passage.

> George Washington emerged out of the American Revolution as an unlikely champion of liberty. On June 14, 1775, the Second Continental Congress created the Continental Army, and John Adams, serving in the Congress, nominated Washington to be its first commander. Washington had fought under the British during the French and Indian War, and his experience and prestige proved instrumental to the American war effort. Washington provided invaluable leadership, training, and strategy during the Revolutionary War. He emerged from the war as the embodiment of liberty and freedom from tyranny.
>
> After vanquishing the heavily favored British forces, Washington could have pronounced himself the autocratic leader of the former colonies without any opposition, but he famously refused and returned to his Mount Vernon plantation. His restraint proved his commitment to the fledgling state's republicanism. Washington was later unanimously elected as the first American president. But it is Washington's farewell address that cemented his legacy as a visionary worthy of study.
>
> In 1796, President Washington issued his farewell address by public letter. Washington enlisted his good friend, Alexander Hamilton, in drafting his most famous address. The letter expressed Washington's faith in the Constitution and rule of law. He encouraged his fellow Americans to put aside partisan differences and establish a national union. Washington warned Americans against meddling in foreign affairs and entering military alliances. Additionally, he stated his opposition to national political parties, which he considered partisan and counterproductive.
>
> Americans would be wise to remember Washington's farewell, especially during presidential elections, when politics hit a fever pitch. They might want to question the political institutions that were not planned by the Founding Fathers, such as the nomination process and political parties themselves.

19. Which of the following is logically based on the information contained in the passage above?
   a. George Washington's background as a wealthy landholder directly led to his faith in equality, liberty, and democracy.
   b. George Washington would have opposed America's involvement in the Second World War.
   c. George Washington would not have been able to write as great a farewell address without the assistance of Alexander Hamilton.
   d. George Washington would probably not approve of modern political parties.

20. Which of the following is the best description of the author's purpose in writing this passage about George Washington?
   a. To inform American voters about a Founding Father's sage advice on a contemporary issue and explain its applicability to modern times
   b. To introduce George Washington to readers as a historical figure worthy of study
   c. To note that George Washington was more than a famous military hero
   d. To convince readers that George Washington is a hero of republicanism and liberty

21. In which of the following materials would the author be the most likely to include this passage?
    a. A history textbook
    b. An obituary
    c. A fictional story
    d. A newspaper editorial

The next question is based on the following conversation between a scientist and a politician.

> Scientist: Last year was the warmest ever recorded in the last 134 years. During that time period, the 10 warmest years have all occurred since 2000. This correlates directly with the recent increases in carbon dioxide as large countries like China, India, and Brazil continue developing and industrializing. No longer do just a handful of countries burn massive amounts of carbon-based fossil fuels; it is quickly becoming the case throughout the whole world as technology and industry spread.
>
> Politician: Yes, but there is no causal link between increases in carbon emissions and increasing temperatures. The link is tenuous and nothing close to certain. We need to wait for all of the data before drawing hasty conclusions. For all we know, the temperature increase could be entirely natural. I believe the temperatures also rose dramatically during the dinosaurs' time, and I do not think they were burning any fossil fuels back then.

22. What is one point on which the scientist and politician agree?
    a. Burning fossil fuels causes global temperatures to rise.
    b. Global temperatures are increasing.
    c. Countries must revisit their energy policies before it's too late.
    d. Earth's climate naturally goes through warming and cooling periods.

23. Raul is going to Egypt next month. He has been looking forward to this vacation all year. Since childhood, Raul has been fascinated with pyramids, especially the Great Pyramid of Giza, which is the oldest of the Seven Wonders of the Ancient World. According to religious custom, Egyptian royalty is buried in the tombs located within the pyramid's great labyrinths. Since it has been many years since Raul read about the pyramid's history, he wants to read a book describing how and why the Egyptians built the Great Pyramid thousands of years ago. Which of the following guides would be the best for Raul?
    a. *A Beginner's Guide to Giza*, a short book describing the city's best historical sites, published by the Egyptian Tourism Bureau (2015)
    b. *The Life of Zahi Hawass*, the autobiography of one of Egypt's most famous archaeologists who was one of the first explorers at Giza (2014)
    c. *A History of Hieroglyphics*, an in-depth look at how archaeologists first broke the ancient code, published by the University of Giza's famed history department (2013)
    d. *Who Built the Great Pyramids?*, a short summary of the latest research and theories on the ancient Egyptians' religious beliefs and archaeological skills, written by a team of leading experts in the field (2015)

The next five questions are based on the following passage.

> Christopher Columbus is often credited with discovering America. This is a matter of perspective; America was unknown to fifteenth-century Europe, but bear in mind that the places he "discovered" were already filled with people who had been living there for centuries. What's more, Christopher Columbus was not the first European explorer to reach the Americas! Rather, it was Leif Erikson who first came to the New World and contacted the natives nearly 500 years before Christopher Columbus.

Leif Erikson, the son of Erik the Red (a famous Viking outlaw and explorer in his own right), was born in either 970 or 980, depending on which historian you read. His own family, though, did not raise Leif, which was a Viking tradition. Instead, one of Erik's prisoners taught Leif reading and writing, languages, sailing, and weaponry. At age 12, Leif was considered a man and returned to his family. He killed a man during a dispute shortly after his return, and the council banished the Erikson clan to Greenland.

In 999, Leif left Greenland and traveled to Norway, where he would serve as a guard to King Olaf Tryggvason. It was there that he became a convert to Christianity. Leif later tried to return home with the intention of taking supplies and spreading Christianity to Greenland, but his ship was blown off course and he arrived in a strange new land: present-day Newfoundland, Canada.

When he finally returned to his adopted homeland of Greenland, Leif consulted with a merchant who had also seen the shores of this previously unknown land. The son of the legendary Viking explorer then gathered a crew of 35 men and set sail. Leif became the first European to step foot in the New World as he explored present-day Baffin Island and Labrador, Canada. His crew called the land Vinland since it was plentiful with grapes.

During their time in present-day Newfoundland, Leif's expedition made contact with the natives, whom they referred to as Skraelings (which translates to "wretched ones" in Norse). There are several secondhand accounts of their meetings. Some contemporaries described trade between the peoples. Other accounts describe clashes where the Skraelings defeated the Viking explorers with long spears, while still others claim the Vikings dominated the natives. Regardless of the circumstances, it seems that the Vikings made contact of some kind. This happened around the year 1000, nearly five hundred years before Columbus famously sailed the ocean blue.

Eventually, in 1003, Leif set sail for home and arrived at Greenland with a ship full of timber.

In 1020, 17 years later, the legendary Viking died. Many believe that Leif Erikson should receive more credit for his contributions in exploring the New World.

24. Which of the following best describes how the author generally presents the information?
    a. Chronological order
    b. Comparison-contrast
    c. Cause-effect
    d. Conclusion-premises

25. Which of the following is an opinion, rather than a historical fact, expressed by the author?
    a. Leif Erikson was definitely the son of Erik the Red; however, historians debate the year of his birth.
    b. Leif Erikson's crew called the land Vinland since it was plentiful with grapes.
    c. Leif Erikson deserves more credit for his contributions in exploring the New World.
    d. Leif Erikson explored the Americas nearly 500 years before Christopher Columbus.

26. Which of the following most accurately describes the author's main conclusion?
    a. Leif Erikson is a legendary Viking explorer.
    b. Leif Erikson deserves more credit for exploring America hundreds of years before Columbus.
    c. Spreading Christianity motivated Leif Erikson's expeditions more than any other factor.
    d. Leif Erikson contacted the natives nearly five hundred years before Columbus.

27. Which of the following best describes the author's intent in the passage?
    a. To entertain
    b. To inform
    c. To alert
    d. To suggest

28. Which of the following can be logically inferred from the passage?
    a. The Vikings disliked exploring the New World.
    b. Leif Erikson's banishment from Iceland led to his exploration of present-day Canada.
    c. Leif Erikson never shared his stories of exploration with the King of Norway.
    d. Historians have difficulty definitively pinpointing events in the Vikings' history.

The next question refers to the following paragraph.

> The Brookside area is an older part of Kansas City, developed mainly in the 1920s and '30s, and is considered one of the nation's first "planned" communities, with shops, restaurants, parks, and churches all within a quick walk. A stroll down any street reveals charming two-story Tudor and Colonial homes with smaller bungalows sprinkled throughout the beautiful tree-lined streets. It is common to see lemonade stands on the corners and baseball games in the numerous "pocket" parks tucked neatly behind rows of well-manicured houses. The Brookside shops on 63rd street between Wornall Road and Oak Street are a hub of commerce and entertainment where residents freely shop and dine with their pets (and children) in tow. This is also a common "hangout" spot for younger teenagers because it is easily accessible by bike for most. In short, it is an idyllic neighborhood just minutes from downtown Kansas City.

29. In what kind of publication might you read the above paragraph?
    a. Fictional novel
    b. Community profile
    c. Newspaper article
    d. Movie review

30. If you were asked to write a comprehensive research paper about life during the Great Depression in the United States, which of the following would be a reliable primary source?
    a. Wikipedia article titled "Life in Depression America."
    b. Diary entry from Elsie May Long published in the article "The Great Depression: Two Kansas Diaries" by C. Robert Haywood in *Great Plains Quarterly*.
    c. Article titled "The Great Depression Begins: the Stock Market Crash of 1929," found at http://www.history.com/topics/great-depression
    d. Book by Glen H. Elder, Jr., titled *Children of the Great Depression: Social Change in Life Experience*, published in 1999 by the American Psychological Association

Question 31 is based on the following table.

Ship 1	Ship 2	Ship 3	Ship 4
Depart: 1:10 p.m.	Depart: 1:00 p.m.	Depart: 1:30 p.m.	Depart: 12:30 p.m.
Arrive: 2:30 p.m.	Arrive: 2:45 p.m.	Arrive: 2:20 p.m.	Arrive: 1:50 p.m.
Return: 4:40 p.m.	Return: 5:30 p.m.	Return: 5:30 p.m.	Return: 5:45 p.m.

31. Lucy and Bob both enjoy fishing and want to take a charter ship to an island, but they have different schedules. Lucy, who works mornings, can't leave until 12:45 p.m. She needs thirty minutes to arrive at the dock. Bob, on the other hand, starts work at 6:30 p.m. and needs an hour to get from the docks to his job. There are four different charter ships available. Based on their schedules, which ship would meet both Lucy and Bob's needs?
   a. Ship 1
   b. Ship 2
   c. Ship 3
   d. Ship 4

The next two questions are based on the following table.

Cooking Oils	Smoking Point F°	Neutral Taste?
Clarified Butter	485°	No
Peanut Oil	450°	Yes
Lard	374°	No
Safflower Oil	510°	Yes
Coconut Oil	350°	No

32. Zack is getting ready to heat some cooking oil. He knows that if an oil goes above its smoking point, it doesn't taste good. For his recipe, he must get the oil to reach 430° F. Zack has a peanut allergy and would prefer a neutral-tasting oil. Which oil should he use?
   a. Clarified butter
   b. Peanut oil
   c. Safflower oil
   d. Coconut oil

33. If Zack still needed the oil to reach 430° F but he didn't have a peanut allergy and preferred a flavored oil, which oil would he use?
   a. Clarified butter
   b. Peanut oil
   c. Safflower oil
   d. Coconut oil

The next two questions are based on the graphic that follows a brief introduction to the topic.

The United States Constitution directs Congress to conduct periodic censuses to determine the country's population. The United States Census Bureau carries out the surveys and collects both population numbers and demographic information. In 1790, then Secretary of State Thomas Jefferson conducted the first census, and the most recent US census was in 2020. The last US census was the first to be issued primarily through the internet.

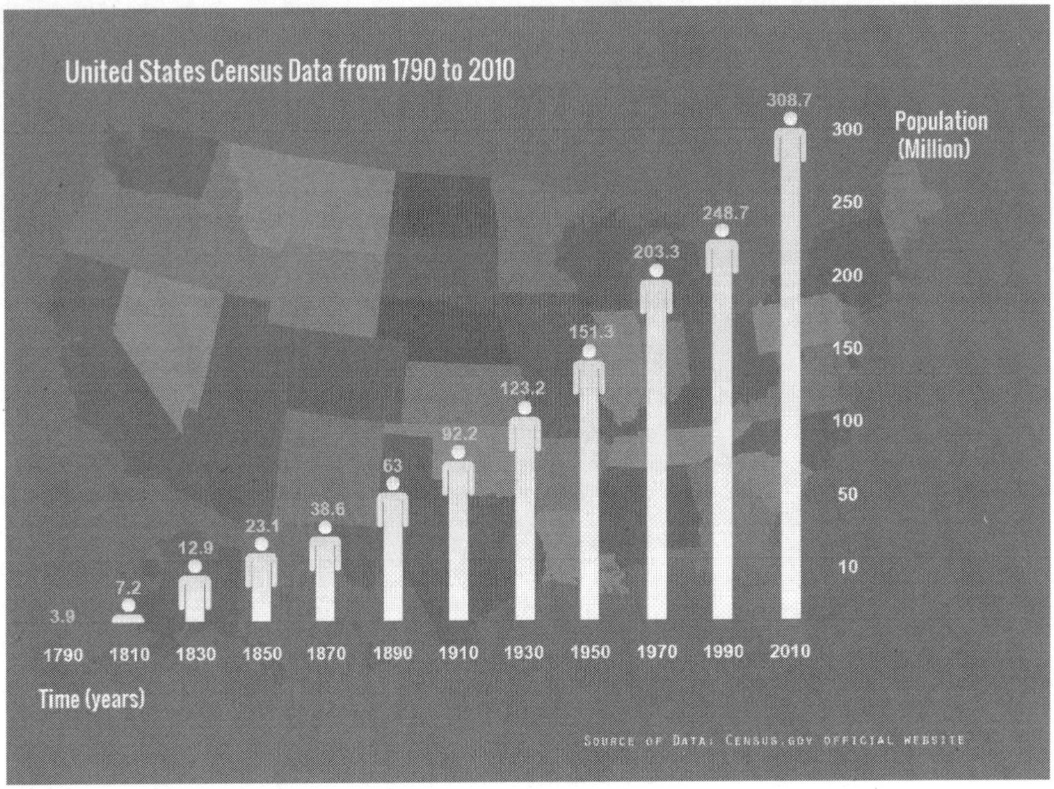

34. Which year marker on the graph first shows the population exceeding 200,000,000 people?

____

35. In what twenty-year interval did the population increase the most?
   a. From 1930 to 1950
   b. From 1950 to 1970
   c. From 1970 to 1990
   d. From 1990 to 2010

The next question is based on the following two passages.

Passage 1

In the modern classroom, cell phones have become indispensable. Cell phones, which are essentially handheld computers, allow students to take notes, connect to the web, perform complex computations, teleconference, and participate in surveys. Most importantly, though, due to their mobility and excellent reception, cell phones are necessary in emergencies. Unlike tablets, laptops, or computers, cell phones are a readily available and free resource—most school district budgets are already strained to begin with—and since today's student is already strongly rooted in technology, when teachers incorporate cell phones, they're "speaking" the student's language, which increases the chance of higher engagement.

Passage 2

As with most forms of technology, there is an appropriate time and place for the use of cell phones. Students are comfortable with cell phones, so it makes sense when teachers allow cell phone use at their discretion. Allowing cell phone use can prove advantageous if done correctly. Unfortunately, if that's not the case—and often it isn't—then a sizable percentage of students pretend to pay attention while *surreptitiously* playing on their phones. This type of disrespectful behavior is often justified by the argument that cell phones are not only a privilege but also a right. Under this logic, confiscating phones is akin to rummaging through students' backpacks. This is in stark contrast to several decades ago when teachers regulated where and when students accessed information.

36. With which of the following statements would both the authors of Passages 1 and 2 agree?
    a. Teachers should incorporate cell phones into curriculum whenever possible.
    b. Cell phones are useful only when an experienced teacher uses them properly.
    c. Cell phones and, moreover, technology are a strong part of today's culture.
    d. Despite a good lesson plan, cell phone disruptions are impossible to avoid.

The next three questions are based on the graphic following a brief introduction to the topic.

A food chain is a diagram used by biologists to better understand ecosystems. It represents the interrelationships between different plants and animals. The energy is derived from the sun and converted into stored energy by plants through photosynthesis, which travels up the food chain. The energy returns to the ecosystem after the organisms die and decompose back into the Earth. This process is an endless cycle.

In food chains, living organisms are grouped into categories called primary producers and consumers, which come in multiple tiers. For example, secondary consumers feed on primary consumers, while tertiary consumers feed on secondary consumers. Apex predators are the animals at the top of the food chain. They are the highest category consumer in an ecosystem, and apex predators do not have natural predators.

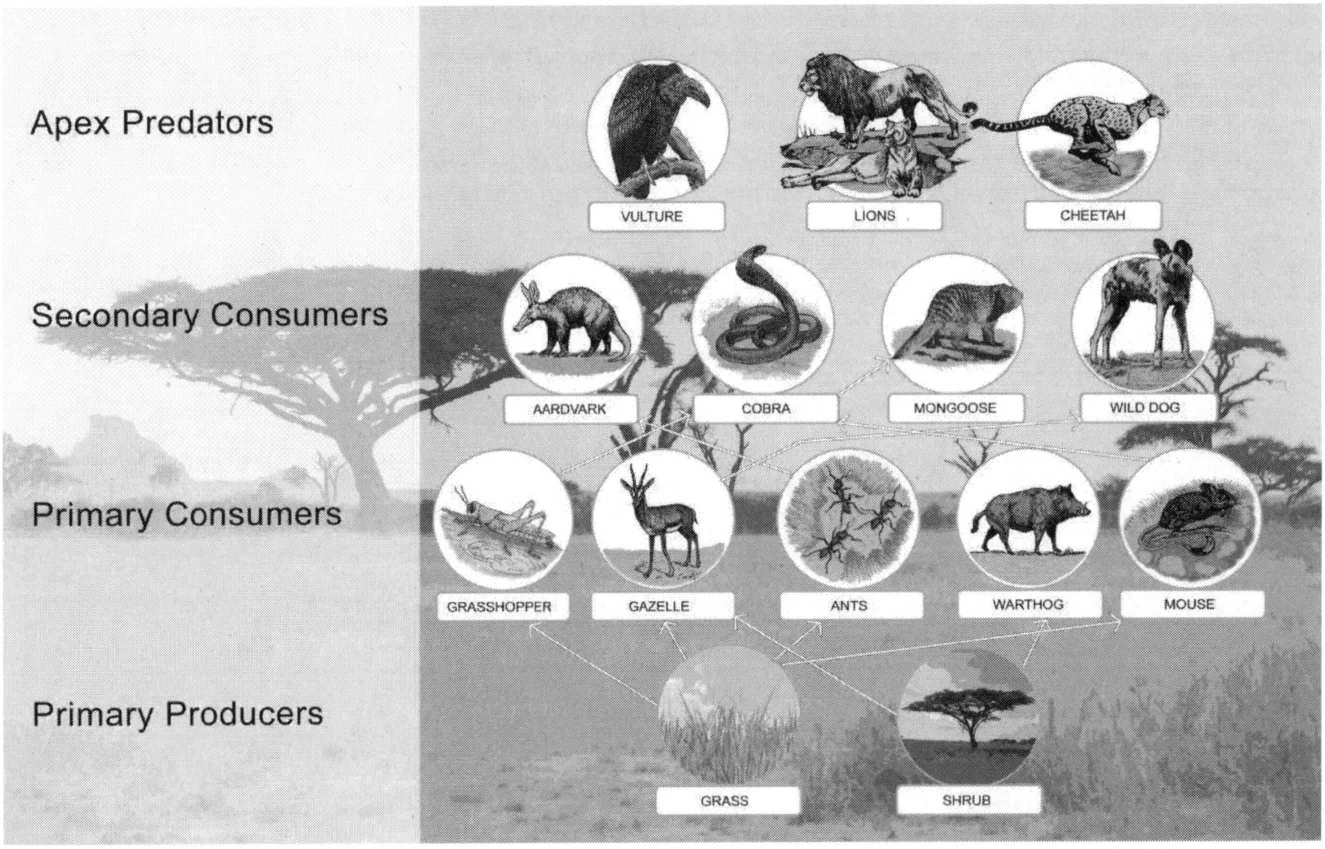

37. Which of the following animals eats primary producers according to the food chain diagram?
   a. Cobra
   b. Gazelle
   c. Wild dog
   d. Aardvark

38. Which of the following animals has no natural predators according to the food chain diagram?
   a. Vulture
   b. Cobra
   c. Mongoose
   d. Aardvark

39. Which of the following is something that the mongoose would eat?
   a. Shrub
   b. Aardvark
   c. Vulture
   d. Mouse

40. Which of the following statements would make the best conclusion to an essay about civil rights activist Rosa Parks?
   a. On December 1, 1955, Rosa Parks refused to give up her bus seat to a white passenger, setting in motion the Montgomery bus boycott.
   b. Rosa Parks was a hero to many and came to symbolize the way that ordinary people could bring about real change in the civil rights movement.
   c. Rosa Parks died in 2005 in Detroit, having moved from Montgomery shortly after the bus boycott.
   d. Rosa Parks' arrest was an early part of the civil rights movement and helped lead to the passage of the Civil Rights Act of 1964.

41. The following exchange occurred after the baseball coach's team suffered a heartbreaking loss in the final inning:

Reporter: The team clearly did not rise to the challenge. I'm sure that getting zero hits in 20 at-bats with runners in scoring position hurt the team's chances at winning the game. What are your thoughts on this devastating loss?

Baseball Coach: Hitting with runners in scoring position was not the reason we lost this game. We made numerous errors in the field, and our pitchers gave out too many free passes. Also, we did not even need a hit with runners in scoring position. Many of those at-bats could have driven in the run by simply making contact. Our team did not deserve to win the game.

Which of the following best describes the main point of dispute between the reporter and baseball coach?
   a. The loss was heartbreaking.
   b. Getting zero hits in 20 at-bats with runners in scoring position caused the loss.
   c. Numerous errors in the field and pitchers giving too many free passes caused the loss.
   d. The team deserved to win the game.

42. The question is based on the following passage: Which option best expresses the symbolic meaning of the "road" and the overall theme?

> Two roads diverged in a yellow wood,
> And sorry I could not travel both
> And be one traveler, long I stood
> And looked down one as far as I could
> To where it bent in the undergrowth;
>
> Then took the other, as just as fair,
> And having perhaps the better claim,
> Because it was grassy and wanted wear;
> Though as for that the passing there
> Had worn them really about the same,
>
> And both that morning equally lay
> In leaves no step had trodden black.
> Oh, I kept the first for another day!
> Yet knowing how way leads on to way,

I doubted if I should ever come back.

I shall be telling this with a sigh
Somewhere ages and ages hence:
Two roads diverged in a wood, and I—
I took the one less traveled by,
And that has made all the difference
—Robert Frost, *The Road Not Taken*

a. A spot where the traveler had to choose between two paths
b. A choice between good and evil that the traveler needs to make
c. The traveler's feelings about a lost love and future prospects
d. Life's journey and the choices with which humans are faced

43. Dwight works at a mid-sized regional tech company. He approaches all tasks with unmatched enthusiasm and leads the company in annual sales. The top salesman is always the best employee. Therefore, Dwight is the best employee.

Which of the following most accurately describes how the argument proceeds?

a. The argument proceeds by first stating a conclusion and then offering several premises to justify that conclusion.
b. The argument proceeds by stating a universal rule and then proceeds to show how this situation is the exception.
c. The argument proceeds by stating several facts that serve as the basis for the conclusion at the end of the argument.
d. The argument proceeds by stating several facts, offering a universal rule, and then drawing a conclusion by applying the facts to the rule.

44. Read the following passage:

> After looking for our perfect pet for several months, we adopted a dog from the local animal shelter last week. We wanted a dog that was not too old, but also past the puppy stage, so that training would be less time-intensive and we could give an older animal a home. Robin, as she's called, was a perfect match. We filled out our application and were approved to bring her home. Her physical exam and lab work all confirmed she was healthy. We went to the pet store and bought all sorts of bedding, food, toys, and treats to outfit our house as a dog-friendly and fun place. The shelter told us she liked dry food only, which is a relief because wet food is expensive and pretty off-putting. We even got fencing and installed a dog run in the backyard for Robin to roam unattended. Then we took her to the vet to make sure she was healthy. Next week, she starts the dog obedience class that we enrolled her in with a discount coupon from the shelter. It will be a good opportunity to bond with her and establish commands and dominance. When we took her to the park the afternoon after we adopted her, it was clear that she is a sociable and friendly dog, easily playing cohesively with dogs of all sizes and dispositions.

Which of the following is out of sequence in the story?

a. After looking for our perfect pet for several months, we adopted a dog from the local animal shelter last week.
b. Robin, as she's called, was a perfect match. We filled out our application and were approved to bring her home.
c. Her physical exam and lab work all confirmed she was healthy.
d. Next week, she starts the dog obedience class that we enrolled her in with a discount coupon from the shelter.

45. You are a high school math teacher and one of your students, Marcus, emailed asking to come see you after the latest exam. His email said he was disappointed and surprised with his grade and wanted to inquire about extra credit work to recoup points he lost on the exam. You decided to look over the details of his performance in your course to find any potential causes for his poor marks and to offer him informed tips to improve for the next exam. Thankfully, you keep detailed records to tracks each student's grades. You have four pieces of information to evaluate before he comes in to meet with you: a graph of his scores on the four exams he's taken so far, a graph of the number of absences he's had each week thus far in the course, a graph of the percentage of homework assignments he's completed each week, and an email from his basketball coach.

> From: William Cooper, Boys Varsity Basketball Coach
> To: All academic teachers
> Re: Marco
>
> Marco will be competing in the Northeast Regional Basketball tournament next week and will be absent from classes Tuesday through Friday. The student athletes will be responsible for obtaining their assignments and making arrangements to complete any missed material. If you have any questions, please don't hesitate to reach out to me. While I understand that this is not ideal so close to final exams, this is the first time our Ravens have made it so far in the tournament, and we are excited to see how well they will perform.
>
> Thanks,
> Coach William Cooper

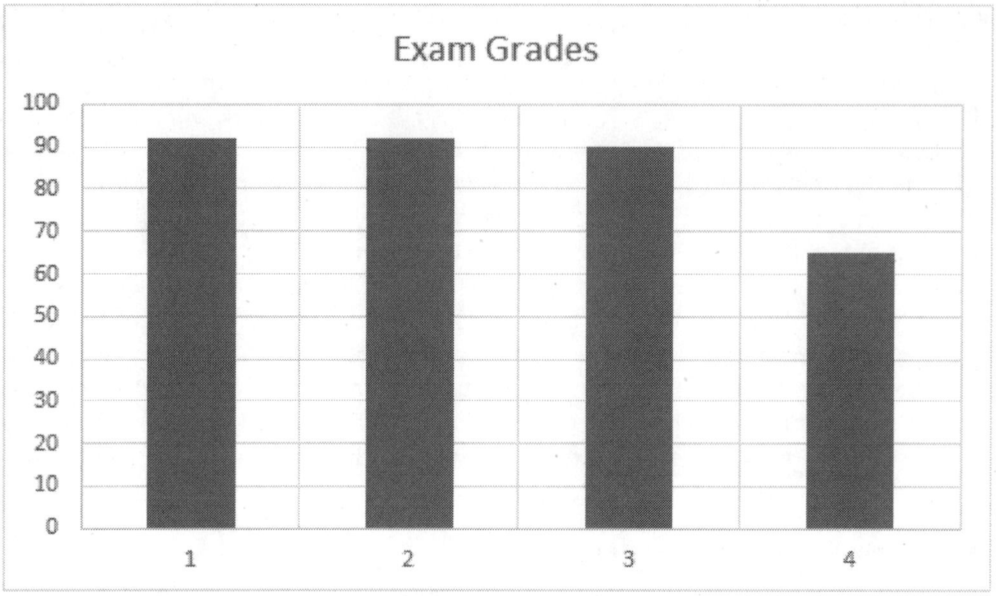
Exam Grades
100
90
80
70
60
50
40
30
20
10
0
1
2
3
4

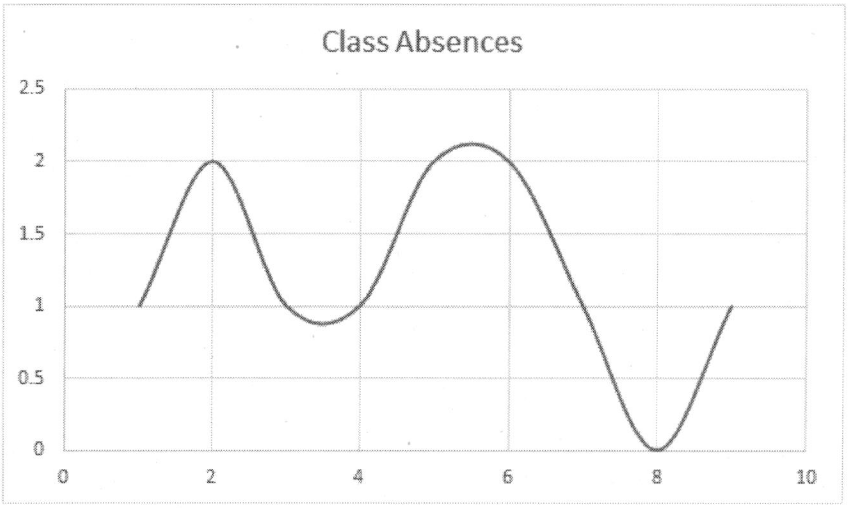
Class Absences
2.5
2
1.5
1
0.5
0
0
2
4
6
8
10

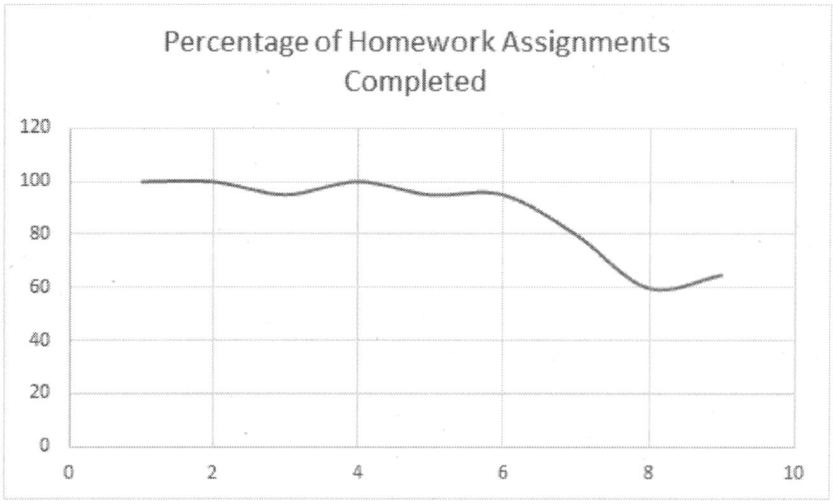
Percentage of Homework Assignments Completed
120
100
80
60
40
20
0
0
2
4
6
8
10

Which of the given information sources provides a possible explanation for a Marco's recent poor exam grade?

a. The email from his basketball coach about the tournament
b. The graph of his exam marks
c. The graph of his class absences each week
d. The graph of the percentage of homework assignments completed

Mathematics

1. Which of the following numbers has the greatest value?

a. 1.43785
b. 1.07548
c. 1.43592
d. 0.89409

2. The value of 6×12 is the same as:

a. $2 \times 4 \times 4 \times 2$
b. $7 \times 4 \times 3$
c. $6 \times 6 \times 3$
d. $3 \times 3 \times 4 \times 2$

3. This chart indicates how many sales of CDs, vinyl records, and MP3 downloads occurred over the last year. Approximately what percentage of the total sales was from CDs?

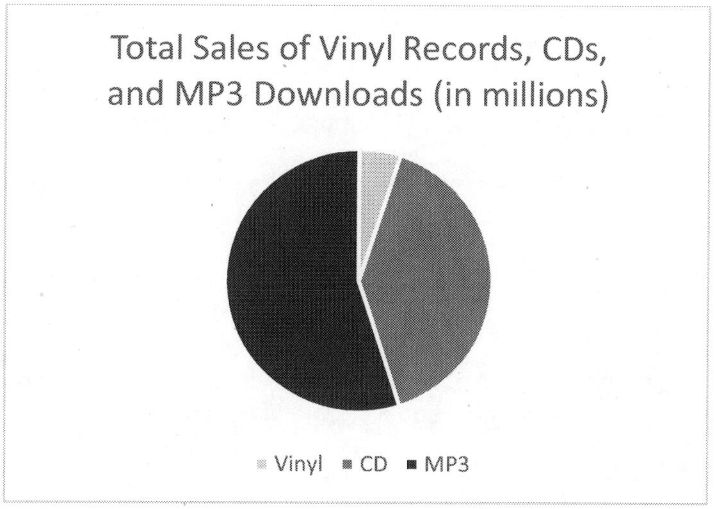

a. 55%
b. 25%
c. 40%
d. 5%

4. After a 20% sale discount, Frank purchased a new refrigerator for $850. How much did he save compared to the original price?

a. $170
b. $212.50
c. $105.75
d. $200

5. Which of the following values is the largest?
   a. 0.45
   b. 0.096
   c. 0.3
   d. 0.313

6. The value of b in this equation is ______.

$$5b - 4 = 2b + 17$$

7. A school's faculty consists of 15 teachers and 20 teaching assistants. They have 200 students. What is the ratio of faculty to students?
   a. $3 : 20$
   b. $4 : 17$
   c. $3 : 2$
   d. $7 : 40$

8. Express the following in decimal form:

$$\frac{3}{5} \times \frac{7}{10} \div \frac{1}{2}$$

   a. 0.042
   b. 84%
   c. 0.84
   d. 0.42

9. A student gets an 85% on a test with 20 questions. How many questions did the student solve correctly? _____

10. If Sarah reads at an average rate of 21 pages in 4 nights, how long will it take her to read 140 pages?
   a. 6 nights
   b. 26 nights
   c. 8 nights
   d. 27 nights

11. Alan currently weighs 200 pounds, but he wants to lose weight to get down to 175 pounds. What is this difference in kilograms? (1 pound is approximately equal to 0.45 kilograms.)
   a. 9 kg
   b. 11.25 kg
   c. 78.75 kg
   d. 90 kg

12. Johnny earns $2,334.50 from his job each month. He pays $1,437 for monthly expenses and saves the rest. Johnny is planning a vacation in 3 months that he estimates will cost $1,750 total. How much will Johnny have left over from 3 months of saving once he pays for his vacation?
   a. $948.50
   b. $584.50
   c. $852.50
   d. $942.50

13. $\frac{420}{98}$ rounded to the nearest integer is _____.

14. Consider a four-year private institution that you would like to attend for college. The tuition per year is $22,000, and it is estimated that room and board will be $5,000 per year and books will cost you $500 per year. Your family is expected to pay for 25% of your total expenses, and you will be paying for the rest. How much will you have to have in a savings account to cover your portion if you would like to have the total amount for all four years available before you even attend?

a. $82,500
b. $110,000
c. $88,000
d. $27,500

15. The total perimeter of a rectangle is 36 cm. If the length is 12 cm, then the width is ________.

16. Dwayne has received the following scores on his math tests: 78, 92, 83, 97. What score must Dwayne get on his next math test to have an overall average of 90?

a. 89
b. 98
c. 95
d. 100

17. What is the overall median of Dwayne's current scores: 78, 92, 83, 97?

a. 80.5
b. 85
c. 90
d. 87.5

18. Solve the following:

$$(\sqrt{36} \times \sqrt{16}) - 3^2$$

a. 30
b. 21
c. 15
d. 13

19. In Jim's school, there are a total of 650 boys and girls. There are three girls for every two boys. How many students are girls?

a. 260
b. 130
c. 65
d. 390

20. What is $4 \times 7 + (25 - 21)^2 \div 2$?

a. 512
b. 36
c. 60.5
d. 22

21. Kimberley earns \$10 an hour babysitting, and after 10 p.m., she earns \$12 an hour. The time she works is rounded to the nearest hour for pay purposes. On her last job, she worked from 5:30 p.m. to 11:00 p.m. In total, how much did Kimberley earn on her last job?

a. \$45
b. \$57
c. \$62
d. \$42

22. What value of x would solve the following equation?

$$9x + x - 7 = 16 + 2x$$

a. $x = -4$
b. $x = 3$
c. $x = \frac{9}{8}$
d. $x = \frac{23}{8}$

23. Arrange the following numbers from least to greatest value:

$$0.85, \frac{4}{5}, \frac{2}{3}, \frac{91}{100}$$

a. $0.85, \frac{4}{5}, \frac{2}{3}, \frac{91}{100}$
b. $\frac{4}{5}, 0.85, \frac{91}{100}, \frac{2}{3}$
c. $\frac{2}{3}, \frac{4}{5}, 0.85, \frac{91}{100}$
d. $0.85, \frac{91}{100}, \frac{4}{5}, \frac{2}{3}$

24. Keith's bakery had 252 customers go through its doors last week. This week, that number increased to 378. Express this increase as a percentage.

a. 26%
b. 50%
c. 35%
d. 12%

25. According to building code regulations, the roof of a house has to be set at a minimum angle of 39° up to a maximum angle of 48° to ensure snow and rain will properly slide off it. What is the maximum incline in terms of radians?

a. $\frac{\pi}{4}$
b. $\frac{\pi}{15}$
c. $\frac{4\pi}{15}$
d. $\frac{3\pi}{4}$

26. Simplify the following fraction:

$$\frac{\left(\frac{5}{7}\right)}{\left(\frac{9}{11}\right)}$$

a. $\frac{55}{63}$
b. $\frac{7}{1{,}000}$
c. $\frac{13}{15}$
d. $\frac{5}{11}$

27. The following graph compares the various test scores of the top three students in each of these teachers' classes. Based on the graph, which teacher's students had the lowest range of test scores?

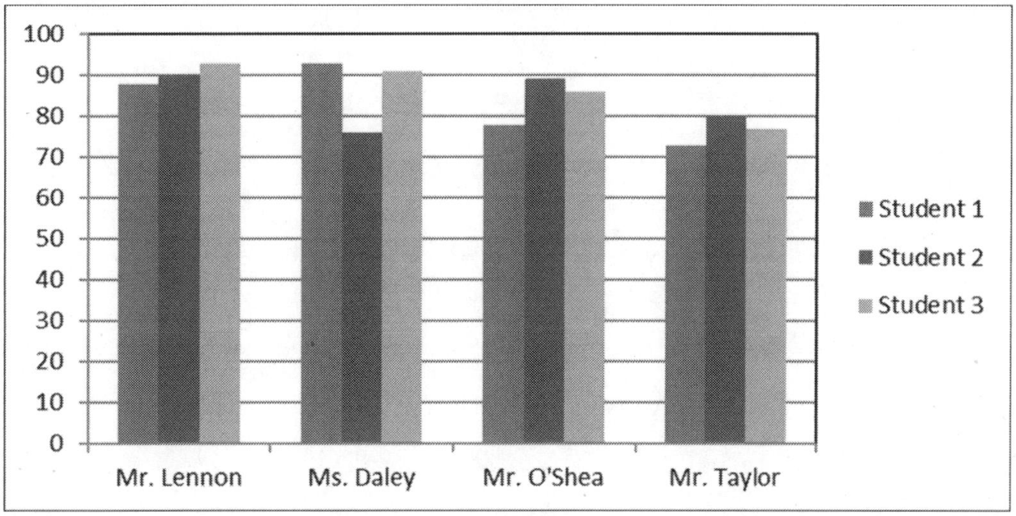

a. Mr. Lennon
b. Mr. O'Shea
c. Mr. Taylor
d. Ms. Daley

28. Bernard can make \$80 per day. If he needs to make \$300 and only works full days, it will take _____ days.

29. Five of six numbers have a sum of 25. The average of all six numbers is 6. What is the sixth number?
a. 8
b. 10
c. 11
d. 12

30. Which measure for the center of a small sample set would be most affected by outliers?
a. Mean
b. Median
c. Mode
d. None of the above

31. A line that travels from the lower left of a graph to the upper right of the graph indicates what kind of relationship between an independent and a dependent variable?
   a. Positive
   b. Negative
   c. Exponential
   d. Logarithmic

32. Approximately how many kilometers is 4,382 feet? There are 0.3048 meters in 1 foot.
   a. 1.336 kilometers
   b. 14,376 kilometers
   c. 1.437 kilometers
   d. 13,336 kilometers

33. Which of the following is the best description of the relationship between x and y?

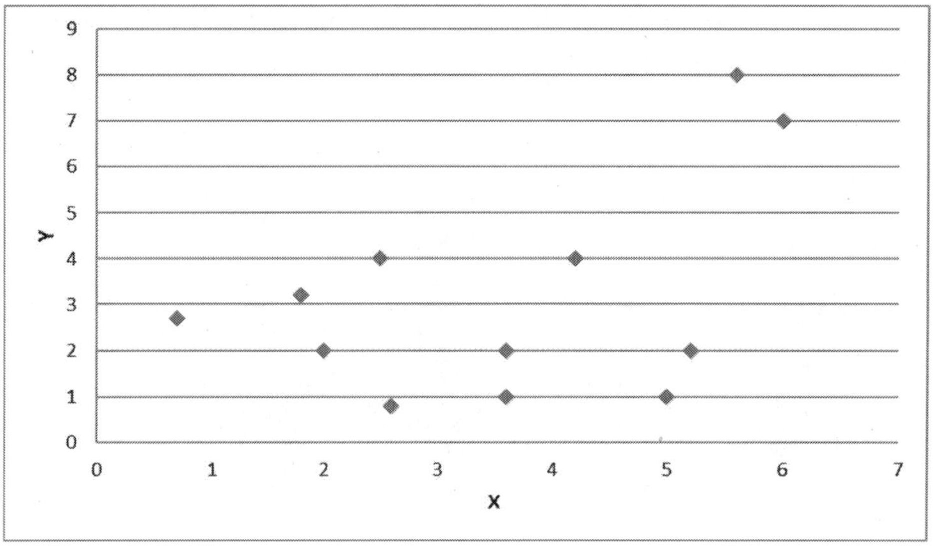

   a. The data has normal distribution.
   b. x and y have a negative relationship.
   c. x and y have no apparent relation.
   d. x and y have a positive relationship.

34. What is the slope of this line?

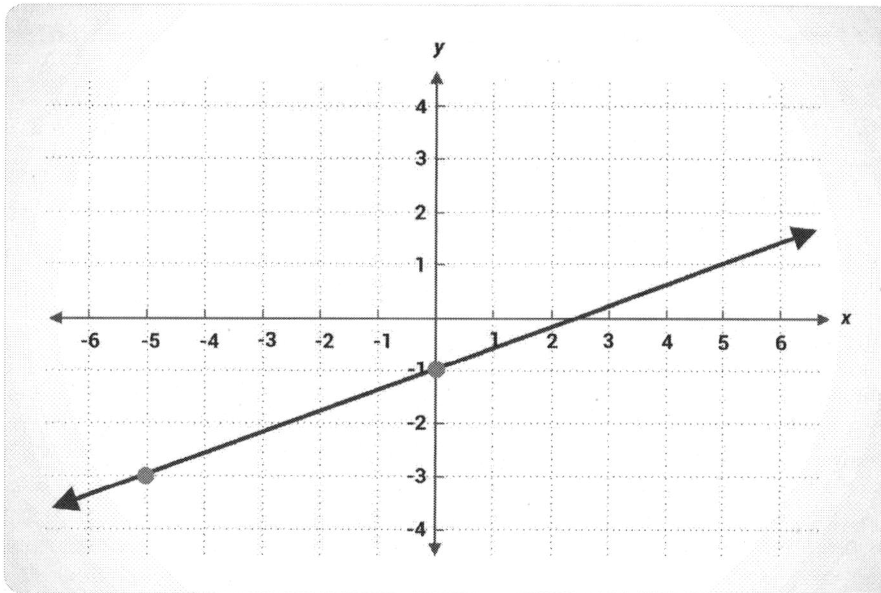

a. 2
b. $\frac{5}{2}$
c. $\frac{1}{2}$
d. $\frac{2}{5}$

35. What is the perimeter of the figure below? Note that the solid outer line is the perimeter.

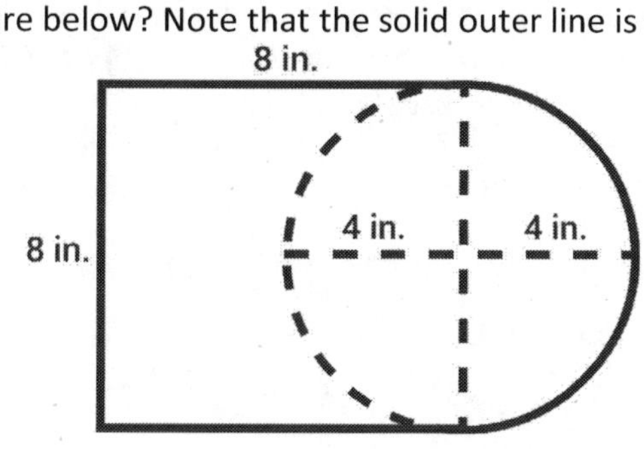

a. 48.565 in
b. 36.565 in
c. 39.78 in
d. 39.565 in

36. Which of the following equations best represents the problem below?

The width of a rectangle is 2 centimeters less than the length. If the perimeter of the rectangle is 44 centimeters, then what are the dimensions of the rectangle?

a. $2l + 2(l - 2) = 44$
b. $(l + 2) + (l + 2) + l = 48$
c. $l \times (l - 2) = 44$
d. $(l + 2) + (l + 2) + l = 44$

37. An equilateral triangle has a perimeter of 18 feet. The sides of a square have the same length as the triangle's sides. What is the area of the square?

a. 6 square feet
b. 36 square feet
c. 256 square feet
d. 1,000 square feet

38. A cube has sides that are 7 inches long. What is the cube's volume?

a. 49 in^3
b. 343 in^3
c. 294 in^3
d. 28 in^3

Science

1. Which statement about white blood cells is true?

a. B cells are responsible for antibody production.
b. White blood cells are made in the white/yellow cartilage before they enter the bloodstream.
c. Platelets, a special class of white blood cell, function to clot blood and stop bleeding.
d. The majority of white blood cells only activate during the age of puberty, which explains why children and the elderly are particularly susceptible to disease.

2. Identify the aorta by placing an "X" on its location:

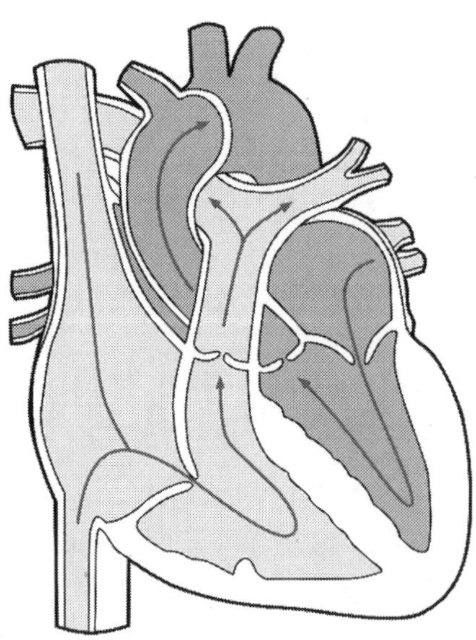

3. Which of the following are functions of the urinary system? *Select all that apply.*
   a. Synthesizing calcitriol and secreting erythropoietin
   b. Regulating the concentrations of sodium, potassium, chloride, calcium, and other ions
   c. Reabsorbing or secreting hydrogen ions and bicarbonate
   d. Detecting reductions in blood volume and pressure

4. Jackson wants to open a dog training business. He wants to see which dog treat is most effective in training dogs to sit. If he wants to design an experiment that tests 20 dogs to figure out which treats are the best to use, what would be a good dependent variable?
   a. Type of food
   b. A good dependent variable would be the time in seconds that the dogs sit.
   c. How many times the dog wags its tail
   d. Shape of food

5. Which cellular organelle is used for digestion to recycle materials?
   a. The Golgi apparatus
   b. The lysosome
   c. The centrioles
   d. The mitochondria

6. What is the sensory threshold?
   a. The smallest amount of stimulus required for an individual to feel a sensation
   b. The amount of stimulus required for an individual to feel pain
   c. The amount of stimulus required to cause an individual to move away from the stimulus
   d. The place where the stimulus is coming from

7. Why do arteries have valves?
   a. They have valves to maintain high blood pressure so that capillaries diffuse nutrients properly.
   b. Their valves are designed to prevent backflow due to their low blood pressure.
   c. They have valves due to a leftover trait from evolution that, like the appendix, are useless.
   d. They do not have valves, but veins do have valves.

8. If the pressure in the pulmonary artery is increased above normal, which chamber of the heart will be affected first?
   a. The right atrium
   b. The left atrium
   c. The right ventricle
   d. The left ventricle

9. What is the last phase of mitosis?
   a. Prophase
   b. Telophase
   c. Anaphase
   d. Metaphase

10. Which of the following describes a reflex arc?
   a. The storage and recall of memory
   b. The maintenance of visual and auditory acuity
   c. The autoregulation of heart rate and blood pressure
   d. A stimulus and response controlled by the spinal cord

11. Describe the synthesis of the lagging strand of DNA.
    a. DNA polymerases synthesize DNA continuously after initially attaching to a primase.
    b. DNA polymerases synthesize DNA discontinuously in pieces called Okazaki fragments after initially attaching to primases.
    c. DNA polymerases synthesize DNA discontinuously in pieces called Okazaki fragments after initially attaching to RNA primers.
    d. DNA polymerases synthesize DNA discontinuously in pieces called Okazaki fragments which are joined together in the end by a DNA helicase.

12. Using anatomical terms, what is the relationship of the sternum relative to the deltoid?
    a. Medial
    b. Lateral
    c. Superficial
    d. Posterior

13. Ligaments connect what?
    a. Muscle to muscle
    b. Bone to bone
    c. Bone to muscle
    d. Muscle to tendon

Use the following image to answer the next question:

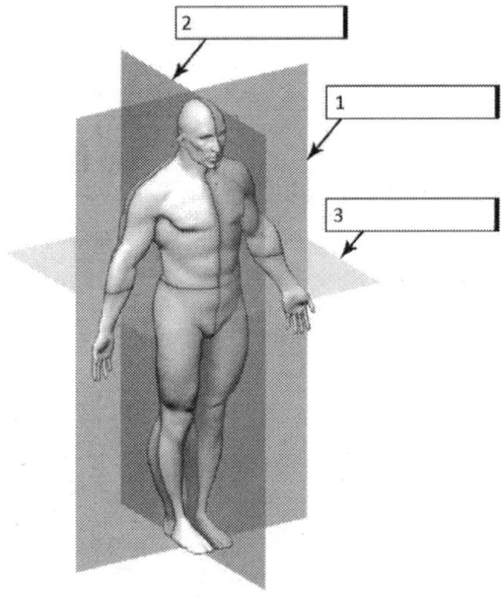

14. Identify the correct sequence of the 3 primary body planes as numbered 1, 2, and 3 in the above image.
    a. Plane 1 is coronal, plane 2 is sagittal, and plane 3 is transverse.
    b. Plane 1 is sagittal, plane 2 is coronal, and plane 3 is medial.
    c. Plane 1 is coronal, plane 2 is sagittal, and plane 3 is medial.
    d. Plane 1 is sagittal, plane 2 is coronal, and plane 3 is transverse.

15. Which of the following is NOT a major function of the respiratory system in humans?
    a. It provides a large surface area for gas exchange of oxygen and carbon dioxide.
    b. It helps regulate the blood's pH.
    c. It helps cushion the heart against jarring motions.
    d. It is responsible for vocalization.

16. Which of the following structures is unique to eukaryotic cells?
    a. Cell walls
    b. Nuclei
    c. Cell membranes
    d. Organelles

17. What is the major difference between somatic and germline mutations?
    a. Somatic mutations usually benefit the individual, while germline mutations usually harm them.
    b. Since germline mutations only affect one cell, they are less noticeable than the rapidly dividing somatic cells.
    c. Somatic mutations are not expressed for several generations, but germline mutations are expressed immediately.
    d. Germline mutations are usually inherited while somatic mutations will affect only the individual.

18. A child complains of heavy breathing even when relaxing. They are an otherwise healthy child with no history of respiratory problems. What might be the issue?
    a. Asthma
    b. A blood clot
    c. Hyperventilation
    d. Exercising too hard

19. How is a theory different from a hypothesis?
    a. Theories are predictions based on previous research, and hypotheses are proven.
    b. Hypotheses can change, while theories cannot.
    c. Theories are accepted by scientists, while hypotheses remain to be proven.
    d. Hypotheses are always wrong, while theories are always true.

20. The following are steps in the scientific method. Put them in the correct order.

- Accept or reject the hypothesis
- Create or propose a hypothesis
- Ask a question
- Make observations
- Test the hypothesis
- Formulate an experiment

1. ______________________
2. ______________________
3. ______________________
4. ______________________
5. ______________________
6. ______________________

21. Most catalysts found in biological systems are which of the following?
    a. Special lipids called cofactors
    b. Special proteins called enzymes
    c. Special lipids called enzymes
    d. Special proteins called cofactors

22. Which statement is true about the pH of a solution?
    a. A solution cannot have a pH less than 1.
    b. The more hydroxide ions in the solution, the higher the pH.
    c. If an acid has a pH greater than 2, it is considered a weak base.
    d. A solution with a pH of 2 has ten times more hydrogen ions than a solution with a pH of 1.

23. Salts like sodium iodide (NaI) and potassium chloride (KCl) use what type of bond?
    a. Ionic bonds
    b. Disulfide bridges
    c. Covalent bonds
    d. London dispersion forces

24. Which of the following is unique to covalent bonds?
    a. Most covalent bonds are formed between the elements H, F, N, and O.
    b. Covalent bonds are dependent on forming dipoles.
    c. Bonding electrons are shared between two or more atoms.
    d. Molecules with covalent bonds tend to have a crystalline solid structure.

25. Which of the following describes a typical gas?
    a. Indefinite shape and indefinite volume
    b. Indefinite shape and definite volume
    c. Definite shape and definite volume
    d. Definite shape and indefinite volume

26. Which of the following areas of the body has the highest density of sweat glands?
    a. Upper back
    b. Arms
    c. Palms/soles of the feet
    d. Head

27. A patient's body is not properly filtering blood. Which of the following body parts is most likely malfunctioning?
    a. Medulla
    B. Heart
    C. Nephrons
    D. Renal cortex

28. A pediatrician notes that an infant's cartilage is disappearing and being replaced by bone. What process has the doctor observed?
    a. Mineralization
    b. Ossification
    c. Osteoporosis
    d. Calcification

29. Which of the following correctly matches a category of protein with a physiologic example?
    a. Keratin is a structural protein.
    b. Antigens are hormonal proteins.
    c. Channel proteins are marker proteins.
    d. Actin is a transport protein.

30. Which of the following is directly transcribed from DNA and represents the first step in protein building?
    a. siRNA
    b. rRNA
    c. mRNA
    d. tRNA

31. What information does a genotype give that a phenotype does not?
    a. The genotype necessarily includes the proteins coded for by its alleles.
    b. The genotype will always show an organism's recessive alleles.
    c. The genotype must include the organism's physical characteristics.
    d. The genotype shows what an organism's parents looked like.

32. Which statement is supported by the Punnett square below, if "T" = Tall and "t" = short?

	T	*t*
T		
t		

    a. Both parents are homozygous tall.
    b. 100% of the offspring will be tall because both parents are tall.
    c. There is a 25% chance that an offspring will be short.
    d. The short allele will soon die out.

33. Which of the following is a chief difference between evaporation and boiling?
   a. Liquids boil only at the surface, while they evaporate equally throughout the liquid.
   b. Evaporating substances change from gas to liquid, while boiling substances change from liquid to gas.
   c. Evaporation happens in nature, while boiling is a man-made phenomenon.
   d. Evaporation can happen below a liquid's boiling point.

34. Which of the following is NOT be found in a human cell's genes?
   a. Sequences of amino acids to be transcribed into mRNA
   b. Lethal recessive traits like sickle cell anemia
   c. Mutated DNA
   d. DNA that codes for proteins the cell doesn't use

35. Which of the following is a special property of water?
   a. Water easily flows through phospholipid bilayers.
   b. A water molecule's oxygen atom allows fish to breathe.
   c. Water is highly cohesive which explains its high boiling point
   d. Water can self-hydrolyze and decompose into hydrogen and oxygen.

36. For any given element, an isotope is an atom with which of the following?
   a. A different atomic number
   b. A different number of protons
   c. A different number of electrons
   d. A different mass number

37. What is the electrical charge of the nucleus?
   a. A nucleus always has a positive charge.
   b. A stable nucleus has a positive charge, but a radioactive nucleus may be neutral with no charge.
   c. A nucleus is always neutral with no charge.
   d. A stable nucleus is neutral with no charge, but a radioactive nucleus may have a charge.

38. A student believes that there is an inverse relationship between sugar consumption and test scores. To test this hypothesis, he recruits several people to eat sugar, wait one hour, and take a short aptitude test afterwards. The student will compile the participants' sugar intake levels and test scores. How should the student conduct the experiment?
   a. One round of testing, where each participant consumes a different level of sugar.
   b. Two rounds of testing: The first, where each participant consumes a different level of sugar, and the second, where each participant consumes the same level as they did in round 1.
   c. Two rounds of testing: The first, where each participant consumes the same level of sugar as each other, and the second, where each participant consumes the same level of sugar as each other but at higher levels than in round 1.
   d. One round of testing, where each participant consumes the same level of sugar.

39. Which of the following creates sperm?
   a. Prostate gland
   b. Seminal vesicles
   c. Scrotum
   d. Seminiferous tubules

40. A researcher is exploring factors that contribute to the GPA of college students. While the sample is small, the researcher is trying to determine what the data shows. What can be reasoned from the table below?

Student	Maintains a Calendar?	Takes Notes?	GPA
A	Sometimes	Often	3.1
B	Never	Always	3.9
C	Never	Never	2.0
D	Sometimes	Often	2.7

a. No college students consistently maintain a calendar of events.
b. There is an inverse correlation between maintaining a calendar and GPA, and there is a positive correlation between taking notes and GPA.
c. There is a positive correlation between maintaining a calendar and GPA, and there is no correlation between taking notes and GPA.
d. There is no correlation between maintaining a calendar and GPA, and there is a positive correlation between taking notes and GPA.

41. Four different groups of the same species of peas are grown and exposed to differing levels of sunlight, water, and fertilizer as documented in the table below. The data in the water and fertilizer columns indicates how many times the peas are watered or fertilized per week, respectively. Group 2 is the only group that withered. What is a reasonable explanation for this occurrence?

Group	Sunlight	Water	Fertilizer
1	Partial sun	4 mL/hr	1
2	Full sun	7 mL/hr	1
3	No sun	14 mL/hr	2
4	Partial sun	3 mL/hr	2

a. Insects gnawed away the stem of the plant.
b. The roots rotted due to poor drainage.
c. The soil type had nutrition deficiencies.
d. This species of peas does not thrive in full sunlight.

42. Which of the following functions corresponds to the parasympathetic nervous system?
a. It stimulates the fight-or-flight response.
b. It increases heart rate.
c. It stimulates digestion.
d. It increases bronchiole dilation.

43. The following elements all are found on the right side of the periodic table, in the p-block:

Fluorine
Oxygen
Neon
Tin

List them from least reactive to most reactive below:

1. ____________________
2. ____________________
3. ____________________
4. ____________________

44. The Human Genome Project is a worldwide research project launched in 1990 to map the entire human genome. Although the Project was faced with the monumental challenge of analyzing tons and tons of data, its objective was completed in 2003 and ahead of its deadline by two years. Which of the following inventions likely had the greatest impact on this project?

a. The sonogram
b. X-ray diffraction
c. The microprocessor
d. Magnetic Resonance Imaging (MRI)

45. Which of the following inventions likely had the greatest improvement on the ability to combat nutrition deficiencies in developing countries?

a. Food products fortified with dietary vitamins and minerals
b. Integrated statistical models of fish populations
c. Advances so that microscopes can use thicker tissue samples
d. Refrigerated train cars for transportation of food

46. Anya was paid by Company X to analyze dwindling honeybee populations of the Southwest. After measuring hive populations over several months, she noticed no patterns in the geographic distributions of the deaths after comparisons with local maps of interest. This supported her hypothesis, so she took samples of the honey and the bees from the hives and performed dozens of dissections to confirm her suspicions. Which of the following is the most likely hypothesis upon which this research was performed?

a. Honeybees are being killed off and having their hives destroyed by other extremely aggressive species of bees from the South.
b. Honeybees are contracting parasites in large droves.
c. Honeybees are so sensitive to certain pesticides that they die on contact.
d. Honeybees die in larger numbers around cell phone towers.

47. Which of the following is the best unit to measure the amount of blood in the human body?

a. Ounces
b. Liters
c. Milliliters
d. Pounds

48. Which of the following systems does NOT include a transportation system throughout the body?
   a. Cardiovascular system
   b. Endocrine system
   c. Immune system
   d. Nervous system

49. Which of the following correctly identifies a difference between the primary and secondary immune responses?
   a. In the secondary response, macrophages migrate to the lymph nodes to present the foreign microorganism to helper T lymphocytes.
   b. The humeral immunity that characterizes the primary response is coordinated by T lymphocytes.
   c. The primary response is quicker and more powerful than the secondary response.
   d. Suppressor T cells activate in the secondary response to prevent an overactive immune response.

50. Eosinophils are best described as which of the following?
   a. A type of granulocyte that secretes histamine, which stimulates the inflammatory response
   b. The most abundant type of white blood cell, which secretes substances that are toxic to pathogens
   c. A type of granulocyte found under mucous membranes that defends against multicellular parasites
   d. A type of circulating granulocyte that is aggressive and has high phagocytic activity

English and Language Usage

1. Which of the following sentences has an error in capitalization?
   a. The East Coast has experienced very unpredictable weather this year.
   b. My Uncle owns a home in Florida, where he lives in the winter.
   c. I am taking English Composition II on campus this fall.
   d. There are several nice beaches we can visit on our trip to the Jersey Shore this summer.

2. Julia Robinson, an avid photographer in her spare time, was able to capture stunning shots of the local wildlife on her last business trip to Australia.

Which of the following is an adjective in the preceding sentence?
   a. Time
   b. Capture
   c. Avid
   d. Photographer

3. Which of the following sentences uses correct punctuation?
   a. Carole is not currently working; her focus is on her children at the moment.
   b. Carole is not currently working and her focus is on her children at the moment.
   c. Carole is not currently working, her focus is on her children at the moment.
   d. Carole is not currently working her focus is on her children at the moment.

4. Which of these examples is a compound sentence?
   a. Alex and Shane spent the morning coloring and later took a walk down to the park.
   b. After coloring all morning, Alex and Shane spent the afternoon at the park.
   c. Alex and Shane spent the morning coloring, and then they took a walk down to the park.
   d. After coloring all morning and spending part of the day at the park, Alex and Shane took a nap.

5. Which of these examples shows INCORRECT use of subject-verb agreement?
   a. Neither of the cars are parked on the street.
   b. Both of my kids are going to camp this summer.
   c. Any of your friends are welcome to join us on the trip in November.
   d. Each of the clothing options is appropriate for the job interview.

6. Compared to other students, twelve-year-old Dave is somewhat of an oddity at six feet, two inches (tallness runs in his family). The parentheses here indicate what?
   a. The information within is essential to the paragraph.
   b. The information, though relevant, carries less emphasis.
   c. The information is redundant and should be eliminated.
   d. The information belongs elsewhere.

7. Which example shows correct comma usage for dates?
   a. The due date for the final paper in the course is Monday, May 16, 2016.
   b. The due date for the final paper in the course is Monday, May 16 2016.
   c. The due date for the final project in the course is Monday, May, 16, 2016.
   d. The due date for the final project in the course is Monday May 16, 2016.

8. Which of the following passages best displays clarity, fluency, and parallelism?
   a. Ernest Hemingway is probably the most noteworthy of expatriate authors. Hemingway's concise writing style, void of emotion and stream of consciousness, had a lasting impact, one which resonates to this very day. In Hemingway's novels, much like in American cinema, the hero acts without thinking, is living in the moment, and is repressing physical and emotional pain.
   b. Ernest Hemingway is probably the most noteworthy of expatriate authors since his concise writing style is void of emotion and stream of consciousness and has had a lasting impact on Americans which has resonated to this very day, and Hemingway's novels are much like in American cinema. The hero acts. He doesn't think. He lives in the moment. He represses physical and emotional pain.
   c. Ernest Hemingway is probably the most noteworthy of authors. His concise writing style, void of emotion and consciousness, had a lasting impact, one which resonates to this very day. In Hemingway's novels, much like in American cinema, the hero acts without thinking, lives in the moment, and represses physical and emotional pain.
   d. Ernest Hemingway is probably the most noteworthy of expatriate authors. His concise writing style, void of emotion and stream of consciousness, had a lasting impact, one which resonates to this very day. In Hemingway's novels, much like in American cinema, the hero acts without thinking, lives in the moment, and represses physical and emotional pain.

9. At last night's company function, in honor of Mr. Robertson's retirement, several employees spoke kindly about his career achievements.

In the following sentence, what part of speech is the word *function*?
   a. Adjective
   b. Adverb
   c. Verb
   d. Noun

10. Which of the examples use the correct plural form? *Select all that apply.*
   a. Tomatos
   b. Analysis
   c. Cacti
   d. Criterion

11. When giving a presentation, one should have three to five bullet points per slide. It is impossible for a presenter to memorize an entire speech, but if you can memorize the main ideas connected to the bullet points, then your speech will be more natural and fluid.

The point(s) of view represented in this passage is/are:

a. First person only
b. Third person only
c. Second person and third person
d. First person and third person

12. Based on the words *transfer*, *transact*, *translation*, and *transport*, what is the meaning of the prefix *trans*?

a. Separation
b. All or everywhere
c. Forward
d. Across, beyond, or over

13. An antibiotic is prescribed to eliminate bacterial infections; someone who is antisocial ignores society and laws. Based on these two definitions, the Latin prefix *anti-* would most likely mean:

a. Reduce
b. Revolt
c. Oppose
d. Without

14. *Conform* means to adjust one's behavior to better fit in with social norms. *Inform* means to communicate new knowledge to another. Based on these definitions, the Latin suffix *-form* most likely means:

a. Match
b. Relay
c. Negate
d. Shape

15. Which of the following sentences uses second person point of view?

a. I don't want to make plans for the weekend before I see my work schedule.
b. She had to miss the last three yoga classes due to illness.
c. Pluto is no longer considered a planet because it is not gravitationally dominant.
d. Be sure to turn off all of the lights before locking up for the night.

16. As the tour group approached the bottom of Chichen Itza, the prodigious Mayan pyramid, they became nervous about climbing its distant peak.

Based on the context of the preceding sentence, which of the following words shows the correct meaning of the word prodigious?

a. Very large
b. Famous
c. Very old
d. Fancy

17. Which of the following sentences correctly uses a hyphen?

a. Last-year, many of the players felt unsure of the coach's methods.
b. Some of the furniture she selected seemed a bit over - the - top for the space.
c. Henry is a beagle-mix and is ready for adoption this weekend.
d. Geena works to maintain a good relationship with her ex-husband to the benefit of their children.

18. Every week, Cindy volunteers time at the local shelter. She always has a smile on her face, and she always talks to others with kindness and patience. Considering that her current job is very taxing, that two of her three children are still in diapers, and that her husband, Steve, the old curmudgeon, is the opposite of her in temperament, it's amazing that no one has ever seen her angry.

Based on the context in this passage, the best substitute for *curmudgeon* would be:

a. Stingy
b. Surly
c. Scared
d. Shy

19. Which of the following sentences shows correct word usage?

a. It's often been said that work is better then rest.
b. Its often been said that work is better then rest.
c. It's often been said that work is better than rest.
d. Its often been said that work is better than rest.

20. Glorify, fortify, gentrify, acidify

Based on the preceding words, what is the correct meaning of the suffix *–fy*?

a. Marked by, given to
b. Doer, believer
c. Make, cause, cause to have
d. Process, state, rank

21. Which of the following uses correct spelling?

a. Jed was disatisfied with the acommodations at his hotel, so he requested another room.
b. Jed was dissatisfied with the accommodations at his hotel, so he requested another room.
c. Jed was dissatisfied with the accomodations at his hotel, so he requested another room.
d. Jed was disatisfied with the accommodations at his hotel, so he requested another room.

22. Most mammals in the New World have prehensile tails while most in Africa do not. Almost all primatologists would agree that animals in places like South America evolved this way to deal with denser vegetation. By moving to a loftier position, animals could avoid predators and move through foliage, unimpeded. On the other hand, it would be less advantageous for a mammal to have a prehensile tail on the African plains. On the long expanses of African savannah, movement is critical for survival, but mammals there would rely on other appendages.

Based on this passage, the best word describing what a *prehensile tail* can do would be:

a. Grasp
b. Punch
c. Move
d. Walk

23. After a long day at work, Tracy had dinner with her family, and then took a walk to the park.

What are the transitional words in the preceding sentence?

a. After, then
b. At, with, to
c. Had, took
d. A, the

24. Which of the following examples is a compound sentence?
    a. Shawn and Jerome played soccer in the backyard for two hours.
    b. Marissa last saw and spoke to Elena this morning.
    c. The baby was sick, so I decided to stay home from work.
    d. Denise, Kurt, and Eric went for a run after dinner.

25. Robert needed to find at least four sources for his final project, so he searched several library databases for reliable academic research.

Which words function as nouns in the preceding sentence? *Select all that apply.*
    a. Robert
    b. Sources
    c. Final
    d. Project
    e. He
    f. Library
    g. Databases
    h. Academic
    i. Research

26. We went on vacation this summer to Arizona. Mom had always wanted to see the Grand Canyon. Dad, on the other hand, wanted to see Saguaro National Park and Hoover Dam. Other than the flat tire our car got, it was a fantastic time.

The point(s) of view represented in this passage is/are:
    a. First person only
    b. Third person only
    c. Second person and third person
    d. First person and third person

27. Polls show that more and more people in the US distrust the government and view it as dysfunctional and corrupt. Every election, the same people are voted back into office.

Which word or words would best link these sentences?
    a. Not surprisingly,
    b. Understandably,
    c. And yet,
    d. Therefore,

28. The realtor showed __________ and __________ a house on Wednesday afternoon.

Which of the following pronoun pairs should be used in the blanks above?
    a. she, I
    b. she, me
    c. me, her
    d. her, me

29. Using the context clues in the following sentence, which of the following is the correct meaning of the word *foliage*?

> Walking through the heavily wooded park by the river in October, I was amazed at the beautiful colors of the foliage, the bright blue sky, and the crystal-clear water.

a. Leaves of the trees
b. Feathers of the birds
c. Tree bark
d. Rocks on the path

30. Select the correct meaning of the underlined word in the following sentence:

> The graduate student's thesis was focused on gerontology.

a. The study of diseases
b. The study of growth
c. The study of genes
d. The study of aging

31. A student wants to rewrite the following sentence:

> Entrepreneurs use their ideas to make money.

He wants to use the word *money* as a verb, but he isn't sure which word ending to use. What is the appropriate suffix to add to *money* to complete the following sentence?

> *Entrepreneurs __________ their ideas.*

a. –ize
b. –ical
c. –en
d. –ful

32. A teacher notices that when students are talking to each other between classes, they are using their own unique vocabulary words and expressions to talk about their daily lives. When the teacher hears these non-standard words that are specific to one age or cultural group, what type of language is she listening to?
a. Slang
b. Jargon
c. Dialect
d. Vernacular

33. A teacher wants to counsel a student about using the word *ain't* in a research paper for a high school English class. What advice should the teacher give?
a. *Ain't* is not in the dictionary, so it isn't a word.
b. Because the student isn't in college yet, *ain't* is an appropriate expression for a high school writer.
c. *Ain't* is incorrect English and should not be part of a serious student's vocabulary because it sounds uneducated.
d. *Ain't* is a colloquial expression, and while it may be appropriate in a conversational setting, it is not standard in academic writing.

Directions for the next two questions: Rewrite each sentence, following the directions given below.

34. Student loan debt is at an all-time high, which is why many politicians are using this issue to gain the attention and votes of students, or anyone with student loan debt.

Rewrite, beginning with <u>Student loan debt is at an all-time high</u>. The next words will be which of the following:

a. because politicians want students' votes.
b. , so politicians are using the issue to gain votes.
c. , so voters are choosing politicians who care about this issue.
d. , and politicians want to do something about it.

35. Seasoned runners often advise new runners to get fitted for better quality running shoes because new runners often complain about minor injuries like sore knees or shin splints.

Rewrite, beginning with <u>Seasoned runners often advise new runners to get fitted for better quality running shoes</u>. The next words will be which of the following:

a. to help them avoid minor injuries
b. because they know better
c. , so they can run further
d. to complain about running injuries

36. What does the suffix *-itis* mean?
a. Pain
b. Disease
c. Inflammation
d. Tumor

37. Which of the following is a dependent clause? *Select all that apply.*
a. he walked his dog
b. because it was raining
c. when it is Saturday
d. they came with us

Answer Explanations #1

Reading

1. B: To *propagate* means to spread, disseminate, promote, or otherwise make known an idea, thought, or belief. Xavier is clearly communicating his belief in dragons to his friends. Choices *A* and *D*, *whispered* and *shouted*, denote a lowered and raised decibel, respectively. Choice *C*, *persuaded*, means to cause someone to believe something in a convincing fashion. Although *persuaded* is a better answer than *whispered* or *shouted*, *expressed* is the best answer because *express* means to convey or communicate information. Choice *B* is the correct answer.

2. D: Choice *A* says that the GDP increased by 2% last year, which supports a claim of health. Choice *B* relays that unemployment is the lowest it's been in over a decade, a sign of a strong economy. Choice *C* states that average household income is at a historical high point, also a sign of a strong economy. In contrast, a declining manufacturing sector is a sign of an unhealthy economy, making Choice *D* is the correct answer.

3. C: The question tells us that Noam Chomsky is a linguist, philosopher, social scientist, cognitive scientist, historian, social critic, and political activist. Choice *A* lists section 700, arts and recreation, which is not relevant. Choice *B* lists section 800, literature, which does not correspond to the answer. Choice *D* lists 200, religion, which is not applicable. Thus, Choice *C* is the correct answer since 100, 400, and 900 are areas of Chomsky's expertise: philosophy, languages, and history.

4. C: This question is asking you the best section to find information about anarchism. Choice *A* is not relevant. Anarchism is not a religion, so Choice *B* is not appropriate. Choice *D* would include history and perhaps provide some appropriate resources. However, anarchism is by nature and definition a theory of social science; therefore, it best fits within the social science section. The correct section is 300, Choice *C*.

5. B: We are looking for the section where we would find books on Judaism, which is a religion. Choice *A* is about philosophy and psychology; this is not relevant, nor is Choice *C* which covers social sciences. Choice *D*, history, could be helpful, but overall, Judaism is a religion. Thus, Choice *B*, religion, is the correct answer.

6. B: Samuel wants to write an academic paper based on his 24 students. His best students come from homes where parental supervision is minimal, while the worst come from parents with extensive involvement. His conclusion is counterintuitive and probably the result of a small sample size. Choices A and D having to do with bias, is not the issue, nor is Choice *C*. Samuel's experience with these students is not applicable to students in general; rather, it is a tiny sample size relative to the millions of school children in the United States. The correct answer is B since the sample contains too few members to make meaningful claims applicable to a large group.

7. B: The passage indicates that Annabelle has a fear of going outside into the daylight. Thus, *heliophobia* must refer to a fear of bright lights or sunlight.

8. C: After removing the first and last letter, *OATHIN* remains. Next, we eliminate all the vowels, except *I*, to get *THIN*. Finally, we remove the *H* to get *TIN*; thus, Choice *C* is the correct answer.

9. C: The answer we seek has both the most detailed and objective information; thus, Choice *C* is the correct answer. The number of incidents and their relationship to a possible cause are both detailed and objective information. Choice *A* describing a television commercial with a dramatized reenactment is not particularly detailed. Choice *B*, a notice to the public informing them of additional drinking and driving units on patrol, is not detailed and objective information. Choice *D*, a highway bulletin, does not present the type of information required.

10. C: We are looking for an inference—a conclusion that is reached on the basis of evidence and reasoning. Choice *A* is wrong because the statement is false according to the passage. Choice *B* is wrong because, although the passage says the author has a graduate degree on the subject, it would be an unrealistic leap to infer that she is the foremost expert on Antebellum America. Choice *D* is wrong because there is nothing in the passage to lead us to infer that people generally prefer a children's series to historical fiction. In contrast, Choice *C* can be logically inferred since the passage speaks of the great success of the children's series and the declaration that the fame of the author's name causes the children's books to "fly off the shelves." Thus, we can infer that she did not receive any bump from her name since she published the historical novel under a pseudonym, which makes Choice *C* correct.

11. B: Narrative, Choice *A*, means a written account of connected events. Think of narrative writing as a story. Choice *C*, expository writing, generally seeks to explain or describe some phenomenon, whereas Choice *D*, technical writing, includes directions, instructions, and/or explanations. This passage is persuasive writing, which hopes to change someone's beliefs based on an appeal to reason or emotion. The author is aiming to convince the reader that smoking is terrible. They use health, price, and beauty in their argument against smoking, so Choice *B*, persuasive, is the correct answer.

12. B: The author is opposed to tobacco. The author cites disease and deaths associated with smoking and points to the monetary expense and aesthetic costs. Choice *A* is wrong because alternatives to smoking are not addressed in the passage. Choice *C* is wrong because it does not summarize the passage but rather is just a premise. Choice *D* is wrong because, while these statistics are a premise in the argument, they do not represent a summary of the piece. Choice *B* is the correct answer because it states the three critiques offered against tobacco and expresses the author's conclusion.

13. C: We are looking for something the author would agree with, so it should be anti-smoking or an argument in favor of quitting smoking. Choice *A* is wrong because the author does not speak against means of cessation. Choice *B* is wrong because the author does not reference other substances but does speak of how addictive nicotine, a drug in tobacco, is. Choice *D* is wrong because the author would not encourage reducing taxes to encourage a reduction of smoking costs, thereby helping smokers to continue the habit. Choice *C* is correct because the author is attempting to persuade smokers to quit smoking.

14. D: Here, we are looking for the author's opinion rather than a fact or statistic. Choice *A* is wrong because quoting statistics from the CDC is stating facts, not opinions. Choice *B* is wrong because it expresses the fact that cigarettes sometimes cost more than a few gallons of gas. It would be an opinion if the author said that cigarettes were not affordable. Choice *C* is incorrect because yellow stains are a known possible adverse effect of smoking. Choice *D* is correct as an opinion because smell is subjective. Some people might like the smell of smoke rather than considering it "a pervasive nastiness," so this is the expression of an opinion.

15. D: Outspending other countries on education could have other benefits, but there is no reference to this in the passage, so Choice *A* is incorrect. Choice *B* is incorrect because the author does not mention corruption. Choice *C* is incorrect because there is nothing in the passage stating that the tests are not genuinely representative. Choice *D* is accurate because spending more money has not brought success. The United States already spends the most money, but the country is not excelling on these tests. Choice *D* is the correct answer.

16. A: The guide words indicate that all of the other words on the page will be found between those words when listed alphabetically. The two guide words are *kingcraft* and *klieg light*, so the correct answer will fit between the two when ordering them alphabetically. Choice *B*, *knead*, comes after *klieg light*; Choice *C*, *kinesthesia*, and Choice *D*, *kickback*, both come before *kingcraft*. The correct answer is Choice *A*, *kleptomania*.

17. C: A primary source is an artifact, document, recording, or other source of information that is created at the time under study. Think of a primary source as the original representation of the information. In contrast, secondary sources make conclusions or draw inferences based on primary sources, as well as other secondary sources. Choice *C* is correct because a personal journal from World War II is a historical document and is, therefore, a primary source. Choice *A*, a critic's summary and review of a new book, is a secondary source. Choice *B*, a table of contents, is a secondary source, since it refers to other information. Choice *D* is also a secondary source.

18. D: Cynthia needs to select the meal with the least vegetarian options. Although the breakfast menu, Choice *A*, includes bacon, there is also coffee, tea, French toast, and eggs available. Choice *B*, lunch, includes an option for vegetarian sandwiches along with the French fries and baked beans. The cocktail hour, Choice *C*, does not contain meat or fish. In contrast, the dinner is a vegetarian's nightmare: nothing suitable is offered. Thus, dinner, Choice *D*, is the best answer.

19. D: Although Washington was from a wealthy background, the passage does not say that his wealth led to his republican ideals, so Choice *A* is not supported. Choice *B* also does not follow from the passage. Washington's warning against meddling in foreign affairs does not mean that he would oppose wars of every kind, so Choice *B* is wrong. Choice *C* is also unjustified since the author does not indicate that Alexander Hamilton's assistance was absolutely necessary. Choice *D* is correct because the passage states that Washington's farewell address clearly opposes political parties and partisanship. The author then notes that presidential elections often hit a fever pitch of partisanship. Thus, it follows that George Washington would probably not approve of modern political parties and their involvement in presidential elections.

20. A: The author finishes the passage by applying Washington's farewell address to modern politics, so the purpose probably includes this application. The other descriptions also fit the passage to some degree, but they do not describe the author's main purpose, which is revealed in the final paragraph.

21. D: Choice *A* is wrong because the last paragraph is not appropriate for a history textbook. Choice *B* is false because the piece is not a notice or announcement of Washington's death. Choice *C* is false because it is not fiction, but a historical writing. Choice *D* is correct. The passage is most likely to appear in a newspaper editorial because it cites information that is relevant and applicable to the present day, a popular subject in editorials.

22. B: The scientist and politician largely disagree, but the question asks for a point where the two are in agreement. The politician would not concur that burning fossil fuels causes global temperatures to rise; thus, Choice *A* is wrong. He would not agree with Choice *C* suggesting that countries must revisit their energy policies. By inference from the given information, the scientist would likely not concur that earth's climate naturally goes through warming and cooling cycles; so Choice *D* is incorrect. However, both the scientist and politician would agree that global temperatures are increasing. The reason for this is in dispute. The politician thinks it is part of the earth's natural cycle; the scientist thinks it is from the burning of fossil fuels. However, both acknowledge an increase, so Choice *B* is the correct answer.

23. D: Raul wants a book that describes how and why ancient Egyptians built the Great Pyramid of Giza. Choice *A* is incorrect because it focuses more generally on Giza as a whole, rather than the Great Pyramid itself. Choice *B* is close but incorrect because it is an autobiography that will largely focus on the archaeologist's life. Choice C is wrong because it focuses on hieroglyphics, not the pyramids. Choice *D*, the book directly covering the building of the Great Pyramids, should be most helpful.

24. D: The passage does not proceed in chronological order since it begins by pointing out Christopher Columbus's explorations in America, so Choice *A* does not work. Although the author compares and contrasts Erikson with Columbus, this is not the main way the information is presented; therefore, Choice *B* does not work. Choice *C* is also incorrect because there is no mention of or reference to cause and effect in the passage. However, the passage does offer a conclusion (Leif Erikson deserves more credit) and premises (first European to set foot in the New World and first to contact the natives) to substantiate Erikson's historical importance. Thus, Choice *D* is correct.

25. C: Choice *A* is wrong because it describes facts: Leif Erikson was the son of Erik the Red and historians debate Leif's date of birth. These are not opinions. Choice *B* is wrong; Erikson calling the land Vinland is a verifiable fact, as is Choice *D,* because he did contact the natives almost 500 years before Columbus. Choice *C* is the correct answer because it is the author's opinion that Erikson deserves more credit. Another person could argue that Columbus or another explorer deserves more credit, which makes it an opinion rather than a historical fact.

26. B: Choice A is wrong because the author aims to go beyond describing Erikson as merely a legendary Viking. Choice *C* is wrong because the author does not focus on Erikson's motivations, let alone name the spreading of Christianity as his primary objective. Although it's true that Erikson contacted the natives 500 years before Columbus, Choice *D* is wrong because it isn't the author's main conclusion, it is simply a fact used to support the main conclusion. Choice *B* is correct because it accurately identifies the author's statement that Erikson deserves more credit than he has received for being the first European to explore the New World.

27. B: Choice *B* is correct because the author wants the reader to be informed about Leif Erikson's contribution to exploring the new world. While several other answers are possible options, Choice *B* is the strongest. Choice *A* is incorrect because the author is not in any way trying to entertain the reader. Choice *C* is incorrect because the nature of the writing does not indicate the author would be satisfied with the reader merely being alerted to Erikson's exploration; instead, the author is making an argument about the credit he should receive. Choice *D* is incorrect because the author goes beyond merely a suggestion; *suggest* is too vague.

28. D: Choice *A* is wrong because the author never addresses the Vikings' state of mind or emotions. Choice *B* is wrong because the author does not elaborate on Erikson's exile and whether he would have become an explorer if not for his banishment. Choice *C* is wrong because there is not enough information to support this premise. It is unclear whether Erikson informed the King of Norway of his findings. Although it is true that the king did not send a follow-up expedition, he could have simply chosen not to expend the resources after receiving Erikson's news. It is not possible to logically infer whether Erikson told him. Choice *D* is correct because the uncertainty about Leif Erikson's birth year is an example of how historians have trouble pinning down important details in Viking history.

29. B: A passage like this one would likely appear in some sort of community profile, highlighting the benefits of living or working there. Choice *A* is incorrect because nothing in this passage suggests that it is fictional. It reads as non-fiction, if anything. Choice *C* is incorrect because it does not report anything particularly newsworthy, and Choice *D* is incorrect because it has absolutely nothing to do with a movie review.

30. B: Primary sources are original, firsthand accounts of events or time periods as they are happening or very close to the time they occurred. Diary entries are excellent primary sources, as are newspaper articles, works of art and literature, interviews, and live recordings. Choice *A* is incorrect because a Wikipedia article is not a reliable source due to the fact that multiple authors can access and manipulate the information. Choices *C* and *D* are incorrect because they are examples of secondary sources. While they might be very reliable and useful, they are not primary sources.

31. C: To arrive at the correct answer, first calculate the actual times Lucy and Bob could arrive at and depart from the dock. Lucy needs an additional thirty minutes after leaving work, so that equates to 1:15 p.m. Bob works at 6:30 p.m. and needs an hour to get to work on time, so that means he would have to leave the dock by 5:30 p.m. Ship 3 leaves at 1:30 p.m., which gives Lucy an additional fifteen minutes' leeway, then returns at 5:30 p.m., which gives Bob the hour he needs to arrive at work on time. None of the other ships would work with their schedules.

32. C: Safflower oil has a smoking point of 510° Fahrenheit. Since Zack's recipe doesn't exceed 430° F, it won't reach the smoking point. In addition, safflower oil doesn't contain peanuts, and safflower oil has a neutral taste. Though clarified butter has a high smoke point, too, it doesn't have a neutral taste. Zack is allergic to peanut oil. Lard, at 374° F, has too low a smoking point and doesn't have a neutral taste. Coconut oil has a smoking point of 350° F and doesn't have a neutral taste.

33. A: Clarified butter has a high smoke point (485°), which would be well above 430° F and doesn't have a neutral taste, which in this scenario Zack prefers. Here, peanut oil is a neutral flavor. Lard, at 374° F, has too low a smoking point. Safflower oil has a smoking point of 510° F, but, here, the flavor is neutral, and he wants a flavored oil. Coconut oil is not neutral, but the smoking point of 350° F is too low.

34. 1970: Note that the population numbers on the graph are in millions. If you are looking for 200,000,000 on the graph, you need to find a number close to 200. The population label for 1970 shows the population as 203.3 which means 203,300,000 people. Now, the population might have exceeded 200,000,000 slightly before 1970, but the question asked for the first-year marker showing it over 200,000,000.

35. D: The population increased the most between 1990 and 2010. The question is asking you to identify the rate of change for each interval. Between 1990 and 2010, the population increased by approximately 60 million. Thus, Choice *D* is the correct answer. The slope of the graph is also the steepest in this interval, which represents its highest increase. Choice *A* is incorrect because between 1930 and 1950, the population increased by approximately 28 million. Choice *B* is incorrect because between 1950 and 1970, the population increased by approximately 52 million. Choice *C* is incorrect because between 1970 and 1990, the population increased by approximately 45 million.

36. C: Despite the opposite stances in Passages 1 and 2, both authors establish that cell phones are a strong part of culture. In Passage 1 the author states, "Today's student is already strongly rooted in technology." In Passage 2 the author states, "Students are comfortable with cell phones." The author of Passage 2 states that cell phones have a "time and place." The author of Passage 2 would disagree with the statement that teachers should incorporate cell phones into curriculum whenever possible. While Passage 2 implies that cell phones are useful only when an experienced teacher uses them properly, the author in Passage 1 says cell phones are "indispensable." In other words, no teacher can do without them. The statement from Choice *D* is not supported by either passage. Even though the author in the second passage is more cautionary, the author states, "This can prove advantageous if done correctly." Therefore, there is a possibility that a classroom can run properly with cell phones.

37. B: Primary producers make up the base of the food chain, so the correct answer will be in the level just above: a primary consumer. The cobra, wild dog, and aardvark are all secondary consumers. The gazelle is a primary consumer, so B is the correct answer.

38. A: According to the passage preceding the food chain, the apex predators do not have natural predators. So, the question is really asking which of the answer choices is an apex predator. The cobra, mongoose, and aardvark are all secondary consumers. The vulture is an apex predator; thus, a vulture has no natural predators, making A the correct answer.

39. D: A mongoose is a secondary consumer; thus, the mongoose consumes primary consumers. The shrub is a primary producer. The aardvark is a secondary consumer. The vulture is an apex predator. The mouse is a primary consumer, so Choice *D* is the correct answer.

40. B: Choices *A*, *C*, and *D* all relate facts but do not present the kind of general statement that would serve as an effective summary or conclusion. Choice *B* is correct.

41. B: Choice *A* uses similar language, but it is not the main point of disagreement. The reporter calls the loss devastating, and there's no reason to believe that the coach would disagree with this assessment, so it can be eliminated.

Choice *B* is strong since both passages mention the at-bats with runners in scoring position. The reporter asserts that the team lost due to the team failing to get such a hit. In contrast, the coach identifies several other reasons for the loss, including fielding and pitching errors. Additionally, the coach disagrees that the team even needed a hit in those situations.

Choice *C* is mentioned by the coach but not by the reporter. It is unclear whether the reporter would agree with this assessment, so it can be eliminated.

Choice *D* is mentioned by the coach but not by the reporter. It is not stated whether the reporter believes that the team deserved to win, so it can be eliminated.

Therefore, Choice *B* is the correct answer.

42. D: Choice *A* is literal, not symbolic. Choice *B* is incorrect because the traveler deems both roads to be equally "fair" or pleasant. Choice *C* deals with the past and the future, but the traveler is considering two paths forward.

43. D: Choice *A* is clearly incorrect. The argument does not start with a conclusion, so it can be eliminated.

Choice *B* is incorrect. Although the argument states a universal rule—the top salesman is always a company's best employee—it does not argue that Dwight is the exception, so it can be eliminated.

Choice *C* is fairly strong. The argument does state several facts and offers a conclusion based on those facts. Leave this choice for now.

Choice *D* looks extremely promising. The argument first states several facts—Dwight works at a mid-sized regional tech company and leads the company in sales—then states a rule. Lastly, the argument applies the facts to the rule and concludes that Dwight is the best employee. This is a better fit than Choice *C* since it includes the rule and its application.

Therefore, Choice *D* is the correct answer.

44. C: The passage is told in chronological order, detailing the steps the family took to adopt their dog. The narrator mentions that Robin's physical exam and lab work confirmed she was healthy before discussing that they brought her to the vet to evaluate her health. It is illogical that lab work would confirm good health prior to an appointment with the vet when, presumably, the lab work would be collected.

45. D: The graph displaying the percentage of weekly homework assignments Marco completed clearly shows a recent decline. It is likely that test performance may suffer without adequate practice, which is one of the primary purposes of homework assignments. Choice *A,* the email, would not necessarily substantiate a poor mark because the absences have not yet occurred and therefore, would not factor into the prior exam. Choice *B,* the graph of test scores simply demonstrates that indeed his score was lower than it had been. Choice *C* is also incorrect because his absences have no obvious trend that would lend to decreased performance. They seem to have bounced around over the duration of the course.

Mathematics

1. A: Compare each number after the decimal point to figure out which overall number is greatest. In Choices *A* (1.43785) and *C* (1.43592), both have the same tenths place (4) and hundredths place (3). However, the thousandths place is greater in Choice *A* (7), so it has the greatest value overall.

2. D: By rearranging and grouping the factors in Choice *D*, we can notice that $3 \times 3 \times 4 \times 2 = (3 \times 2) \times (4 \times 3) = 6 \times 12$, which is what we were looking for.

3. C: The total percentage of a pie chart equals 100%. CD sales make up less than half of the chart (50%) but more than a quarter (25%), and the only answer choice that meets these criteria is Choice *C*, 40%.

4. B: Since \$850 is the price after a 20% discount, \$850 represents 80% (or 0.8) of the original price. In other words, $850 = 0.8x$ (where x is the original price). Solving this leaves the answer $x = \frac{850}{0.8} = 1{,}062.5$. Now, to find the savings, calculate the original price minus the sale price: $\$1{,}062.50 - \$850 = \$212.50$.

5. A: To figure out which value is the largest, look at the first nonzero digits. Choice *B*'s first nonzero digit is in the hundredths place. The other three all have nonzero digits in the tenths place, so it must be Choice *A*, *C*, or *D*. Of these, Choice *A*'s first nonzero digit is the largest.

6. 7: To solve for the value of b, isolate the variable b on one side of the equation.

Start by moving the lower value of –4 to the other side by adding 4 to both sides:

$$5b - 4 = 2b + 17$$

$$5b - 4 + 4 = 2b + 17 + 4$$

$$5b = 2b + 21$$

Then, subtract $2b$ from both sides:

$$5b - 2b = 2b + 21 - 2b$$

$$3b = 21$$

Then, divide both sides by 3 to get the value of b:

$$\frac{3b}{3} = \frac{21}{3}$$

$$b = 7$$

7. D: The total faculty is:

$$15 + 20 = 35$$

So, the ratio is $35 : 200$. Then, divide both of these numbers by 5, since 5 is a common factor to both, with a result of $7 : 40$.

8. C: The first step in solving this problem is expressing the result in fraction form. Multiplication and division are typically performed in order from left to right, but they can be performed in any order. For this problem, start with the division operation between the last two fractions. When dividing one fraction by another, invert—or flip—the second fraction and then multiply the numerators and denominators.

$$\frac{7}{10} \times \frac{2}{1} = \frac{14}{10}$$

Next, multiply the first fraction by this value:

$$\frac{3}{5} \times \frac{14}{10} = \frac{42}{50}$$

In this instance, to find the decimal form, multiply the numerator and denominator by 2 to get 100 in the denominator.

$$\frac{42}{50} \times \frac{2}{2} = \frac{84}{100}$$

In decimal form, this would be expressed as 0.84.

9. 17: To find what 85% of 20 questions is, multiply 20 by 0.85:

$$20 \text{ x } .85 = 17 \text{ questions}$$

10. D: This problem can be solved by setting up a proportion involving the given information and the unknown value. The proportion is:

$$\frac{21 \text{ pages}}{4 \text{ nights}} = \frac{140 \text{ pages}}{x \text{ nights}}$$

Cross-multiply to get $21x = 4 \times 140$. Solving this leaves $x \approx 26.67$. Since this is not an integer, round up to 27 nights because 26 nights would not give Sarah enough time to finish.

11. B: Using the conversion rate, multiply the projected weight loss of 25 lb by $0.45\frac{\text{kg}}{\text{lb}}$ to get the amount in kilograms (11.25 kg).

12. D: First, subtract $1,437 from $2,334.50 to find Johnny's monthly savings; this equals $897.50. Then, multiply this amount by 3 to find out how much he will have (in 3 months) before he pays for his vacation; this equals $2,692.50. Finally, subtract the cost of the vacation ($1,750) from this amount to find how much Johnny will have left: $942.50.

13. 4: Dividing by 98 can be approximated by dividing by 100, which would mean shifting the decimal point of the numerator to the left by 2. The result is 4.2, which rounds to 4.

14. A: Total tuition for 4 years is:

$$\$22{,}000 \times 4 = \$88{,}000$$

Total room and board for 4 years is:

$$\$5{,}000 \times 4 = \$20{,}000$$

Total cost of books for four years is $\$500 \times 4 = \$2{,}000$. Therefore, it is estimated that you will spend $88,000+$20,000+$2,000=$110,000 on college. Your family is going to pay 25% of this cost, which is:

$$0.25 \times \$110{,}000 = \$27{,}500$$

Therefore, you will be responsible for:

$$\$110{,}000 - \$27{,}500 = \$82{,}500$$

Therefore, to obtain your goal, you will need to have $82,500 in your account before college starts.

15. 6 cm: The formula for the perimeter of a rectangle is $P = 2L + 2W$, where P is the perimeter, L is the length, and W is the width. The first step is to substitute all of the data into the formula:

$$36 = 2(12) + 2W$$

Simplify by multiplying 2×12:

$$36 = 24 + 2W$$

Simplifying this further by subtracting 24 on each side gives:

$$36 - 24 = 24 - 24 + 2W$$

$$12 = 2W$$

Divide by 2:

$$6 = W$$

The width is 6 cm. Remember to test this answer by substituting this value into the original formula:

$$36 = 2(12) + 2(6)$$

16. D: To find the average of a set of values, add the values together and then divide by the total number of values. In this case, include the unknown value of what Dwayne needs to score on his next test, in order to solve it.

$$\frac{78 + 92 + 83 + 97 + x}{5} = 90$$

Then multiply each side by 5 to simplify the equation, resulting in:

$$78 + 92 + 83 + 97 + x = 450$$

$$350 + x = 450$$

$$x = 100$$

Dwayne would need to get a perfect score of 100 in order to get an average of at least 90.

Test this answer by substituting 100 back into the original formula.

$$\frac{78 + 92 + 83 + 97 + 100}{5} = 90$$

17. D: For an even number of total values, the median is calculated by finding the mean, or average, of the two middle values once all values have been arranged in order from least to greatest. In this case, $\frac{83+92}{2}$ would equal the median 87.5, Choice *D*.

18. C: Follow the order of operations in order to solve this problem. Solve the parentheses first, following the order of operations inside the parentheses as well. First, simplify the square roots:

$$(6 \times 4) - 3^2$$

Then, simplify the multiplication inside the parentheses:

$$24 - 3^2$$

Next, simplify the exponent:

$$24 - 9$$

Finally, subtract. This equals $24 - 9 = 5$, Choice C.

19. D: Three girls for every two boys can be expressed as a ratio, 3 : 2. This can be visualized as splitting the school into five groups: three girl groups and two boy groups. The number of students that are in each group can be found by dividing the total number of students by five:

$$\frac{650 \text{ students}}{5 \text{ groups}} = \frac{130 \text{ students}}{\text{group}}$$

To find the total number of girls, multiply the number of students per group (130) by the number of girl groups in the school (3). This equals 390, Choice *D*.

20. B: To solve this correctly, keep in mind the order of operations with the mnemonic PEMDAS (Please Excuse My Dear Aunt Sally). This stands for Parentheses, Exponents, Multiplication & Division, Addition & Subtraction. Taking it step by step, start with the parentheses:

$$4 \times 7 + (4)^2 \div 2$$

Then, apply the exponent:

$$4 \times 7 + 16 \div 2$$

Multiplication and division are both performed next:

$$28 + 8$$

Then finally, addition:

$$28 + 8 = 36$$

21. C: Kimberley worked 4.5 hours at the rate of $10 / h and 1 hour at the rate of $12 / h. The problem states that her time is rounded to the nearest hour, so the 4.5 hours would round up to 5 hours at the rate of $10 / h.

$$(5 \text{ hours}) \times \left(\frac{\$10}{\text{hour}}\right) + (1 \text{ hour}) \times \left(\frac{\$12}{\text{hour}}\right) = \$50 + \$12 = \$62$$

22. D:

$9x + x - 7 = 16 + 2x$	Combine $9x$ and x
$10x - 7 = 16 + 2x$	
$10x - 7 + 7 = 16 + 2x + 7$	Add 7 to both sides to remove the −7.
$10x = 23 + 2x$	
$10x - 2x = 23 + 2x - 2x$	Subtract $2x$ from both sides to move it to the other side of the equation.
$8x = 23$	
$\frac{8x}{8} = \frac{23}{8}$	Divide by 8 to get x by itself.
$x = \frac{23}{8}$	

23. C: For each fraction, we can divide the numerator by the denominator to find a decimal value. $\frac{4}{5} = 0.8$, $\frac{2}{3} \approx 0.67$, and $\frac{91}{100} = 0.91$. Ordering these from least to greatest gives us 0.67, 0.8, 0.85, and 0.91, which matches Choice *C*.

24. B: First, calculate the difference between the larger value and the smaller value:

$$378 - 252 = 126$$

To calculate this difference as a percentage of the original value, which is the percentage *increase*, divide 126 by 252 to get 0.5, then multiply by 100 to reach the percentage 50%, Choice *B*.

25. C: To find the angle in radians, multiply by pi and divide by 180. When you simplify $\frac{48° \times \pi}{180}$, you get $\frac{4\pi}{15}$. Choice *A* is not the correct answer because $\frac{\pi}{4}$ is 45°. Choice *B* is not the correct answer because $\frac{\pi}{15}$ is 12°. Choice *D* is not the correct answer because $\frac{3\pi}{4} = 135°$.

26. A: First, simplify the larger fraction by separating it into two. When dividing one fraction by another, remember to invert the second fraction and multiply, like so:

$$\frac{5}{7} \times \frac{11}{9}$$

The resulting fraction $\frac{55}{63}$ cannot be simplified further, so this is the answer to the problem.

27. A: To calculate the range in a set of data, subtract the highest value with the lowest value. In this graph, the range of Mr. Lennon's students is 5, which can be seen physically in the graph as having the smallest difference between the highest value and the lowest value when compared with the other teachers.

28. 4: The number of days can be found by taking the total amount Bernard needs to make and dividing it by the amount he earns per day:

$$\frac{300}{80} = \frac{30}{8} = \frac{15}{4} = 3.75$$

But Bernard is only working full days, so he will need to work 4 days, since 3 days is not a sufficient amount of time.

29. C: The average is calculated by adding all six numbers, then dividing by 6. The first five numbers have a sum of 25. This scenario can be expressed by the equation $\frac{25+n}{6} = 6$, where n is the unknown number. After multiplying both sides by 6, we get $25 + n = 36$, which means $n = 11$.

30. A: An outlier is a data value that's either far above or below the majority of values in a sample set. The mean is the average of all values in the set. In a small sample, a very high or low number could greatly change the average. The median is the middle value when arranged from lowest to highest. Outliers would have no more of an effect on the median than any other value. Mode is the value that repeats most often in a set. Assuming that the same outlier doesn't repeat, outliers would have no effect on the mode of a sample set.

31. A: This kind of line indicates a positive relationship. A negative relationship would match a line traveling from the upper left of the graph to the lower right. Exponential and logarithmic functions aren't linear—their graphs do not make a straight line.

32. A: The conversion can be obtained by setting up and evaluating the following expression:

$$4{,}382 \text{ ft} \times \frac{0.3048 \text{ m}}{1 \text{ ft}} \times \frac{1 \text{ km}}{1{,}000 \text{ m}} = 1.336 \text{ km}$$

33. C: The data points do not appear to form any sort of line, even approximately, as we would expect for a positive or negative relation. They also do not form the characteristic bell-shaped curve of a normal distribution. No relation is apparent.

34. D: The slope is given by the change in y divided by the change in x. Specifically, it's:

$$slope = \frac{y_2 - y_1}{x_2 - x_1}$$

The first point is $(-5, -3)$, and the second point is $(0, -1)$. Work from left to right when identifying coordinates. Thus the point on the left is point 1 $(-5, -3)$ and the point on the right is point 2 $(0, -1)$.

Now we just need to plug those numbers into the equation:

$$slope = \frac{-1 - (-3)}{0 - (-5)}$$

It can be simplified to:

$$slope = \frac{-1 + 3}{0 + 5}$$

$$slope = \frac{2}{5}$$

35. B: The figure is composed of three sides of a square and a semicircle. The sides of the square are simply added:

$$8 \text{ in} + 8 \text{ in} + 8 \text{ in} = 24 \text{ in}$$

The circumference of a circle is found by the equation $C = 2\pi r$. The radius is 4 in, so the circumference of the circle is 25.13 in. Only half of the circle makes up the outer border of the figure (part of the perimeter), and half of 25.13 in is 12.565 in. Therefore, the total perimeter is:

$$24 \text{ in} + 12.565 \text{ in} = 36.565 \text{ in}$$

The other answer choices use the incorrect formula or fail to include all of the necessary sides.

36. A: The perimeter of a rectangle is $P = 2l + 2w$. We are told $P = 44$, so $2l + 2w = 44$. We are also told that the width is 2 cm less than the length: $w = l - 2$. Substituting this for w in the perimeter equation, we get $2l + 2(l - 2) = 44$, which is Choice *A*.

Although it's not necessary to answer the test question, we could solve the equation to find the length and width. The equation simplifies to $4l - 4 = 44$, or $l = 12$, and since $w = l - 2$, we find $w = 10$.

37. B: An equilateral triangle has 3 sides of equal length, so if the total perimeter is 18 feet, each side must be 6 feet long. A square with sides of 6 feet will have an area of $6^2 = 36$ square feet.

38. B: The formula for the volume of a cube is $V = s^3$. Substitute the side length of $7in$ to get:

$$V = 7^3 = 343in^3$$

Science

1. A: When activated, B cells create antibodies against specific antigens. White blood cells are generated in the red bone marrow, not in cartilage. Platelets are not a type of white blood cell and are typically cell fragments produced by megakaryocytes. White blood cells are active throughout nearly all of one's life and have not been shown to specially activate or deactivate because of life events like puberty or menopause.

2. The aorta leads directly from the left ventricle and to the systemic circuit:

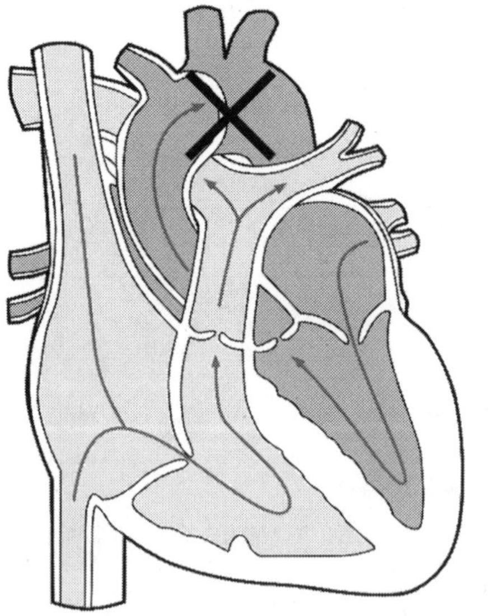

3. A, B, C, D: The urinary system has many functions, the primary of which is removing waste products and balancing water and electrolyte concentrations in the blood. It also plays a key role in regulating ion concentrations, such as sodium, potassium, chloride, and calcium, in the filtrate. The urinary system helps maintain blood pH by reabsorbing or secreting hydrogen ions and bicarbonate as necessary. Certain kidney cells can detect reductions in blood volume and pressure and then can secrete renin to activate a hormone that causes increased reabsorption of sodium ions and water. This serves to raise blood volume and pressure. Kidney cells secrete erythropoietin under hypoxic conditions to stimulate red blood cell production. They also synthesize calcitriol, a hormone derivative of vitamin D3, which aids in calcium ion absorption by the intestinal epithelium.

4. B: The time in seconds that the dogs sit is a better choice than Choice *C* (tail wagging) because it is a measurable, meaningful, and relevant dependent variable. Tail wagging, although quantitative, is not a valid measure of anything. Choices *A* and *D* could be independent variables in the experiment.

5. B: The cell structure responsible for cellular storage, digestion, and waste removal is the lysosome. Lysosomes are like recycle bins. They are filled with digestive enzymes that facilitate catabolic reactions to regenerate monomers. The Golgi apparatus is designed to tag, package, and ship out proteins destined for other cells or locations. The centrioles typically play a large role only in cell division when they ratchet the chromosomes from the mitotic plate to the poles of the cell. The mitochondria are involved in energy production and are the powerhouses of the cell.

6. A: The sensory threshold is the smallest amount of stimulus that is required for an individual to experience one of the senses. For example, during a hearing test, the sensory threshold would be the quietest sound that a person could detect. This threshold is an important indicator of whether a person's senses are working within a normal range.

7. D: Veins have valves, but arteries do not. Valves in veins are designed to prevent backflow since they are the furthest blood vessels from the pumping action of the heart and steadily increase in volume (which decreases the available pressure). Capillaries diffuse nutrients properly because of their thin walls and high surface area and are not particularly dependent on positive pressure.

8. C: The blood leaves the right ventricle through a semi-lunar valve and goes through the pulmonary artery to the lungs. Any increase in pressure in the artery will eventually affect the contractibility of the right ventricle. Blood enters the right atrium from the superior and inferior vena cava, and blood leaves the right atrium through the tricuspid valve to the right ventricle. Blood enters the left atrium from the right ventricle. Blood enters the left atrium from the pulmonary veins carrying oxygenated blood from the lungs. Blood flows from the left atrium to the left ventricle through the mitral valve and leaves the left ventricle through a semi-lunar valve to enter the aorta.

9. B: During telophase, two nuclei form at each end of the cell and nuclear envelopes begin to form around each nucleus. The nucleoli reappear, and the chromosomes become less compact. The microtubules are broken down by the cell, and mitosis is complete. The process begins with prophase as the mitotic spindles begin to form from centrosomes. Prometaphase follows, with the breakdown of the nuclear envelope and the further condensing of the chromosomes. Next, metaphase occurs when the microtubules are stretched across the cell and the chromosomes align at the metaphase plate. Finally, in the last step before telophase, anaphase occurs as the sister chromatids break apart and form chromosomes.

10. D: A reflex arc is a simple nerve pathway involving a stimulus, a synapse, and a response that is controlled by the spinal cord—not the brain. The knee-jerk reflex is an example of a reflex arc. The stimulus is the hammer hitting the tendon, reaching the synapse in the spinal cord by an afferent pathway. The response is the resulting muscle contraction reaching the muscle by an efferent pathway. None of the remaining processes is a simple reflex. Memories are processed and stored in the hippocampus in the limbic system. The visual center is located in the occipital lobe, while auditory processing occurs in the temporal lobe. The sympathetic and parasympathetic divisions of the autonomic nervous system control heart rate and blood pressure.

11. C: The lagging strand of DNA falls behind the leading strand because of its discontinuous synthesis. DNA helicase unzips the DNA helices so that synthesis can take place, and RNA primers are created by the RNA primase for the polymerases to attach to and build from. The lagging strand is synthesizing DNA in a direction that is hard for the polymerase to build, so multiple primers are laid down so that the entire length of DNA can be synthesized simultaneously. These short pieces of DNA being synthesized are known as Okazaki fragments and are joined together by DNA ligase.

12. A: The sternum is medial to the deltoid because it is much closer to (typically right on) the midline of the body, while the deltoid is lateral at the shoulder cap. Superficial means that a structure is closer to the body surface and posterior means that it falls behind something else. For example, skin is superficial to bone and the kidneys are posterior to the rectus abdominis.

13. B: Ligaments connect bone to bone. Tendons connect muscle to bone. Both are made of dense, fibrous connective tissue (primary Type 1 collagen) to give strength. However, tendons are more organized, especially in the long axis direction like muscle fibers themselves, and they have more collagen. This arrangement makes sense because muscles have specific orientations of their fibers, so they contract in somewhat predictable directions. Ligaments are less organized and have more of a woven pattern because bone connections are not as organized as bundles of muscle fibers, so ligaments must have strength in multiple directions to protect against injury.

14. A: The three primary body planes are coronal, sagittal, and transverse. The coronal or frontal plane, named for the plane in which a corona or halo might appear in old paintings, divides the body vertically into front and back sections. The sagittal plane, named for the path an arrow might take when shot at the body, divides the body vertically into right and left sections. The transverse plane divides the body horizontally into upper or superior and lower or inferior sections. There is no medial plane, per se. The anatomical direction medial simply references a location close or closer to the center of the body than another location.

15. C: Although the lungs may provide some cushioning for the heart when the body is violently struck, this is not a major function of the respiratory system. Its most notable function is that of gas exchange for oxygen and carbon dioxide, but it also plays a vital role in the regulation of blood pH. The aqueous form of carbon dioxide, carbonic acid, is a major pH buffer of the blood, and the respiratory system directly controls how much carbon dioxide stays and is released from the blood through respiration. The respiratory system also enables vocalization and forms the basis for the mode of speech and language used by most humans.

16. B: The structure exclusively found in eukaryotic cells is the nucleus. Animal, plant, fungi, and protist cells are all eukaryotic. DNA is contained within the nucleus of eukaryotic cells, and they also have membrane-bound organelles that perform complex intracellular metabolic activities. Prokaryotic cells (archaea and bacteria) do not have a nucleus or other membrane-bound organelles and are less complex than eukaryotic cells.

17. D: Germline mutations in eggs and sperm are permanent, can be on the chromosomal level, and will be inherited by offspring. Somatic mutations cannot affect eggs and sperm, and therefore are not inherited by offspring. Mutations of either kind are rarely beneficial to the individual but do not necessarily harm them. Germline cells divide much more rapidly than do somatic cells, and a mutation in a sex cell would promulgate and affect many thousands of its daughter cells.

18. A: It is most likely asthma. Any of the answer choices listed can cause heavy breathing. A blood clot in the lung (*B*) could cause this, but this would be very uncommon for a child. Choices *C* and *D* can both be ruled out because the question mentions that it occurs even when the patient is relaxing. Hyperventilation is usually caused by a panic attack or some sort of physical activity. Asthma often develops during childhood. It would stand to reason then that the child may have not yet been diagnosed. While asthma attacks can be caused by exercise, they can also occur when a person is not exerting themselves.

19. C: Theories are accepted by scientists, while hypotheses remain to be proven, making Choice *C* correct. Choice *A* is incorrect because theories are far more than predictions; they are actually highly supported and accepted as truth. Choice *B* is incorrect because theories can change with new technology and understanding. Choice *D* is also incorrect because theories may not always be true and can change. Also, hypotheses can be and often are supported.

20.

1. **Make observations**
2. **Ask a question**
3. **Create or propose a hypothesis**
4. **Formulate an experiment**
5. **Test the hypothesis**
6. **Accept or reject the hypothesis**

While there is no consensus on the exact number of steps in the scientific process, it is agreed that those six elements are needed and in that order.

21. B: Biological catalysts are termed *enzymes*, which are proteins with conformations that specifically manipulate reactants into positions which decrease the reaction's activation energy. Lipids do not usually affect reactions, and cofactors, while they can aid or be necessary to the proper functioning of enzymes, do not make up the majority of biological catalysts.

22. B: Substances with higher amounts of hydrogen ions will have lower pHs, while substances with higher amounts of hydroxide ions will have higher pHs. Choice *A* is incorrect because it is possible to have an extremely strong acid with a pH less than 1, as long as its molarity of hydrogen ions is greater than 1. Choice *C* is false because a weak base is determined by having a pH lower than some value, not higher. Substances with pHs greater than 2 include anything from neutral water to extremely caustic lye. Choice *D* is false because a solution with a pH of 2 has ten times fewer hydrogen ions than a solution of pH 1.

23. A: Salts are formed from compounds that use ionic bonds. Disulfide bridges are special bonds in protein synthesis which hold the protein in their secondary and tertiary structures. Covalent bonds are strong bonds formed through the sharing of electrons between atoms and are typically found in organic molecules like carbohydrates and lipids. London dispersion forces are fleeting, momentary bonds which occur between atoms that have instantaneous dipoles but quickly disintegrate.

24. C: Covalent bonds are special because they share electrons between multiple atoms. Most covalent bonds are formed between the elements H, F, N, O, S, and C, while hydrogen bonds are formed nearly exclusively between H and either O, N, or F of other molecules. Covalent bonds may inadvertently form dipoles, but this does not necessarily happen. For instance, dipoles do not form with similarly electronegative atoms, like carbon and hydrogen. Crystal solids are typically formed by substances with ionic bonds like the salts sodium iodide and potassium chloride.

25. A: Gases like air will move and expand to fill their container, so they are considered to have an indefinite shape and indefinite volume. Liquids like water will move and flow freely, so their shapes change constantly, but they do not change volume or density on their own. Solids change neither shape nor volume without external forces acting on them, so they have definite shapes and volumes.

26. C: The relative density of eccrine sweat glands varies in different areas of the body. The palms and soles of the feet have the highest density, reaching values of approximately 400 sweat glands per square centimeter of epidermis. The head also has a high density of sweat glands, though significantly less than on the palms and soles. Areas such as the upper arms and thighs have only around 80 eccrine sweat glands per square inch of skin.

27. C: Nephrons are responsible for filtering blood. When functioning properly they allow blood cells and nutrients to go back into the bloodstream while sending waste to the bladder. However, nephrons can fail at doing this, particularly when blood flood to the kidneys is limited. The medulla (also called the renal medulla) (*A*) and the renal cortex (*D*) are both parts of the kidney but are not specifically responsible for filtering blood. The medulla is in the inner part of the kidney and contains the nephrons. The renal cortex is the outer part of the kidney. The heart (*B*) is responsible for pumping blood throughout the body rather than filtering it.

28. B: Ossification is the process by which cartilage, a soft, flexible substance is replaced by bone throughout the body. All humans regardless of age have cartilage, but cartilage in some areas is replaced by bones as a person grows.

29. A: Keratin is a structural protein, and it is the primary constituent of things like hair and nails. Choice B is incorrect; antigens are immune proteins that help fight disease. Hormonal proteins are responsible for initiating the signal transduction cascade to regulate gene expression. Choice *C* is incorrect because channel proteins are transport proteins that help move molecules into and out of a cell. Marker proteins help identify or distinguish a cell. Lastly, Choice *D* is incorrect because actin, like myosin, is a motor protein because it is involved in the process of muscle contraction.

30. C: mRNA is directly transcribed from DNA before being taken to the cytoplasm and translated by rRNA into a protein. tRNA transfers amino acids from the cytoplasm to the rRNA for use in building these proteins. siRNA is a special type of RNA which interferes with other strands of mRNA, typically by causing them to get degraded by the cell rather than translated into protein.

31. B: Since the genotype is a depiction of the specific alleles that an organism's genes code for, it includes recessive genes that may or may not be otherwise expressed. The genotype does not have to name the proteins that its alleles code for; indeed, some of them may be unknown. The phenotype is the physical, visual manifestations of a gene, not the genotype. The genotype does not necessarily include any information about the organism's physical characteristics. Although some information about an organism's parents can be obtained from its genotype, its genotype does not actually show the parents' phenotypes.

32. C: One in four offspring (or 25%) will be short, so all four offspring cannot be tall. Although both of the parents are tall, they are hybrid or heterozygous tall, not homozygous. Although it may seem intuitive that the short allele will be expressed by lower numbers of the population than the tall allele, it still appears in 75% of the offspring (although its effects are masked in $\frac{2}{3}$ of those). Besides, conditions could favor the recessive allele and kill off the tall offspring.

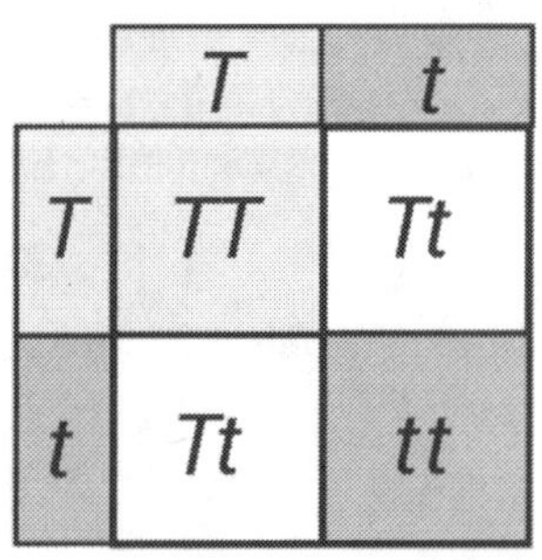

Both parents are mixed hybrids so offspring are a 3:1 ratio

33. D: Evaporation takes place at the surface of a fluid, while boiling takes place throughout the fluid. The liquid will boil when it reaches its boiling or vaporization temperature, but evaporation can happen due to a liquid's volatility. Volatile substances often coexist as a liquid and as a gas, depending on the pressure forced on them. The phase change from gas to liquid is condensation, and both evaporation and boiling take place in nature.

34. A: Human genes are strictly DNA and do not include proteins or amino acids. A human's genome and collection of genes will include even their recessive traits, mutations, and unused DNA.

35. C: Water's polarity lends it to be extremely cohesive and adhesive; this cohesion keeps its atoms very close together. Because of this, it takes a large amount of energy to boil its liquid form. Phospholipid bilayers are made of nonpolar lipids; water, a polar liquid, cannot easily flow through it. Cell membranes use proteins called aquaporins to solve this issue and let water flow in and out. Fish breathe by capturing dissolved oxygen through their gills. Water can self-ionize, wherein it decomposes into a hydrogen ion (H^+) and a hydroxide ion (OH^-), but it cannot self-hydrolyze.

36. D: An isotope of an element has an atomic number equal to its number of protons, but a different mass number because of the additional neutrons. Even though there are differences in the nucleus, the behavior and properties of isotopes of a given element are identical. Atoms with different atomic numbers also have different numbers of protons and are different elements, so they cannot be isotopes.

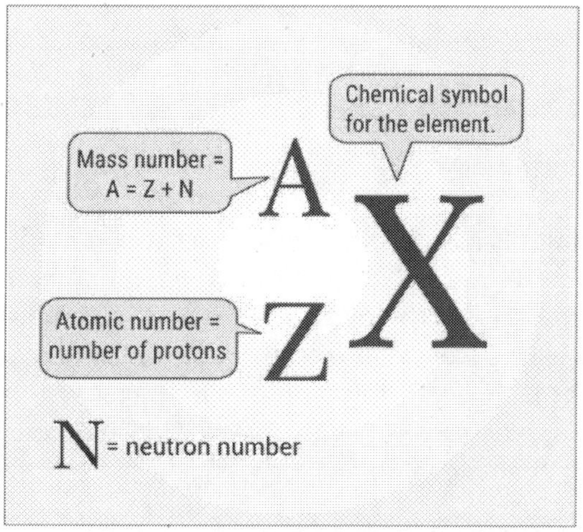

37. A: The neutrons and protons make up the nucleus of the atom. The nucleus is positively charged due to the presence of the protons. The negatively charged electrons are attracted to the positively charged nucleus by the electrostatic or Coulomb force; however, the electrons are not contained in the nucleus. The positively charged protons create the positive charge in the nucleus, and the neutrons are electrically neutral, so they have no effect. Radioactivity does not directly have a bearing on the charge of the nucleus.

38. C: To gather accurate data, the student must be able compare a participant's test score from round 1 with their test score from round 2. The differing levels of intellect among the participants means that comparing participants' test scores to those of other participants would be inaccurate. This requirement excludes Choices *A* and *D*, which involve only one round of testing. The experiment must also involve different levels of sugar consumption from round 1 to round 2. In this way, the effects of different levels of sugar consumption can be seen on the same subjects. Thus, Choice *B* is incorrect because the experiment provides for no variation of sugar consumption. Choice *C* is the correct answer because it allows the student to compare each participant's test score from round 1 with their test score from round 2 after different levels of sugar consumption.

39. D: The seminiferous tubules are responsible for sperm production. Had *testicles* been an answer choice, it would also have been correct since it houses the seminiferous tubules. The prostate gland (*A*) secretes enzymes that help nourish sperm after creation. The seminal vesicles (*B*) secrete some of the components of semen. The scrotum (*C)* is the pouch holding the testicles.

40. D: Based on this table, it can be reasoned that there is not a correlation between maintaining a calendar and GPA since Student B never maintains a calendar but has the highest GPA of the cohort. Furthermore, it can be reasoned that there is a positive correlation between taking notes and GPA since the more notes a student takes, the higher the GPA they have. Thus, Choice *D* is the correct answer. Choice *A* offers an absolute that cannot be proven based on this study; thus, it is incorrect. Choices *B* and *C* are incorrect because they have at least one incorrect correlation.

41. D: Choice *D* is the correct answer because excess sunlight is a common cause of plant wilting. Choices *A, B,* and *C* are all possible but unlikely to be a cause for wilting. Given that the test question asks for a reasonable explanation, sunlight is by far the most reasonable answer.

42. C: The parasympathetic nervous system is related to calm, peaceful times without stress that require no immediate decisions. It relaxes the fight-or-flight response, slows heart rate to a comfortable pace, and decreases bronchiole dilation to a normal size. On the other hand, the sympathetic nervous system is in charge of the fight-or-flight response and works to increase blood pressure and oxygen absorption.

43.

1. **Neon**
2. **Tin**
3. **Oxygen**
4. **Fluorine**

Neon, one of the noble gases, is chemically inert or not reactive because it contains eight valence electrons in the outermost shell. The atomic number is 10, with a 2.8 electron arrangement, meaning that there are 2 electrons in the inner shell and the remaining 8 electrons in the outer shell. This is extremely stable for the atom, so it will not want to add or subtract any of its electrons and will not react under typical circumstances. In contrast, fluorine is the most reactive halogen owing to its high electronegativity, so it is placed at the bottom. Oxygen is slightly less reactive, possessing a lower affinity for electrons, while tin, a post-transition metal, is relatively unreactive (although not inert like neon), placing them at #3 and #2 respectively.

44. C: Because of the vast amounts of data that needed to be processed and analyzed, technological breakthroughs like innovations to the microprocessor were directly responsible for the ease of computing handled by the Human Genome Project. Although the sonogram and MRI technology are helpful to the healthcare industry in general, they would not have provided a great deal of help for sequencing and comprehending DNA data, in general. X-ray diffraction is a technique that helps visualize the structures of crystallized proteins, but it cannot determine DNA bases with enough precision to help sequence DNA.

45. A: Many foods from developed countries are grown from plants which have been processed or bioengineered to include increased amounts of nutrients like vitamins and minerals that otherwise would be lost during manufacturing or are uncommon to the human diet. White rice, for example, is typically enriched with niacin, iron, and folic acid, while salt has been fortified with iodine for nearly a century. These help to prevent nutrition deficiencies. While it can be useful for fisheries to maintain models of fish populations so that they don't overfish their stock, this is not as immediately important to nutrition as are fortified and enriched foods. Although innovations to microscopes could lead to improved healthcare, this also has no direct effect on nutrition deficiency. Refrigerated train carts were historically a crucial invention around Civil War times and were used to transport meat and dairy products long distances without spoiling, but dietary deficiencies could be more easily remedied by supplying people with fortified foods containing those nutrients rather than spoilable meats.

46. B: The most likely hypothesis that Anya is testing has something to with the pathophysiology of the bees, as she performed dissections on some of her samples. These dissections would be unnecessary if the bees were being killed off by another species, as the destruction of the hives would be obvious. As the deaths did not seem linked in any particular way geographically, it is also safe to assume that there was no correlation to cell phone towers, as maps of cell phone coverage would be readily available to her. If the pesticides were so toxic that the bees died on contact, then they wouldn't make it back to the hive to be available for her dissections or to drop off chemicals in the honey. The most likely of the choices is that parasites are killing off the bees, which would be easily communicable.

47. B: For measuring blood, we're looking for a unit that measures volume. Choices *A, B,* and *C*, are all measures of volume, but pounds (*D*) is a measure of weight. The correct answer is liters, as the average adult has about 5 liters of blood in their body. Blood can certainly be measured in ounces or milliliters; however, 5 liters is equal to 5,000 milliliters or 176 ounces. Thus, liters seems to be the more rational measuring unit.

48. B: The endocrine system's organs are glands which are spread throughout the body. The endocrine system itself does not connect the organs or transport the hormones they secrete. Rather, the various glands secrete the hormone into the bloodstream and lets the cardiovascular system pump it throughout the body. The other three body systems each include a network throughout the body:

- Cardiovascular system: veins and arteries
- Immune system: lymphatic vessels (it also uses the circulatory system)
- Nervous system: nerve networks

49. D: In the secondary immune response, suppressor T lymphocytes are activated to negate the potential risk of damage to healthy cells brought on by an unchecked, overactive immune response. Choice *A* is incorrect because this activity is characteristic of the primary response, not the secondary response. Choice *B* is incorrect because humeral immunity is mediated by antibodies produced by B, not T, lymphocytes. Choice *C* is wrong because the secondary response is faster than the primary response because the primary response entails the time-consuming process of macrophage activation.

50. C: Eosinophils, like neutrophils, basophils, and mast cells, are a type of leukocyte in a class called granulocytes. They are found underneath mucous membranes in the body and they primarily secrete destructive enzymes and defend against multicellular parasites like worms. Choice *A* describes basophils and mast cells, and Choice *B* and *D* describe neutrophils. Unlike neutrophils, which are aggressive phagocytic cells, eosinophils have low phagocytic activity.

English and Language Usage

1. B: In Choice *B* the word Uncle should not be capitalized because it is not functioning as a proper noun. If the word named a specific uncle, such as *Uncle Jerry*, then it would be considered a proper noun and should be capitalized. Choice *A* correctly capitalizes the proper noun *East Coast*, and does not capitalize winter, which functions as a common noun in the sentence. Choice *C* correctly capitalizes the name of a specific college course, which is considered a proper noun. Choice *D* correctly capitalizes the proper noun *Jersey Shore*.

2. C: In Choice *C*, avid is functioning as an adjective that modifies the word photographer. *Avid* describes the photographer Julia Robinson's style. The words *time* and *photographer* are functioning as nouns, and the word *capture* is functioning as a verb in the sentence. Other words functioning as adjectives in the sentence include *local*, *business*, and *spare*, as they all describe the nouns they precede.

3. A: Choice *A* is correct because it uses a semicolon to join the two independent clauses (clauses that could function as independent sentences). Choice *B* is incorrect because the conjunction is not preceded by a comma. A comma and conjunction should be used together to join independent clauses. Choice *C* is incorrect because a comma should only be used to join independent sentences when it also includes a coordinating conjunction such as *and* or *so*. Choice *D* does not use punctuation to join the independent clauses, so it is considered a fused (same as a run-on) sentence.

4. C: Choice *C* is a compound sentence because it joins two independent clauses with a comma and the coordinating conjunction *and*. The sentences in Choices *B* and *D* include one independent clause and one dependent clause, so they are complex sentences, not compound sentences. The sentence in Choice *A* has both a compound subject, *Alex and Shane*, and a compound verb, *spent and took*, but the entire sentence itself is one independent clause.

5. A: Choice *A* uses incorrect subject-verb agreement because the indefinite pronoun *neither* is singular and must use the singular verb form *is*. In Choice *B*, the pronoun *both* is plural and uses the plural verb form of *are*. The pronoun *any* can be either singular or plural. In Choice *C*, it is plural, so the plural verb form *are* is used. The pronoun *each* is singular and uses the singular verb form *is*, as seen in Choice *D*.

6. B: Parentheses indicate that the information contained within carries less weight or importance than the surrounding text. The word *essential* makes Choice *A* false. The information, though relevant, is not essential, and the paragraph could survive without it. For Choice *C*, the information is not repeated at any point, and, therefore, is not redundant. For Choice *D*, the information is placed next to his height, which is relevant. Placing it anywhere else would make it out of place.

7. A: It is necessary to put a comma between the date and the year. It is also required to put a comma between the day of the week and the month. Choice *B* is incorrect because it is missing the comma between the day and year. Choice *C* is incorrect because it adds an unnecessary comma between the month and date. Choice *D* is missing the necessary comma between day of the week and the month.

8. D: This passage displays clarity (the author states precisely what he or she intended), fluency (the sentences run smoothly together), and parallelism (words are used in a similar fashion to help provide rhythm). Choice *A* lacks parallelism. When the author states, "the hero acts without thinking, is living in the moment, and is repressing physical and emotional pain," the words *acts, is living* and *is repressing* are in different tenses, and, consequently, jarring to one's ears. Choice *B* runs on endlessly in the first half ("Ernest Hemingway is probably the most noteworthy of expatriate authors since his concise writing style is void of emotion and stream of consciousness and has had a lasting impact on Americans which has resonated to this very day, and Hemingway's novels are much like in American cinema."). It demands some type of pause and strains the readers' eyes. The second half of the passage is choppy: "The hero acts. He doesn't think. He lives in the moment. He represses physical and emotional pain." For Choice *C*, leaving out *expatriate* is, first, vague, and second, alters the meaning. The correct version claims that Hemingway was the most notable of the expatriate authors while the second version claims he's the most notable of any author *ever*, a very bold claim indeed. Also, leaving out *stream of* in "stream of consciousness" no longer references the non-sequential manner in which most people think. Instead, this version sounds like all the characters in the novel are in a coma!

9. D: In Choice *D*, the word *function* is a noun. While the word function can also act as a verb, in this particular sentence it is acting as a noun as the object of the preposition at. Choices *A* and *B* are incorrect because the word function cannot be used as an adjective or adverb.

10. C: *Cacti* is the correct plural form of the word *cactus*. Choice *A* (*tomatos*) includes an incorrect spelling of the plural of *tomato*. Both Choice *B* (*analysis*) and Choice *D* (*criterion*) are incorrect because they are in singular form. The correct plural form for these choices would be *criteria* and *analyses*.

11. C: The phrases one should have and impossible for a presenter are in the third person. The phrases containing the the words you and your are in second person, in which the reader or listener is directly addressed.

12. D: The prefix *trans* can mean *across, beyond, or over*. Choices *A*, *B*, and *C* are incorrect because they are the meanings of other prefixes. Choice *A* is a meaning of the prefix *de*. Choice *B* is the meaning of the prefix *omni*. Choice *C* is one of the meanings of the prefix *pro*. The example words are helpful in determining the meaning of *trans*. All of the example words—*transfer, transact, translation*, and *transport*—indicate something being *across*, *beyond*, or *over* something else. For example, *translation* refers to text going across languages. If no example words were given, you could think of words starting with *trans* and then compare their meanings to try to determine a common definition.

13. C: Oppose makes sense in both instances. *Antibiotics* oppose *bacteria*, and *antisocial people* oppose *society.*

14. D: If *conform* means to adjust behavior, *shape* could replace conform, as if to say that the behavior was reshaped or modified. The same goes for *inform*. New information reshapes how one thinks about the world. Also, the word *shape* gives rise to the abstract idea that both behavior and knowledge are malleable, like modeling clay, and can be molded into new forms. Choice *A* (*match*) works for *conform* (matching to society), but it doesn't work for *inform* (one cannot *match* information to a person). Choice *B* (*relay*) doesn't work for *conform* (there's no way to pass on new behavior), but it does work for *inform*, as to pass on new information. Choice *C* (*negate*) works for neither *conform* (the behavior is not being completely cancelled out) nor *inform* (the information is not being rescinded).

15. D: Choice *D* directly addresses the reader, so it is in second person point of view. This is an imperative sentence since it issues a command; imperative sentences have an understood you as the subject. Choice *A* uses first person pronouns *I* and *my*. Choices *B* and *C* are incorrect because they use third person point of view.

16. A: The word *prodigious* is defined as very impressive, amazing, or large. In this sentence, the meaning can be drawn from the words *they became nervous about climbing its distant peak*, as this would be an appropriate reaction upon seeing a very large peak that's far in the distance. Choices *B*, *C*, and *D* do not accurately define the word prodigious, so they are incorrect.

17. D: Choice *D* correctly places a hyphen after the prefix *ex* to join it to the word *husband.* Many words that begin with the prefixes *great, trans, ex, all,* and *self* require a hyphen. Choices *A* and *C* place hyphens in words where they are not needed. *Beagle mix* would only require a hyphen if coming before the word *Henry*, since it would be serving as a compound adjective in that instance. Choice *B* contains hyphens that are in the correct place but are formatted incorrectly since they include spaces between the hyphens and the surrounding words.

18. B: To arrive at the best answer, all the character traits for Cindy must be analyzed. She's described as *happy* ("always has a smile on her face"), *kind* ("volunteers at the local shelter"), and *patient* ("no one has ever seen her angry"). Since Cindy's husband is the *opposite* of her, these adjectives must be converted to antonyms. Someone who is *surly* is *unhappy*, *rude*, and *impatient*. *Stingy*, Choice *A*, is too narrow of a word. Someone could be *happy* and *kind*, for instance, but still be *stingy*. For Choice *C*, *scared*, to be plausible, the rest of the passage would need instances of Cindy being *bold* or *courageous*. *Shy*, Choice *D*, also doesn't match. Someone who is *shy* could still be *happy*, *kind*, and *patient.*

19. C: This question focuses on the correct usage of the commonly confused word pairs of *it's/its* and *then/than. It's* is a contraction for *it is* or *it has*. *Its* is a possessive pronoun. The word *than* shows comparison between two things. *Then* is an adverb that conveys time. Choice *C* correctly uses *it's* and *than*. *It's* is a contraction for *it has* in this sentence, and *than* shows comparison between *work* and *rest*. None of the other answer choices use both of the correct words.

20. C: The suffix *-fy* means to make, cause, or cause to have. Choices *A*, *B*, and *D* are incorrect because they show meanings of other suffixes. Choice *A* shows the meaning of the suffix -ous. Choice B shows the meaning of the suffix –ist, and Choice *D* shows the meaning of the suffix -age.

21. B: *Dissatisfied* and *accommodations* are both spelled correctly in Choice *B*. These are both considered commonly misspelled words. One or both words are spelled incorrectly in Choices *A, C,* and *D.*

22: A: *Grasp* is the best answer. It's important both in the New World and in Africa to ambulate or *move* (the word is used more than once), but only in the New World must mammals deal with dense vegetation and foliage. Choice *B* (*punch*) is incorrect because punching is unrelated to dealing with dense vegetation. *Prehensile tails* are designed to *grasp*. It's established in *both* environments that *movement* is critical to survival. Choice *C* (*move*) applies, again, to both jungle and savannah environments. Choice *D* (*walk*) would be applicable to savannahs, not environments populated with dense vegetation.

23. A: *After* and *then* are transitional words that indicate time or position. Choice *B* is incorrect because the words *at, with,* and *to* are used as prepositions in this sentence, not transitions. Choice *C* is incorrect because the words *had* and *took* are used as verbs in this sentence. In Choice *D, a* and *the* are used as articles in the sentence.

24. C: Choice *C* is a compound sentence because it joins two independent clauses—*The baby was sick* and *I decided to stay home from work*—with a comma and the coordinating conjunction *so*. Choices *A, B,* and *D* are all simple sentences, each containing one independent clause with a complete subject and predicate. Choices *A* and *D* each contain a compound subject, or more than one subject, but they are still simple sentences that only contain one independent clause. Choice *B* contains a compound verb (more than one verb), but it's still a simple sentence.

25. A, B, D, G, I: The other choices are not nouns:

Final: adjective

He: pronoun

Library: adjective. It can function as a noun, but in this sentence, it functions as an adjective modifying the word *databases*.

Academic: adjective

26. A: First person is known as the "I" voice. There are no "I's" in this passage, but the words *we* and *our* indicate first person plural. *We*, logically, includes *I* and other people. *Our*, plural possessive, includes *mine* and *others'*. Even though the narrator is talking about other people (Mom and Dad), the whole passage is still written from the perspective of that same first person narrator.

27. C: The second sentence tells of an unexpected outcome of the first sentence. Choice *A*, Choice *B*, and Choice *D* indicate a logical progression, which does not match this surprise. Only Choice *C* indicates this unexpected twist.

28. D: The object pronouns *her* and *me* act as the indirect objects of the sentence. If *me* is in a series of object pronouns, it should always come last in the series. Choice *A* is incorrect because it uses subject pronouns *she* and *I*. Choice *B* is incorrect because it uses the subject pronoun *she.* Choice *C* uses the correct object pronouns, but they are in the wrong order.

29. A: The word *foliage* is defined as leaves on plants or trees. In this sentence, the meaning can be drawn from the fact that a heavily wooded area in October would be characterized by the beautiful changing colors of the leaves. The other answer choices do not accurately define the word *foliage*, so they are incorrect.

30. D: The prefix *ger*- or *gero*- means old age as in geriatric.

31. A: Only two of these suffixes, *–ize* and *–en*, can be used to form verbs, so *B* and *D* are incorrect. Those choices create adjectives. The suffix –ize can mean "to convert or turn into." Because this sentence is about converting ideas into money, monetize is the appropriate word to use.

32. A: Slang refers to non-standard expressions that are not used in elevated speech and writing. Slang tends to be specific to one group or time period and is commonly used within groups of young people during their conversations with each other. Jargon refers to the language used in a specialized field. The vernacular is the native language of a local area, and a dialect is one form of a language in a certain region. Thus, Choices *B*, *C*, and *D* are incorrect.

33. D: Colloquial language is that which is used conversationally or informally, in contrast to professional or academic language. While *ain't* is common in conversational English, it is a non-standard expression in academic writing. For college-bound students, high school should introduce them to the expectations of a college classroom, so Choice *B* is not the best answer. Teachers should also avoid placing moral or social value on certain patterns of speech. Rather than teaching students that their familiar speech patterns are bad, teachers should help students learn when and how to use appropriate forms of expression, so Choice *C* is wrong. *Ain't* is in the dictionary, so Choice *A* is incorrect, both in the reason for counseling and in the factual sense.

34. B: The original sentence focuses on how politicians are using the student debt issue to their advantage, so Choice *B* is the best answer choice. Choice *A* says politicians want students' votes but suggests that it is the reason for student loan debt, which is incorrect. Choice *C* shifts the focus to voters, when the sentence is really about politicians. Choice *D* is vague and doesn't best restate the original meaning of the sentence.

35. A: This answer best matches the meaning of the original sentence, which states that seasoned runners offer advice to new runners because they have complaints of injuries. Choice *B* may be true, but it doesn't mention the complaints of injuries by new runners. Choice *C* may also be true, but it does not match the original meaning of the sentence. Choice *D* does not make sense in the context of the sentence.

36. C: Inflammation. Tendonitis, conjunctivitis, and colitis are examples of medical conditions that are specific areas of inflammation.

37. B, C: A dependent clause cannot stand by itself as a sentence. The clauses *because it was raining* and *when it is Saturday* are missing information that is necessary to complete the sentences. The remaining choices are independent clauses, meaning they would form complete sentences by themselves.

TEAS 7 Practice Test #2

Reading

The next six questions are based upon the following passage:

My gentleness and good behaviour had gained so far on the emperor and his court, and indeed upon the army and people in general, that I began to conceive hopes of getting my liberty in a short time. I took all possible methods to cultivate this favourable disposition. The natives came, by degrees, to be less apprehensive of any danger from me. I, Gulliver, would sometimes lie down, and let five or six of them dance on my hand; and at last, the boys and girls would venture to come and play at hide-and-seek in my hair. I had now made a good progress in understanding and speaking the language. The emperor had a mind one day to entertain me with several of the country shows, wherein they exceed all nations I have known, both for dexterity and magnificence. I was diverted with none so much as that of the rope-dancers, performed upon a slender white thread, extended about two feet, and twelve inches from the ground. Upon which I shall desire liberty, with the reader's patience, to enlarge a little.

This diversion is only practised by those persons who are candidates for great employments, and high favour at court. They are trained in this art from their youth, and are not always of noble birth, or liberal education. When a great office is vacant, either by death or disgrace (which often happens), five or six of those candidates petition the emperor to entertain his majesty and the court with a dance on the rope; and whoever jumps the highest, without falling, succeeds in the office. Very often the chief ministers themselves are commanded to show their skill, and to convince the emperor that they have not lost their faculty. Flimnap, the treasurer, is allowed to cut a caper on the straight rope, at least an inch higher than any other lord in the whole empire. I have seen him do the summerset several times together, upon a trencher fixed on a rope which is no thicker than a common packthread in England. My friend Reldresal, principal secretary for private affairs, is, in my opinion, if I am not partial, the second after the treasurer; the rest of the great officers are much upon a par.

Excerpt adapted from *Gulliver's Travels into Several Remote Nations of the World* by Jonathan Swift

1. Which of the following statements best summarizes the central purpose of this text?
    a. Gulliver details his fondness for the archaic, yet interesting, practices of his captors.
    b. Gulliver conjectures about the intentions of the aristocratic sector of society.
    c. Gulliver becomes acquainted with the people and practices of his new surroundings.
    d. Gulliver's differences cause him to become penitent around new acquaintances.

2. What is the word *principal* referring to in the following text?

    My friend Reldresal, principal secretary for private affairs, is, in my opinion, if I am not partial, the second after the treasurer; the rest of the great officers are much upon a par.

    a. Primary or chief
    b. An acolyte
    c. An individual who provides nurturing
    d. One in a subordinate position

3. What can the reader infer from the following text?

> I, Gulliver, would sometimes lie down, and let five or six of them dance on my hand; and at last, the boys and girls would venture to come and play at hide-and-seek in my hair.

a. The children tortured Gulliver.
b. Gulliver traveled because he wanted to meet new people.
c. Gulliver is considerably larger than the children who are playing around him.
d. Gulliver has a genuine love and enthusiasm for people of all sizes.

4. What is the significance of the word *mind* in the following passage?

> The emperor had a mind one day to entertain me with several of the country shows, wherein they exceed all nations I have known, both for dexterity and magnificence.

a. The ability to think
b. A collective vote
c. A definitive decision
d. A mythological question

5. Which of the following assertions does not support the fact that games are a commonplace event in this culture?
a. My gentleness and good behavior... short time.
b. They are trained in this art from their youth...liberal education.
c. Very often the chief ministers themselves are commanded to show their skill...not lost their faculty.
d. Flimnap, the treasurer, is allowed to cut a caper on the straight rope...higher than any other lord in the whole empire.

6. How do Flimnap and Reldresal demonstrate the community's emphasis on physical strength and leadership abilities?
a. Only children used Gulliver's hands as a playground.
b. The two men who exhibited superior abilities held prominent positions in the community.
c. Only common townspeople, not leaders, walk the straight rope.
d. No one could jump higher than Gulliver.

The next question is based on the following outline.

Chapter 5: Outdoor Activities

1. Hiking
   a. Gear
   b. First Aid
2. Camping
   a. Tents & Gear
   b. Camping Activities
3. Cycling
   a. Safety
   b. Finding Cycling Trails
4. Canoeing
   a. Equipment
   b. Tips for Maneuvering

7. What aspect of this outline is inconsistent?
   a. Hiking, which starts with an H, is included with activities that all start with C.
   b. There is no information about gear/equipment for cycling
   c. Rock climbing is not included in the outline.
   d. There is no section for hiking tips.

8. The assassination of Archduke Franz Ferdinand of Austria is often ascribed as the cause of World War I. However, the assassination merely lit the fuse in a combustible situation since many of the world powers were in complicated and convoluted military alliances. For example, England, France, and Russia entered into a mutual defense treaty seven years prior to World War I. Even without Franz Ferdinand's assassination, ______________________

Which of the following most logically completes the passage?
   a. a war between the world powers was extremely likely.
   b. World War I never would have happened.
   c. England, France, and Russia would have started the war.
   d. Austria would have started the war.

The next four questions are based on the timeline of the life of Alexander Graham Bell.

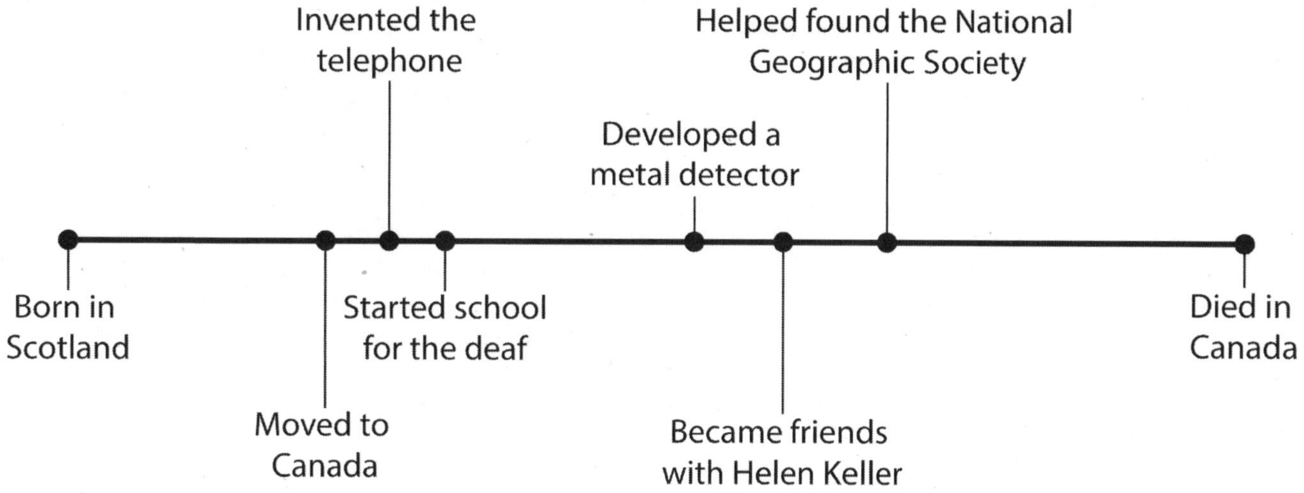

9. Which of the following is the event that occurred fourth on the timeline?
   a. Helped found National Geographic Society
   b. Developed a metal detector
   c. Moved to Canada
   d. Started a school for the deaf

10. Of the pairings in the answer choices, which has the longest gap between the two events?
   a. Moved to Canada and Became friends with Helen Keller
   b. Became friends with Helen Keller and Died in Canada
   c. Started school for the deaf and Developed a metal detector
   d. Born in Scotland and Started school for the deaf

11. Which one of the following statements is accurate based on the timeline?
   a. Bell did nothing significant after he helped found the National Geographic Society.
   b. Bell started a school for the deaf in Canada.
   c. Bell lived in at least two countries.
   d. Developing a metal detector allowed Bell to meet Helen Keller.

12. Which one of the following events occurred most recently?
   a. Bell's invention of the telephone
   b. Bell's founding of the school
   c. Bell's birth
   d. Bell's move to Canada

Questions 13 – 17 are based upon the following passage:

This excerpt is an adaptation of Robert Louis Stevenson's *The Strange Case of Dr. Jekyll and Mr. Hyde*.

> "Did you ever come across a protégé of his—one Hyde?" he asked.
>
> "Hyde?" repeated Lanyon. "No. Never heard of him. Since my time."
>
> That was the amount of information that the lawyer carried back with him to the great, dark bed on which he tossed to and fro until the small hours of the morning began to grow large. It was a night of little ease to his toiling mind, toiling in mere darkness and besieged by questions.

Six o'clock struck on the bells of the church that was so conveniently near to Mr. Utterson's dwelling, and still he was digging at the problem. Hitherto it had touched him on the intellectual side alone; but now his imagination also was engaged, or rather enslaved; and as he lay and tossed in the gross darkness of the night in the curtained room, Mr. Enfield's tale went by before his mind in a scroll of lighted pictures. He would be aware of the great field of lamps in a nocturnal city; then of the figure of a man walking swiftly; then of a child running from the doctor's; and then these met, and that human Juggernaut trod the child down and passed on regardless of her screams. Or else he would see a room in a rich house, where his friend lay asleep, dreaming and smiling at his dreams; and then the door of that room would be opened, the curtains of the bed plucked apart, the sleeper recalled, and, lo! There would stand by his side a figure to whom power was given, and even at that dead hour he must rise and do its bidding. The figure in these two phases haunted the lawyer all night; and if at any time he dozed over, it was but to see it glide more stealthily through sleeping houses, or move the more swiftly, and still the more smoothly, even to dizziness, through wider labyrinths of lamplighted city, and at every street corner crush a child and leave her screaming. And still the figure had no face by which he might know it; even in his dreams it had no face, or one that baffled him and melted before his eyes; and thus it was that there sprung up and grew apace in the lawyer's mind a singularly strong almost an inordinate, curiosity to behold the features of the real Mr. Hyde. If he could but once set eyes on him, he thought the mystery would lighten and perhaps roll altogether away, as was the habit of mysterious things when well examined. He might see a reason for his friend's strange preference or bondage, and even for the startling clauses of the will. And at least it would be a face worth seeing: the face of a man who was without bowels of mercy: a face which had but to show itself to raise up, in the mind of the unimpressionable Enfield, a spirit of enduring hatred.

From that time forward, Mr. Utterson began to haunt the door in the by-street of shops. In the morning before office hours, at noon when business was plenty and time scarce, at night under the face of the fogged city moon, by all lights and at all hours of solitude or concourse, the lawyer was to be found on his chosen post.

"If he be Mr. Hyde," he had thought, "I should be Mr. Seek."

13. What is the setting of the story in this passage?
    a. In the city
    b. On the countryside
    c. In a jail
    d. In a mental health facility

14. What can one infer about the meaning of the word Juggernaut from the author's use of it in the passage?
    a. It is an apparition that appears at daybreak.
    b. It scares children.
    c. It is associated with space travel.
    d. Mr. Utterson finds it soothing.

15. What is the definition of the word *haunt* in the following passage?

> From that time forward, Mr. Utterson began to haunt the door in the by-street of shops. In the morning before office hours, at noon when business was plenty and time scarce, at night under the face of the fogged city moon, by all lights and at all hours of solitude or concourse, the lawyer was to be found on his chosen post.

a. To levitate
b. To constantly visit
c. To terrorize
d. To daunt

16. The phrase *labyrinths of lamp lighted city* contains an example of what?
a. Hyperbole
b. Simile
c. Juxtaposition
d. Alliteration

17. What can one reasonably conclude from the final comment of this passage?

> "If he be Mr. Hyde," he had thought, "I should be Mr. Seek."

a. The speaker is considering a name change.
b. The speaker is experiencing an identity crisis.
c. The speaker has mistakenly been looking for the wrong person.
d. The speaker intends to continue to look for Hyde.

The next five questions are based on the chart following a brief introduction to the topic.

The American Civil War was fought from 1861 to 1865. It is the only civil war in American history. While the South's secession was the initiating event of the war, the conflict grew out of several issues, like slavery and differing interpretations of individual state rights. General Robert E. Lee led the Confederate Army for the South for the duration of the conflict. The North employed a variety of lead generals, but Ulysses S. Grant finished the war as the victorious general. There were more American casualties in the Civil War than any other military conflict in American history.

Civil War Casualties by Battle (approximate)

Battle	**Date**	**Union General**	**Confederate General**	**Union Casualties**	**Confederate Casualties**
Gettysburg	July 1863	George Meade	Robert E. Lee	23,049	28,063
Chancellorsville	May 1863	Joseph Hooker	Robert E. Lee	17,304	13,460
Shiloh	April 1862	Ulysses S. Grant	Albert Sydney Johnston	13,047	10,669
Cold Harbor	May 1864	Ulysses S. Grant	Robert E. Lee	12,737	4,595
Atlanta	July 1864	William T. Sherman	John Bell Hood	3,722	5,500

18. In which of the following battles were there more Confederate casualties than Union casualties?
   a. Cold Harbor
   b. Chancellorsville
   c. Atlanta
   d. Shiloh

19. Which one of the following battles occurred first?
   a. Cold Harbor
   b. Chancellorsville
   c. Atlanta
   d. Shiloh

20. Robert E. Lee did NOT lead the Confederate forces in which one of the following battles?
   a. Atlanta
   b. Chancellorsville
   c. Cold Harbor
   d. Gettysburg

21. In which of the following battles did the Union casualties exceed the Confederate casualties by the greatest number?
    a. Cold Harbor
    b. Chancellorsville
    c. Atlanta
    d. Shiloh

22 The total number of American casualties suffered at the battle of Gettysburg is about double the total number of casualties suffered at which one of the following battles?
    a. Cold Harbor
    b. Chancellorsville
    c. Atlanta
    d. Shiloh

23. A student is starting a research assignment on Japanese American internment camps during World War II, but she is unsure of how to gather relevant resources. Which of the following would be helpful advice for the student? *Select all that apply.*
    a. Conduct a broad internet search to get a wide view of the subject.
    b. Locate digital or print interviews of individuals interned in the camps.
    c. Find websites about Japanese culture such as fashion and politics.
    d. Locate texts in the library related to World War II in America and look for references to internment camps in the index.
    e. Consult an American history textbook.

24. When selecting a career path, it's important to explore the various options available. Many students entering college may shy away from a major because they don't know much about it. For example, many students won't opt for a career as an actuary because they aren't exactly sure what it entails. But in doing so, they are missing out on a career that is very lucrative and in high demand. Actuaries work in the insurance field and assess risks and premiums. The average salary of an actuary is $100,000 per year. Another career option students may avoid, due to lack of knowledge of the field, is a hospitalist. This is a physician that specializes in the care of patients in a hospital, as opposed to those seen in private practices. The average salary of a hospitalist is upwards of $200,000. It pays to do some digging and find out more about these lesser-known career fields.

An actuary is:
    a. A doctor who works in a hospital
    b. The same as a hospitalist
    c. An insurance agent who works in a hospital
    d. A person who assesses insurance risks and premiums

The next five questions are based on the following passages.

Passage I

Lethal force, or deadly force, is defined as the physical means to cause death or serious harm to another individual. The law holds that lethal force is only acceptable when you or another person are in immediate and unavoidable danger of death or severe bodily harm. For example, a person could be beating someone in such a way that the victim is suffering severe trauma that could result in death or serious harm. This would be an instance where lethal force would be acceptable and possibly the only way to save the victim from irrevocable damage.

Another example of when to use lethal force would be when someone enters your home with a deadly weapon. The intruder's presence and possession of the weapon indicate malicious intent and the ability to inflict death or severe injury upon you and your loved ones. Again, lethal force can be used in this situation. Lethal force can also be applied to prevent the harm of another individual. If a woman is being brutally assaulted and is unable to fend off an attacker, lethal force can be used to defend her as a last-ditch effort. If she is in immediate jeopardy of rape, harm, and/or death, lethal force could be the only response that could effectively deter the assailant.

The key to understanding the concept of lethal force is the term *last resort*. Deadly force cannot be taken back; it should be used only to prevent severe harm or death. The law does distinguish whether the means of one's self-defense is fully warranted or if the individual goes out of control in the process. If you continually attack the assailant after they are rendered incapacitated, this would be causing unnecessary harm, and the law can bring charges against you. Likewise, if you kill an attacker unnecessarily after defending yourself, you can be charged with murder. This would move lethal force beyond necessary defense, making it no longer a last resort but rather a use of excessive force.

Passage II

Assault is an unlawful attempt and intentional act that causes reasonable apprehension in another individual, either by an imminent threat or by initiating offensive contact. Assaults can vary, encompassing physical strikes, threatening body language, and even provocative language. In the case of the latter, even if a hand has not been laid, it is still considered an assault because of its threatening nature.

Let's look at an example. A homeowner is angered because his neighbor blows fallen leaves onto his freshly mowed lawn. Irate, the homeowner gestures a fist to his neighbor and threatens to bash his head in for littering on his lawn. The homeowner's physical motions and verbal threats herald a physical threat against the other neighbor. These factors classify the homeowner's reaction as an assault. If the angry neighbor hits the threatening homeowner in retaliation, that would constitute an assault as well because he physically hit the homeowner.

Assault also centers on the involvement of weapons in a conflict. If someone fired a gun at another person, it could be interpreted as an assault, unless the shooter acted in self-defense. If an individual drew a gun or a knife on someone with the intent to harm them, it would be considered assault. However, it's also considered an assault if someone simply aims a weapon, loaded or not, at another person in a threatening manner.

25. What is the purpose of the second passage?
    a. To inform the reader about what assault is and how it is committed
    b. To inform the reader about how assault is a minor example of lethal force
    c. To disprove the previous passage concerning lethal force
    d. To argue that the use of assault is more common than the use of lethal force

26. According to the passages, in which of the following situations would the use of lethal force be permissible?
    a. A disgruntled cashier yells obscenities at a customer.
    b. A thief is seen running away with stolen cash.
    c. A man is attacked in an alley by another man with a knife.
    d. A woman punches another woman in a bar.

27. Given the information in the passages, which of the following must be true about assault?
    a. All assault is considered an expression of lethal force.
    b. There are various forms of assault.
    c. Smaller, weaker people cannot commit assault.
    d. Assault is justified only as a last resort.

28. Which of the following, if true, would most seriously undermine the explanation proposed by the author in the third paragraph of Passage I?
    a. An instance of lethal force in self-defense is not absolutely absolved from blame. The law takes into account the necessary use of force at the time it is committed.
    b. An individual who uses lethal force only in necessary defense is in direct compliance with the law under most circumstances.
    c. Lethal force in self-defense should be forgiven in all cases for the peace of mind of the primary victim.
    d. The use of lethal force is not evaluated on the intent of the user but rather the severity of the primary attack that warranted self-defense.

29. Based on the passages, what can we infer about the relationship between assault and lethal force?
    a. An act of lethal force always leads to a type of assault.
    b. An assault will result in someone using lethal force.
    c. An assault with deadly intent can lead to an individual using lethal force to preserve their well-being.
    d. If someone uses self-defense in a conflict, it is called deadly force; if actions or threats are intended, it is called assault.

30. If you were looking for the most reliable and up-to-date information regarding the safety of travel overseas, which of the following websites would be the most accurate?
    a. http://www.nomadicmatt.com/travel-blog/
    b. https://en.wikipedia.org/wiki/Tourism
    c. http://gizmodo.com/how-to-travel-internationally-for-the-very-first-time
    d. http://www.state.gov/travel/

Use the following pie chart to complete the next question.

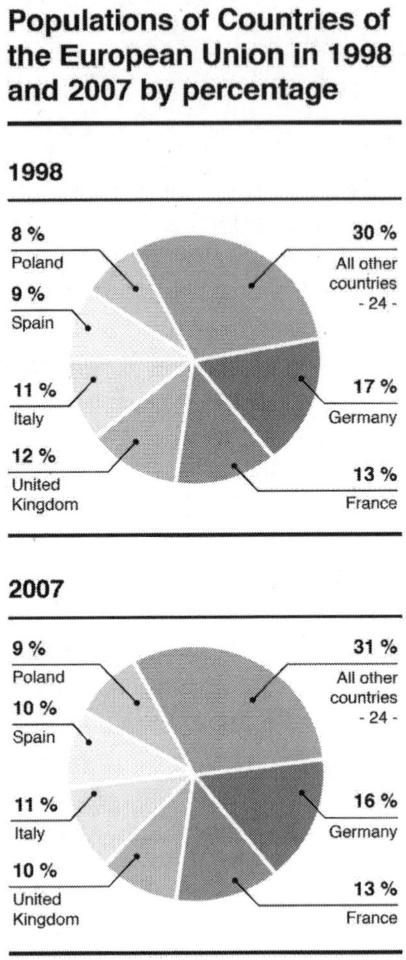

31. According to the pie charts above, how did the population percentage of Germany change from 1998 to 2007?
    a. It decreased one percent.
    b. It increased one percent.
    c. It decreased three percent.
    d. It increased three percent.

32. After reading *To Kill a Mockingbird*, Louise has been asked to write an expository piece that explores the life, significant achievements, and societal impact of Harper Lee, the book's author. Which of the following sources would yield the most information about the author?
    a. A dictionary
    b. A newspaper article about the author
    c. A study guide for *To Kill a Mockingbird*
    d. A biographical account

33. Bobo the clown books more shows and makes more money than Gob the magician. Despite rampant coulrophobia—an irrational fear of clowns—Bobo still books more parties and receives higher rates of compensation per show. Gob's magic shows are no worse than Bobo's clown performances.

Which of the following statements, if true, best explains the apparent paradox?

a. Bobo is an experienced clown.
b. Despite rampant coulrophobia, statistical data shows that people generally prefer clowns to magicians for children's birthday parties.
c. Bobo goes out of his way to appear non-threatening.
d. Bobo works in a densely populated city, while Gob works in a rural town.

34. Read the following words:

mixed
thrown
are
grown
beaten
jumped

Analyze the list and determine which word does not belong.

a. Mixed
b. Are
c. Grown
d. Jumped

The next six questions are based upon the following passage:

This excerpt is adapted from Charles Dickens' speech in Birmingham in England on December 30, 1853 on behalf of the Birmingham and Midland Institute." Questions 35-40 are based on it.

> My Good Friends,—When I first imparted to the committee of the projected Institute my particular wish that on one of the evenings of my readings here the main body of my audience should be composed of working men and their families, I was animated by two desires; first, by the wish to have the great pleasure of meeting you face to face at this Christmas time, and accompany you myself through one of my little Christmas books; and second, by the wish to have an opportunity of stating publicly in your presence, and in the presence of the committee, my earnest hope that the Institute will, from the beginning, recognize one great principle—strong in reason and justice—which I believe to be essential to the very life of such an Institution. It is, that the working man shall, from the first unto the last, have a share in the management of an Institution which is designed for his benefit, and which calls itself by his name.
>
> I have no fear here of being misunderstood—of being supposed to mean too much in this. If there ever was a time when any one class could of itself do much for its own good, and for the welfare of society—which I greatly doubt—that time is unquestionably past. It is in the fusion of different classes, without confusion; in the bringing together of employers and employed; in the creating of a better common understanding among those whose interests are identical, who depend upon each other, who are vitally essential to each other, and who never can be in unnatural antagonism without deplorable results, that one of the chief principles of a Mechanics' Institution should consist. In this world a great deal of the bitterness among us arises from an imperfect understanding of one another. Erect in Birmingham a great Educational Institution, properly

educational; educational of the feelings as well as of the reason; to which all orders of Birmingham men contribute; in which all orders of Birmingham men meet; wherein all orders of Birmingham men are faithfully represented—and you will erect a Temple of Concord here which will be a model edifice to the whole of England.

Contemplating as I do the existence of the Artisans' Committee, which not long ago considered the establishment of the Institute so sensibly, and supported it so heartily, I earnestly entreat the gentlemen—earnest I know in the good work, and who are now among us,—by all means to avoid the great shortcoming of similar institutions; and in asking the working man for his confidence, to set him the great example and give him theirs in return. You will judge for yourselves if I promise too much for the working man, when I say that he will stand by such an enterprise with the utmost of his patience, his perseverance, sense, and support; that I am sure he will need no charitable aid or condescending patronage; but will readily and cheerfully pay for the advantages which it confers; that he will prepare himself in individual cases where he feels that the adverse circumstances around him have rendered it necessary; in a word, that he will feel his responsibility like an honest man, and will most honestly and manfully discharge it. I now proceed to the pleasant task to which I assure you I have looked forward for a long time.

35. Which word is most closely synonymous with the word *patronage* as it appears in the following statement:

> ... that I am sure he will need no charitable aid or condescending patronage

a. Auspices
b. Aberration
c. Acerbic
d. Adulation

36. Which term is most closely aligned with the definition of the term working man as it is used in the following quotation?

> You will judge for yourselves if I promise too much for the working man, when I say that he will stand by such an enterprise with the utmost of his patience, his perseverance, sense, and support...

a. Athlete
b. Viscount
c. Entrepreneur
d. Bourgeois

37. Which of the following statements most closely correlates with the definition of the term *working man* as it is defined in the previous question?

a. A working man is not someone who works for institutions or corporations but rather someone who is well versed in the workings of the soul.
b. A working man is someone who is probably not involved in social activities because the physical demand for work is too high.
c. A working man is someone who works for wages among the middle class.
d. The working man has historically taken to the field, to the factory, and now to the screen.

38. Based upon the contextual evidence provided in the passage above, what is the meaning of the term *enterprise* in the third paragraph?

   a. Company
   b. Courage
   c. Game
   d. Cause

39. The speaker addresses his audience as "My Good Friends." What function does this salutation serve for the speaker?

   a. The speaker is an employer addressing his employees, so the salutation is a way for the boss to bridge the gap between himself and his employees.
   b. The speaker's salutation is one from an entertainer to his audience and uses the friendly language to connect to his audience before a serious speech.
   c. The salutation gives the serious speech that follows a somber tone, as it is used ironically.
   d. The speech is one from a politician to the public, so the salutation is used to grab the audience's attention.

40. According to the passage, what is the speaker's second desire for his time in front of the audience?

   a. To read a Christmas story
   b. To support the idea that the working man should have a say in an institution that is designed for his benefit
   c. To have an opportunity to stand in their presence
   d. For the life of the institution to be essential to the audience as a whole

Use the following table to complete the next two questions.

	D	E	F
1	Payment	T-shirt Color	T-shirt Size
2	1 - Jan	Heather Gray	*Large*
3	1 - Jan	White	*Large*
4	4 - Jan	Dark Red	*X - Large*
5	5 - Jan	Dark Red	*Medium*
6	5 - Jan	Heather Gray	*Large*
7	5 - Jan	Dark Red	*Medium*
8	5 - Jan	Heather Gray	*X - Large*
9	6 - Jan	White	*X - Large*
10	6 - Jan	Dark Red	*X - Large*
11	7 - Jan	Heather Gray	*Small*
12	7 - Jan	Dark Red	*Small*
13	7 - Jan	Heather Gray	*Small*
14	7 - Jan	Heather Gray	*Small*
15	11 - Jan	Dark Red	*Medium*
16	11 - Jan	White	*Medium*
17	11 - Jan	Dark Red	*Medium*

41. In the table above, how many Heather Gray T-shirts were ordered in a size small in the month of January?

____

42. According to the table above, how many more shirts were ordered in size medium than size small in the month of January?

____

43. Which effective writing area engages and connects with the audience, igniting emotion?
   a. Ethos
   b. Logos
   c. Pathos
   d. Kairos

44. Firsthand accounts of an event, subject matter, time period, or individual are referred to as what type of sources?
   a. Primary
   b. Secondary
   c. Direct
   d. Indirect

45. Conservative politician: Social welfare programs are destroying our country. These programs are not only adding to the annual deficit, which increases the national debt, but they also discourage hard work. Our country must continue producing leaders who bootstrap their way to the top. None of our country's citizens truly *need* assistance from the government; rather, the assistance just makes things easier.

Liberal politician: Our great country is founded on the principle of hope. The country is built on the backs of immigrants who came here with nothing, except for the hope of a better life. Our country is too wealthy not to provide basic necessities for the less fortunate. Recent immigrants, single mothers, and people who are elderly, disabled, or have historically been disenfranchised all require an ample safety net.

What is the main point of dispute between the politicians?

a. Whether spending on social welfare programs increases the national debt
b. Whether certain classes of people rely on social welfare programs to meet their basic needs
c. Whether social welfare programs are necessary
d. Whether the country's leaders have bootstrapped their way to the top

Mathematics

1. Simplify: $\frac{4a^{-1}b^3}{a^4b^{-2}} \times \frac{3a}{b}$?

a. $12a^3b^5$
b. $12\frac{b^4}{a^4}$
c. $\frac{12}{a^4}$
d. $7\frac{b^4}{a}$

2. What is the product of two irrational numbers?

a. Irrational
b. Rational
c. Irrational or rational
d. Complex and imaginary

3. The graph shows the position of a car over a 10-second time interval. Which of the following is the correct interpretation of the graph for the interval 1 to 3 seconds?

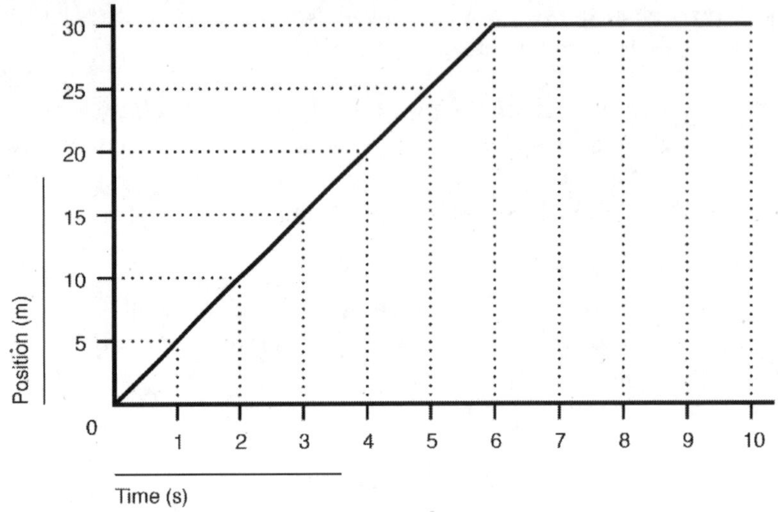

a. The car remains in the same position.
b. The car is traveling at a speed of 5 m/s.
c. The car is traveling up a hill.
d. The car is traveling at 5 mph.

4. The number -4 can be classified as which of the following?
a. Real, rational, integer, whole, natural
b. Real, rational, integer, natural
c. Real, rational, integer
d. Real, irrational

5. $4\frac{5}{7} + 6\frac{5}{8} =$

a. $10\frac{12}{56}$

b. $11\frac{19}{43}$

c. $11\frac{19}{56}$

d. $10\frac{19}{56}$

6. The total circumference of the following diagram, rounding to the nearest decimal place, is ______.

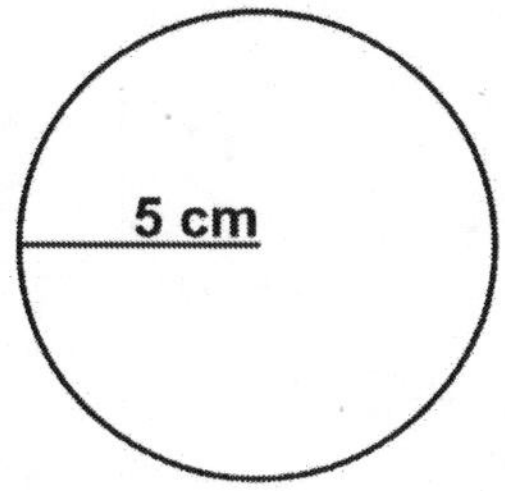

7. 4.67 miles is equivalent to how many kilometers, to three significant digits? Use the conversion 1 mi=1.609 km.

a. 7.514 km
b. 7.51 km
c. 2.90 km
d. 2.902 km

8. If $\frac{5}{2} \div \frac{1}{3} = n$, then n is between:

a. 5 and 7
b. 7 and 9
c. 9 and 11
d. 3 and 5

9. A closet is filled with red, blue, and green shirts. If $\frac{1}{3}$ of the shirts are green and $\frac{2}{5}$ are red, what fraction of the shirts are blue?

a. $\frac{4}{15}$
b. $\frac{1}{5}$
c. $\frac{7}{15}$
d. $\frac{1}{2}$

10. A right triangle has a hypotenuse of 10 inches, and one leg is 8 inches. How long is the other leg in inches?

a. 6 in
b. 18 in
c. 80 in
d. 13 in

11. The chart below shows the average car sales for the months of July through December for two different car dealers. What is the average number of cars sold per month in the given time period for Dealer 1?

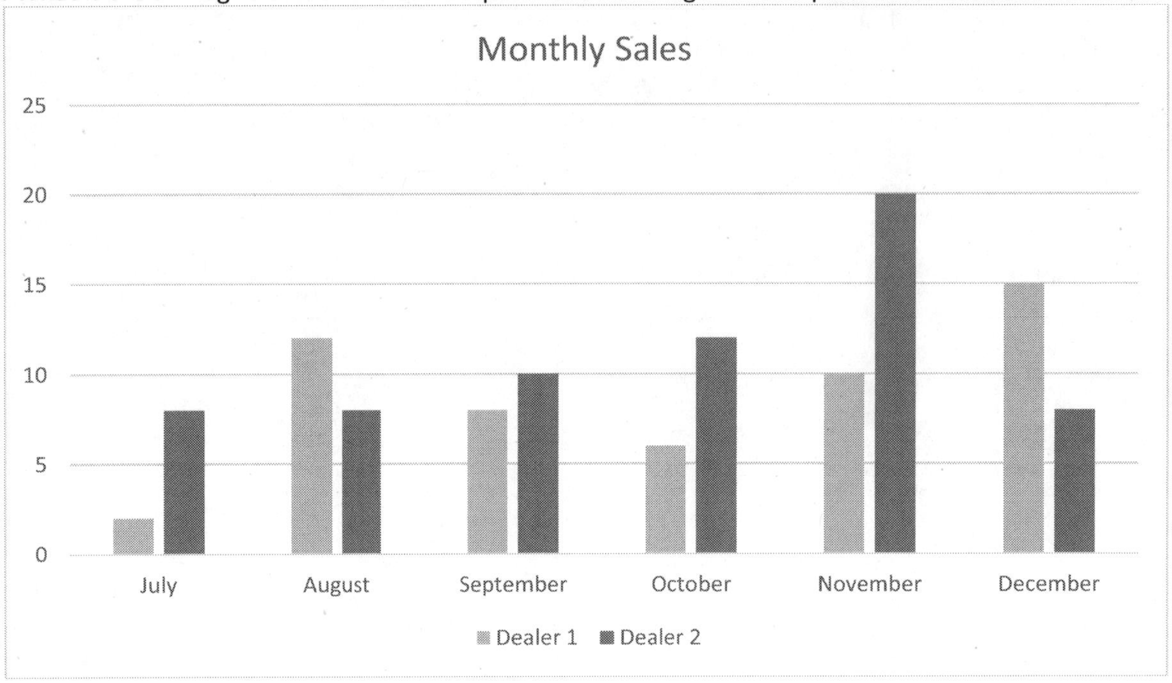

a. 7 cars
b. 11 cars
c. 9 cars
d. 8 cars

12. What are all the factors of 12?

a. 12, 24, 36
b. 1, 2, 4, 6, 12
c. 12, 24, 36, 48
d. 1, 2, 3, 4, 6, 12

13. At the beginning of the day, Xavier has 20 apples. At lunch, he meets his sister Emma and gives her half of his apples. After lunch, he stops by his neighbor Jim's house and gives him six of his apples. He then uses $\frac{3}{4}$ of his remaining apples to make an apple pie for dessert at dinner. At the end of the day, Xavier has ______ apple(s) left?

14. How would the number 847.89632 be written if rounded to the nearest hundredth?

a. 847.90
b. 900
c. 847.89
d. 847.896

15. What is the sum of $\frac{1}{3}$ and $\frac{2}{5}$?

a. $\frac{3}{8}$

b. $\frac{11}{15}$

c. $\frac{11}{30}$

d. $\frac{4}{5}$

16. A rectangle has a length that is 5 feet longer than 3 times its width. If the perimeter is 90 feet, what is the length in feet?

a. 10
b. 20
c. 25
d. 35

17. Five students take a test. The scores of the first four students are 80, 85, 75, and 60. If the median score is 80, which of the following could NOT be the score of the fifth student?

a. 60
b. 80
c. 85
d. 100

18. Express $\frac{54}{15}$ as a mixed number, reduced to lowest terms.

a. $3\frac{3}{5}$

b. $3\frac{1}{15}$

c. $3\frac{3}{54}$

d. $3\frac{1}{54}$

19. In the problem $5 \times 6 + 4 \div 2 - 1$, which operation should be completed first?

a. Multiplication
b. Addition
c. Division
d. Subtraction

20. Express $8\frac{3}{7}$ as an improper fraction.

a. $\frac{11}{7}$

b. $\frac{21}{8}$

c. $\frac{5}{3}$

d. $\frac{59}{7}$

21. An accounting firm charted its income on the following pie graph. If the total income for the year was \$500,000, how much income was received from Audit Services and Taxation Services?

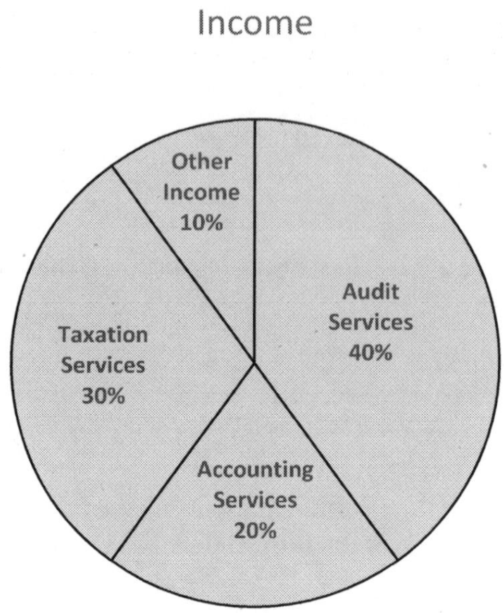

a. \$200,000
b. \$350,000
c. \$150,000
d. \$300,000

22. Ten students take a test. Five students get a 50. Four students get a 70. If the average score is 55, what was the last student's score?

a. 20
b. 40
c. 50
d. 60

23. When rounding 245.2678 to the nearest thousandth, which place value would be used to decide whether to round up or round down?

a. Ten-thousandths
b. Thousandths
c. Hundredths
d. Thousands

24. Simplify $(1.2 \times 10^{12}) \div (3.0 \times 10^{8})$ and write the result in scientific notation.

a. 0.4×10^{4}
b. 4.0×10^{4}
c. 4.0×10^{3}
d. 3.6×10^{20}

25. You measure the width of your door to be 36 inches. The true width of the door is 35.75 inches. What is the relative error in your measurement?
  a. 0.7%
  b. 0.007%
  c. 0.99%
  d. 0.1%

26. The phone bill is calculated each month using the equation $c = 50g + 75$. The cost of the phone bill per month is represented by c, and g represents the gigabytes of data used that month. What is the value and interpretation of the slope of this equation?
  a. 75 dollars per day
  b. 75 gigabytes per day
  c. 50 dollars per day
  d. 50 dollars per gigabyte

27. Mom's car drove 72 miles in 90 minutes. How fast did she drive in feet per second? (There are 5,280 ft. in 1 mile.)
  a. 0.8 feet per second
  b. 48.9 feet per second
  c. 0.009 feet per second
  d. 70.4 feet per second

28. How do you solve $V = lwh$ for h?
  a. $lwV = h$
  b. $h = \frac{V}{lw}$
  c. $h = \frac{Vl}{w}$
  d. $h = \frac{Vw}{l}$

29. 20 is 40% of what number?

______

30. A landscaper is making a circular garden with a radius of 13 feet in his backyard. He needs to compute the area to know how much soil to purchase. What is the area of the circle in terms of π?
  a. $26\,\pi\ \text{ft}^2$
  b. $169\,\pi\ \text{ft}^2$
  c. $130\,\pi\ \text{ft}^2$
  d. $260\,\pi\ \text{ft}^2$

31. What is the domain for the function $y = \sqrt{x}$?
  a. All real numbers
  b. $x \geq 0$
  c. $x > 0$
  d. $y \geq 0$

32. Jessica buys 10 cans of paint. Red paint costs \$1 per can, and blue paint costs \$2 per can. In total, she spends \$16. How many red cans did she buy?

a. 2 red cans
b. 3 red cans
c. 4 red cans
d. 5 red cans

33. What is the volume of a rectangular prism with a height of 3 centimeters, a width of 5 centimeters, and a depth of 11 centimeters?

a. 19 cm^3
b. 165 cm^3
c. 225 cm^3
d. 150 cm^3

34. Four people split a bill. The first person pays for $\frac{1}{5}$, the second person pays for $\frac{1}{4}$, and the third person pays for $\frac{1}{3}$. What fraction of the bill does the fourth person pay?

a. $\frac{13}{60}$
b. $\frac{47}{60}$
c. $\frac{1}{4}$
d. $\frac{4}{15}$

35. What is the length of the hypotenuse of a right triangle with one leg equal to 3 centimeters and the other leg equal to 4 centimeters?

a. 7 cm
b. 5 cm
c. 25 cm
d. 12 cm

36. $52.3 \times 10^{-3} =$

a. 0.00523
b. 0.0523
c. 0.523
d. 523

37. For a group of 20 men, the median weight is 180 pounds, and the range is 30 pounds. If each man gains 10 pounds, which of the following would be true?

a. The median weight will increase, and the range will remain the same.
b. The median weight and range will both remain the same.
c. The median weight will stay the same, and the range will increase.
d. The median weight and range will both increase.

38. What is $\frac{\pi}{5}$ in terms of degrees?

a. 10°
b. 20°
c. 30°
d. 36°

Science

1. A scientist is trying to determine the amount of poison that will kill a rat the fastest. Which of the following statements is an example of an appropriate hypothesis?
   a. Rats that are given lots of poison seem to die quickly.
   b. Does the amount of poison affect how quickly the rat dies?
   c. The more poison a rat is given, the quicker it will die.
   d. Poison is fatal to rats.

2. Which of the following correctly describes the independent and dependent variables in an experiment that tests how quickly a rat dies based on the amount of poison it eats?
   a. How quickly the rat dies is the independent variable; the amount of poison is the dependent variable.
   b. The amount of poison is the independent variable; how quickly the rat dies is the dependent variable.
   c. Whether the rat eats the poison is the independent variable; how quickly the rat dies is the dependent variable.
   d. The cage the rat is kept in is the independent variable; the amount of poison is the dependent variable.

3. Which of the following is a representation of a natural pattern or occurrence that's difficult or impossible to experience directly?
   a. A theory
   b. A model
   c. A law
   d. An observation

4. Which of the following is a standard or series of standards to which the results from an experiment are compared?
   a. A control
   b. A variable
   c. A constant
   d. Collected data

5. "This flower is dead; someone must have forgotten to water it." This statement is an example of which of the following?
   a. A classification
   b. An observation
   c. An inference
   d. A collection

6. Which of the following correctly displays 8,600,000,000,000 in scientific notation (to two significant figures)?
   a. 8.6×10^{12}
   b. 8.6×10^{-12}
   c. 8.6×10^{11}
   d. 8.60×10^{12}

7. The acceleration of a falling object due to gravity has been proven to be 9.8 m/s^2. A scientist drops a cactus four times, measures the acceleration with an accelerometer, and gets the following results: 9.79 m/s^2, 9.81 m/s^2, 9.80 m/s^2, and 9.78 m/s^2. Which of the following accurately describes the measurements?
   a. They're both accurate and precise.
   b. They're accurate but not precise.
   c. They're precise but not accurate.
   d. They're neither accurate nor precise.

8. The atomic mass of Na is 23.0 g/mol and Cl is 35.5 g/mol. The molarity of a solution made by dissolving 4.0 grams of NaCl into enough water to make 120 mL of solution is ________.

9. Consider a gas in a closed system that is kept at a constant volume. What will happen to the temperature if the pressure is increased?
   a. The temperature will stay the same.
   b. The temperature will decrease.
   c. The temperature will increase.
   d. The result cannot be determined with the information given.

10. Which statement is true regarding atomic structure?
   a. Protons orbit around a nucleus.
   b. Neutrons have a positive charge.
   c. Electrons are in the nucleus.
   d. Protons have a positive charge.

11. What types of molecules can move through a cell membrane by passive transport?
   a. Complex sugars
   b. Non-lipid-soluble molecules
   c. Oxygen
   d. Molecules moving from areas of low concentration to areas of high concentration

12. What is the balance of the following chemical equation?

$$\_\,F_2 + \_\,H_2O \rightarrow \_\,HF + \_\,O_2$$

   a. 2:4:2:1
   b. 4:2:8:2
   c. 2:2:4:1
   d. 1:1:2:1

13. What is the purpose of a catalyst?
   a. To increase a reaction's rate by increasing the activation energy
   b. To increase a reaction's rate by increasing the temperature
   c. To increase a reaction's rate by decreasing the activation energy
   d. To increase a reaction's rate by decreasing the temperature

14. How many daughter cells are formed from one parent cell during meiosis?
   a. One
   b. Two
   c. Three
   d. Four

15. Which level of protein structure is defined by the folds and coils of the protein's polypeptide backbone?
   a. Primary
   b. Secondary
   c. Tertiary
   d. Quaternary

16. What type of chemical reaction produces a salt?
    a. An oxidation reaction
    b. A neutralization reaction
    c. A synthesis reaction
    d. A decomposition reaction

17. How many neurons generally make up a sensory pathway?
    a. 1
    b. 2
    c. 3
    d. 4

18. In which part of the eye does visual processing begin?
    a. Cornea
    b. Optic nerve
    c. Retina
    d. Eyelid

19. What kind of energy do plants use in photosynthesis to create chemical energy?
    a. Light
    b. Electric
    c. Nuclear
    d. Cellular

20. The somatic nervous system is responsible for which of the following?
    a. Breathing
    b. Thought
    c. Movement
    d. Fear

21. The process of breaking down large molecules into smaller molecules to provide energy is known as which of the following?
    a. Metabolism
    b. Bioenergetics
    c. Anabolism
    d. Catabolism

22. Which blood component is chiefly responsible for clotting?
    a. Platelets
    b. Red blood cells
    c. Antigens
    d. Plasma cells

23. Which is the first event to happen in a primary immune response?
    a. Macrophages ingest pathogens and present their antigens.
    b. Neutrophils aggregate and act as cytotoxic, nonspecific killers of pathogens.
    c. B lymphocytes make pathogen-specific antibodies.
    d. Helper T cells secrete interleukins to activate pathogen-fighting cells.

24. Where does sperm maturation take place in the male reproductive system?
   a. Seminal vesicles
   b. Prostate gland
   c. Epididymis
   d. Vas deferens

25. Which of the following lists of joint types is in the correct order for increasing amounts of permitted motion (least mobile to most mobile)?
   a. Hinge, condyloid, saddle
   b. Saddle, hinge, condyloid
   c. Saddle, condyloid, hinge
   d. Hinge, saddle, condyloid

26. What is ionization energy?
   a. One-half the distance between the nuclei of atoms of the same element
   b. A measurement of the tendency of an atom to form a chemical bond
   c. The amount of energy needed to remove a valence electron from a gas or ion
   d. The ability or tendency of an atom to accept an electron into its valence shell

27. How many centimeters is 0.78 kilometers?
   a. 7.8 cm
   b. 0.078 cm
   c. 78,000 cm
   d. 780 cm

28. How do organisms maintain homeostasis?
   a. They increase their body temperature, blood pH, and fluid balance.
   b. They undergo biochemical processes and absorb energy to increase entropy.
   c. They undergo biochemical processes to maintain the order of their external environment.
   d. They use free energy and matter via biochemical processes to work against entropy.

29. Which of the following correctly lists the four properties that all types of muscle tissue share? *Select all that apply*
   a. Contractile
   b. Excitable
   c. Elastic
   d. Extensible
   e. Voluntary

30. The following graph demonstrates which type of correlation?

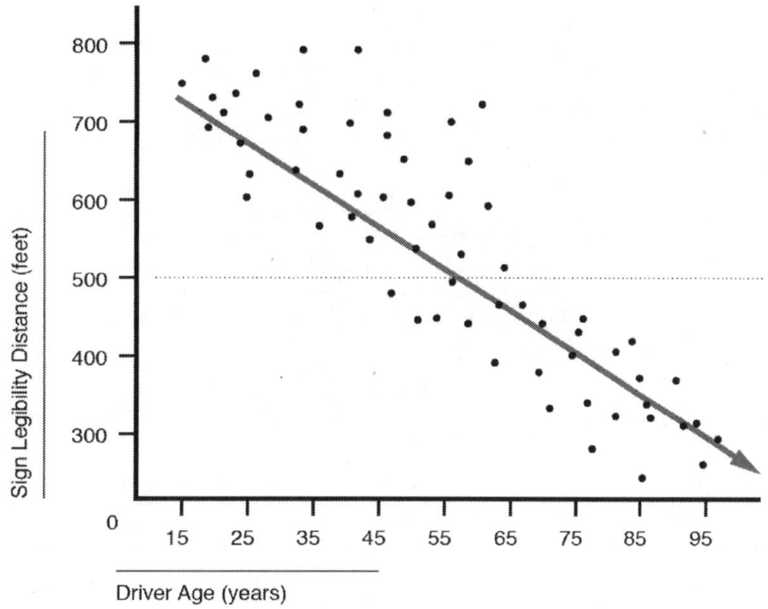

a. Positive correlation
b. No correlation
c. Negative correlation
d. Zero correlation

31. When researching a problem in science, what are the best sources to use?
a. People you have seen on television
b. Anyone with a Ph.D.
c. Accredited laboratories and universities
d. Any source with an internet webpage

32. Which of the following structures acts like a funnel by delivering the urine from the millions of collecting tubules to the ureters?
a. The renal pelvis
b. The renal cortex
c. The renal medulla
d. Bowman's capsule

33. The nurse is looking to locate the lower margin of the liver for assessment. Which abdominal quadrant should the nurse palpate? Place an X to mark your answer.

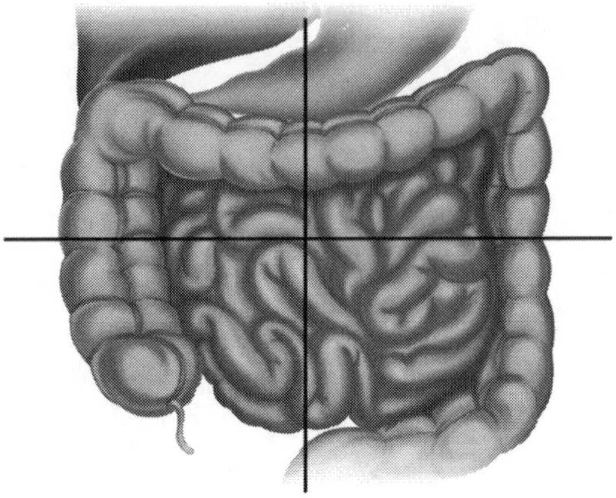

34. Which of the following best defines the term *amphoteric*?
   a. A substance that conducts electricity due to ionization when dissolved in a solvent
   b. A substance that can act as an acid or a base depending on the properties of the solute
   c. A substance that, according to the Brønsted-Lowry Acid-Base Theory, is a proton-donor
   d. A substance that donates its proton and forms its conjugate base in a neutralization reaction

35. Which of the following touch receptors respond to light touch and slower vibrations?
   a. Merkel's discs
   b. Pacinian corpuscles
   c. Meissner's corpuscles
   d. Ruffini endings

36. The muscular tube that connects the outer surface to the cervix in a woman's birth canal is referred to as which of the following?
   a. The uterus
   b. The cervix
   c. The vagina
   d. The ovaries

37. A cluster of capillaries that functions as the main filter of the blood entering the kidney is known as which of the following?
   a. The Bowman's capsule
   b. The loop of Henle
   c. The glomerulus
   d. The nephron

38. What is an alteration in the normal gene sequence called?
   a. DNA mutation
   b. Gene migration
   c. Polygenetic inheritance
   d. Incomplete dominance

39. Blood type is a trait determined by multiple alleles, and two of them are co-dominant: I^A codes for A blood and I^B codes for B blood. The i allele codes for O blood and is recessive to both. If an A heterozygous individual and an O individual have a child, what is the probability that the child will have A blood?

a. 25%
b. 50%
c. 75%
d. 100%

40. Esther is left-handed. Hand dominance is a genetic factor. If being right-handed is a dominant trait over being left-handed, which of the following must NOT be true about Esther's parents?

a. Her parents are both right-handed.
b. Her parents are both left-handed.
c. Only one parent is right-handed.
d. All of the above can be true.

41. What is the process of cell division in somatic (most body) cells called?

a. Mitosis
b. Meiosis
c. Respiration
d. Cytogenesis

42. When human cells divide by meiosis, how many chromosomes do the resulting cells contain?

a. 96
b. 54
c. 46
d. 23

43. What is the name for the sac-shaped structures that facilitate the exchanging of carbon dioxide and oxygen?

a. Kidneys
b. Medulla oblongata
c. Alveoli
d. Bronchioles

44. The following parts of the cardiac system form a pathway of oxygenated blood from the lungs to the tissue:

Left atrium

Aorta

Mitral valve

Arteries and capillaries

Left ventricle

Put them in the correct order below:

1. Lungs
2. ____________________
3. ____________________
4. ____________________
5. ____________________
6. ____________________
7. Tissue

45. Which structure serves as the electrical stimulator of the cardiac muscle?
a. The sinoatrial node
b. The left ventricle
c. The aorta
d. The tricuspid valve

46. The primary function of the endocrine system is to maintain which of the following?
a. Heartbeat
b. Respiration
c. Electrolyte and water balance
d. Homeostasis

47. Which of the following hormones is primarily responsible for regulating metabolism?
a. Insulin
b. Testosterone
c. Adrenaline
d. Thyroid hormone

48. How many grams of solid $CaCO_3$ are needed to make exactly 600 mL of a 0.350 M solution? The atomic masses for the elements are as follows: Ca = 40.07 g/mol; C = 12.01 g/mol; O = 15.99 g/mol.
a. 18.3 g
b. 19.7 g
c. 21.0 g
d. 24.2 g

49. How many mL (to the appropriate number of significant figures) of a 12.0 M stock solution of HCl should be added to water to create exactly 250 mL of a 1.50 M solution of HCl?

a. 31.25 mL
b. 30.3 mL
c. 31.35 mL
d. 31.3 mL

50. There are three ways in which a phenotype can change due to natural selection. Directional selection occurs when one extreme of a phenotype is favored. Disruptive selection occurs when both extremes of a phenotype are favored. Stabilizing selection occurs when an intermediate phenotype is favored over either extreme phenotype. In Cameroon, seeds are either large or small. Finches in Cameroon have either large beaks or small beaks. They are not found with medium-sized beaks. What type of selection is described in the previous scenario?

a. Stabilizing
b. Directional
c. Disruptive
d. Beak-type

English and Language Usage

1. What is the structure of the following sentence?

> The restaurant is unconventional because it serves both Chicago style pizza and New York style pizza.

a. Simple
b. Compound
c. Complex
d. Compound-complex

2. The following sentence contains what kind of error?

> This summer, I'm planning to travel to Italy, take a Mediterranean cruise, going to Pompeii, and eat a lot of Italian food.

a. Parallelism
b. Sentence fragment
c. Misplaced modifier
d. Subject-verb agreement

3. What is the best definition of the word *engorge*?

a. Nourish
b. Squeeze
c. Consume
d. Swell

4. Which of the following refers to what an author wants to express about a given subject?

a. Primary purpose
b. Plot
c. Main idea
d. Characterization

5. A student writes the following in an essay:

Protestors filled the streets of the city. Because they were dissatisfied with the government's leadership.

Which of the following is an appropriately-punctuated correction for this sentence?

a. Protestors filled the streets of the city, because they were dissatisfied with the government's leadership.
b. Protesters, filled the streets of the city, because they were dissatisfied with the government's leadership.
c. Because they were dissatisfied with the government's leadership protestors filled the streets of the city.
d. Protestors filled the streets of the city because they were dissatisfied with the government's leadership.

6. What is the part of speech of the underlined word in the sentence?

We need to come up with a fresh <u>approach</u> to this problem.

a. Noun
b. Verb
c. Adverb
d. Adjective

7. Which of the following are steps in the writing process? *Select all that apply.*

a. Prewriting
b. Revising
c. Sourcing
d. Conferencing

8. The underlined portion of the sentence is an example of which sentence component?

New students should report <u>to the student center</u>.

a. Dependent clause
b. Adverbial phrase
c. Adjective clause
d. Noun phrase

9. What is the noun phrase in the following sentence?

Charlotte's new German Shepherd puppy is energetic.

a. Puppy
b. Charlotte
c. German Shepherd puppy
d. Charlotte's new German Shepherd puppy

10. Emma is writing an essay about Shakespeare's *Macbeth*. She started with a detailed outline and first draft. Her ideas are her own, but she has quoted excerpts from the play to support her main points. She reworked her draft several times and revised her essay based on feedback from a writing center tutor. She asked a few classmates to read the essay and identify mistakes she missed while editing. Which of the following actions does she still need to take at this point in the writing process?

a. Write the introduction and conclusion paragraphs.
b. Rearrange the order of paragraphs.
c. Insert citations where she used quotes.
d. Organize her thoughts.

11. While studying vocabulary, a student notices that the words *circumference*, *circumnavigate*, and *circumstance* all begin with the prefix *circum–*. The student uses her knowledge of affixes to infer that all of these words share what related meaning?

a. Around, surrounding
b. Travel, transport
c. Size, measurement
d. Area, location

12. The following is an example of what type of sentence?

Although I wished it were summer, I accepted the change of seasons, and I started to appreciate the fall.

a. Compound
b. Simple
c. Complex
d. Compound-complex

13. A student reads the following sentence:

A hundred years ago, automobiles were rare, but now cars are ubiquitous.

However, she doesn't know what the word *ubiquitous* means. Which key context clue is essential to decipher the word's meaning?

a. Ago
b. Cars
c. Now
d. Rare

Read the selection about traveling in an RV to answer the next eight questions:

I have to admit that when my father bought a recreational vehicle (RV), I thought he was making a huge mistake. I didn't really know anything about RVs, but I knew that my dad was as big a "city slicker" as there was. <u>In fact, I even thought he might have gone a little bit crazy.</u> On trips to the beach, he preferred to swim at the pool, and whenever he went hiking, he avoided touching any plants for fear that they might be poison ivy. Why would this man, with an almost irrational fear of the outdoors, want a 40-foot camping behemoth?

<u>The RV</u> was a great purchase for our family and brought us all closer together. Every morning <u>we would wake up, eat breakfast, and broke camp.</u> We laughed at our own comical attempts to back The Beast into spaces that seemed impossibly small. <u>We rejoiced as "hackers."</u> When things inevitably went wrong and we couldn't solve the problems on our own, we discovered the incredible helpfulness and friendliness of the RV community. <u>We even made some new friends in the process.</u>

<u>Above all, it allowed us to share adventures. While traveling across America</u>, which we could not have experienced in cars and hotels. Enjoying a campfire on a chilly summer evening with the mountains of Glacier National Park in the background, or waking up early in the morning to see the sun rising over the distant spires of Arches National Park are memories that will always stay with me and our entire family. <u>Those are also memories that my siblings and me</u> have now shared with our own children.

14. Which of the following would be the best choice for this sentence?

In fact, I even thought he might have gone a little bit crazy.

a. Leave it where it is now.
b. Move the sentence so that it comes before the preceding sentence.
c. Move the sentence to the end of the first paragraph.
d. Omit the sentence.

15. Which of the following would be the best choice for this sentence?

The RV

a. NO CHANGE
b. Not surprisingly, the RV
c. Furthermore, the RV
d. As it turns out, the RV

16. Which of the following would be the best choice for this sentence?

we would wake up, eat breakfast, and broke camp.

a. NO CHANGE
b. we would wake up, eat breakfast, and break camp.
c. would we wake up, eat breakfast, and break camp?
d. we are waking up, eating breakfast, and breaking camp.

17. Which of the following would be the best choice for this sentence?

We rejoiced as “hackers.”

a. NO CHANGE
b. To a nagging problem of technology, we rejoiced as “hackers.”
c. We rejoiced when we figured out how to “hack” a solution during a difficult situation.
d. To “hack” our way to a solution, we had to rejoice.

18. Which of the following would be the best choice for this sentence?

We even made some new friends in the process.

a. NO CHANGE
b. In the process was the friends we were making.
c. We are even making some new friends in the process.
d. We will make new friends in the process.

19. Which of the following would be the best choice for this sentence?

Above all, it allowed us to share adventures. While traveling across America

a. NO CHANGE
b. Above all, it allowed us to share adventures while traveling across America
c. Above all, it allowed us to share adventures; while traveling across America
d. Above all, it allowed us to share adventures—while traveling across America

20. Which of the following would be the best choice for this sentence?

Those are also memories that my siblings and me

a. NO CHANGE
b. Those are also memories that me and my siblings
c. Those are also memories that my siblings and I
d. Those are also memories that I and my siblings

21. What is the overall tone of this section?
a. Formal
b. Informal
c. Academic
d. Pessimistic

Read the following section about Fred Hampton and answer Questions 22-30.

Fred Hampton desired to see lasting social change for African American people through nonviolent means and community recognition. In the meantime, he became an African American activist during the American Civil Rights Movement and led the Chicago chapter of the Black Panther Party.

Hampton's Education

Hampton was born and raised in the Maywood neighborhood of Chicago, Illinois in 1948. Gifted academically and a natural athlete, he became a stellar baseball player in high school. After graduating from Proviso East High School in 1966, he later went on to study law at Triton Junior College. While studying at Triton, Hampton joined and became a leader of the National Association for the Advancement of Colored People (NAACP). As a result of his leadership, the NAACP gained more than 500 members. Hampton worked relentlessly to establish recreational facilities in the Maywood neighborhood and improve the educational resources provided to the impoverished black community.

The Black Panthers

The Black Panther Party (BPP) was another that formed around the same time as and was similar in function to the NAACP. Hampton was quickly attracted to the Black Panther Party's approach to the fight for equal rights for African Americans. Hampton eventually joined the chapter and relocated to downtown Chicago to be closer to its headquarters.

His charismatic personality, organizational abilities, sheer determination, and rhetorical skills (26) enable him to quickly rise through the chapter's ranks. Hampton soon became the leader of the Chicago chapter of the BPP where he organized rallies, taught political education classes, and established a free medical clinic. He also took part in the community police supervision project. He played an instrumental role in the BPP breakfast program for impoverished African American children.

Hampton's greatest acheivement as the leader of the BPP may have been his fight against street gang violence in Chicago. In 1969, Hampton held a press conference where he made the gangs agree to a nonaggression pact known as the Rainbow Coalition. As a result of the pact, a multiracial alliance between blacks, Puerto Ricans, and poor youth was developed.

22. Which of the following would be the best choice for this sentence?

    In the meantime, he became an African American activist during the American Civil Rights Movement and led the Chicago chapter of the Black Panther Party.

    a. NO CHANGE
    b. Unfortunately,
    c. Finally,
    d. As a result,

23. Which of the following would be the best choice for this sentence?

    Hampton was born and raised in the Maywood neighborhood of Chicago, Illinois in 1948.

    a. NO CHANGE
    b. in the Maywood neighborhood, of Chicago, Illinois in 1948.
    c. in the Maywood neighborhood of Chicago, Illinois, in 1948.
    d. in Chicago, Illinois of Maywood neighborhood in 1948.

24. Which of these sentences, if any, should begin a new paragraph?

    After graduating from Proviso East High School in 1966, he later went on to study law at Triton Junior College. While studying at Triton, Hampton joined and became a leader of the National Association for the Advancement of Colored People (NAACP). As a result of his leadership, the NAACP gained more than 500 members.

    a. NO CHANGE
    b. After graduating from Proviso East High School in 1966, he later went on to study law at Triton Junior College.
    c. While studying at Triton, Hampton joined and became a leader of the National Association for the Advancement of Colored People (NAACP).
    d. As a result of his leadership, the NAACP gained more than 500 members.

25. Choose the best replacement for the underlined text (reproduced below).

    The Black Panther Party (BPP) was another that formed around the same time as and was similar in function to the NAACP.

    a. NO CHANGE; best as written
    b. was another activist group that
    c. had a lot of members that
    d. was another school that

26. Which of the following would be the best choice for this sentence?

    Hampton was quickly attracted to the Black Panther Party's approach to the fight for equal rights for African Americans.

    a. NO CHANGE
    b. Black Panther Parties approach
    c. Black Panther Partys' approach
    d. Black Panther Parties' approach

27. Which of the following would be the best choice for this sentence?

His charismatic personality, organizational abilities, sheer determination, and rhetorical skills enable him to quickly rise through the chapter's ranks.

a. NO CHANGE
b. are enabling him to quickly rise
c. enabled him to quickly rise
d. will enable him to quickly rise

28. Which of the following would be the best choice for this sentence?

He also took part in the community police supervision project. He played an instrumental role in the BPP breakfast program for impoverished African American children.

a. NO CHANGE
b. He also took part in the community police supervision project but played an instrumental role
c. He also took part in the community police supervision project, he played an instrumental role
d. He also took part in the community police supervision project and played an instrumental role

29. Which word, if any, is misspelled? *Select all that apply.*
a. Seperate
b. Greatest
c. Acheivement
d. Leader

30. What is the tone of this passage?
a. Formal
b. Informal
c. Academic
d. Pessimistic

31. Which of the following sentences gives an example of using specific language?
a. The bucket is for the pens.
b. The red sign says to go left.
c. The decorations are for the party.
d. Lunch will be in the cafeteria.

32. Which of the following sentences provides an example of constructive language?
a. In all my years of teaching, I have never had a student struggle as badly as you.
b. Even though you practice every day, your soccer skills still do not match up to your team's.
c. I understand that you may be having difficulty, but that's ok; the material is challenging.
d. You will never meet the required qualifications for a position like that.

33. Which of the following most clearly completes the sentence?

Annabelle must be ________ to school, meaning, she must arrive on time in order to not be counted late.

a. punctual
b. early
c. tardy
d. premature

34. In which of the following circumstances would a writer need to use a citation?
   a. Stating their own conclusion about the work of another author
   b. Writing an original short story
   c. Stating a fact that is considered common knowledge
   d. Summarizing the work of another author

35. How are the revising and editing processes different?
   a. Revising primarily addresses grammatical issues while editing primarily addresses broader content issues.
   b. Editing primarily addresses grammatical issues while revising primarily addresses broader content issues.
   c. Revising focuses on the entire body of writing while editing focuses on a smaller section.
   d. Editing focuses on the entire body of writing while editing focuses on a smaller section.

36. Which of the following would NOT be an appropriate source for an academic research paper?
   a. Blog post
   b. Government website
   c. Peer-reviewed journal article
   d. Documentary

37. Which step of the writing process involves determining the purpose and topic of writing, researching, and outlining?
   a. Revising
   b. Conferencing
   c. Writing
   d. Prewriting

Answer Explanations #2

Reading

1. C: Choice *C* is the correct answer because it most extensively summarizes the entire passage. While Choices *A* and *B* are reasonable possibilities, they reference portions of Gulliver's experience, not the whole. Choice *D* is incorrect because Gulliver doesn't express repentance or sorrow in this particular passage.

2. A: Principal refers to *chief* or *primary* within the context of this text. Choice *A* is the answer that most closely aligns with this definition. Choices *B* and *D* refer to a helper or follower, while Choice *C* doesn't meet the description of Reldresal from the passage.

3. C: One can reasonably infer that Gulliver is considerably larger than the children who were playing around him because multiple children could fit into his hand. Choice *A* is incorrect because there is no indication of stress in Gulliver's tone. Choices *B* and *D* aren't the best answers because, though Gulliver seems fond of his new acquaintances, he didn't travel there with the intentions of meeting new people, nor does he express a definite love for them in this particular portion of the text.

4. C: The emperor made a definitive decision to expose Gulliver to their native customs. In this instance, the word *mind* was not related to a vote, question, or cognitive ability.

5. A: This assertion does not support the fact that games are a commonplace event in this culture because it mentions conduct, not games. Choices *B*, *C*, and *D* are incorrect because these do support the fact that games are a commonplace event.

6. B: Choice *B* is the only option that mentions the correlation between physical ability and leadership positions. Choices *A* and *D* are unrelated to physical strength and leadership abilities. Choice *C* does not make a deduction that would lead to the correct answer—it only comments upon the abilities of common townspeople.

7. B: Choice *A* is irrelevant as Chapter 5 is for outdoor activities as a whole and not only for ones that start with a particular letter. Choice *C* brings up an omission, not a potential inconsistency; furthermore, Chapter 5 does not have to include all outdoor activities. Choice *D* points out a possible inconsistency; however, it would only be an inconsistency if all the other sections contained tips. The camping section does not contain any tips. Choice B is the correct answer because every segment except cycling contains a section about equipment or gear.

8. A: Choice *A* is consistent with the argument's logic. The argument asserts that the world powers' military alliances amounted to a delicate fuse and that the assassination merely lit it. The main point of the argument is that any event involving the military alliances would have led to a world war. Choice *B* runs counter to the argument's tone and reasoning. It can immediately be eliminated. Choice *C* is also clearly incorrect. At no point does the argument blame any single country or group of countries for World War I. Choice *D* is incorrect for the same reason as Choice *C*, so it can be eliminated.

9. D: This question is testing whether you realize how a timeline illustrates information in chronological order from left to right. "Started school for the deaf" is fourth on the timeline from the left, which means that it is the fourth event on the timeline. Thus, Choice *D* is the correct answer.

10. B: This question is asking you to determine the length of time between the pairs of events listed as answer choices. Events in timelines are arranged proportional to time. To determine the answer to this question, one must find the largest space between two events. Visually, this can be seen between the events of befriending Helen Keller and dying in Canada. Thus, Choice *B* is the correct answer.

11. C: This question is testing whether you can discern accurate conclusions from a timeline. Although the incorrect answer choices can seem correct, they cannot be confirmed from the information presented on the timeline. Choice *A* is incorrect; while it may be reasonable to assume that the timeline documents all major life events, we do not know for certain that Bell did not engage in any notable activities after founding the National Geographic Society. Choice *B* is incorrect because the timeline does not confirm that the school was in Canada; Bell actually started it in the United States. Choice *D* is incorrect because nothing on the timeline shows causation between the two events. Choice *C* is the only verifiable statement based on the timeline, so it must be the correct answer.

12. B: The founding of the school is the event listed farthest to the right of the events in the answer choices. This means it occurred most recently. Thus, Choice *B* is the correct answer.

13. A: The word city appears in the passage several times, thus establishing the location for the reader.

14. B: The passage states that the Juggernaut causes the children to scream. Choices *A* and *D* don't apply because the text doesn't mention either of these instances specifically. Choice *C* is incorrect because there is nothing in the text that mentions space travel.

15. B: The mention of *morning*, *noon*, and *night* make it clear that the word *haunt* refers to frequent appearances at various times. Choice *A* doesn't work because the text makes no mention of levitating. Choices *C* and *D* are not correct because the text mentions Mr. Utterson's anguish and disheartenment because of his failure to find Hyde but does not mention Mr. Utterson's feelings negatively affecting anyone else.

16. D: Choice *D* is the correct answer because of the repetition of the *L*-words. Hyperbole is an exaggeration, so Choice *A* doesn't work. No comparison is being made, so no simile or juxtaposition is being used, thus eliminating Choices B and C.

17. D: One can conclude that the speaker intends to continue to look for Hyde. Choices *A* and *B* are not possible answers because the text doesn't refer to any name changes or an identity crisis, despite Mr. Utterson's extreme obsession with finding Hyde. The text also makes no mention of a mistaken identity when referring to Hyde, so Choice *C* is also incorrect.

18. C: There were more Confederate casualties than Union casualties at the Battles of Gettysburg and Atlanta. Of the two, only Atlanta is listed as an answer choice. Thus, Choice *C*, Atlanta, is the correct answer.

19. D: The question is asking you to find where the dates are located in the table and to identify the earliest battle. Choice *D*, Shiloh, occurred in April 1862, and no other battle listed on the table happened until May 1863.

20. A: Robert E. Lee led the Confederate Army in all battles listed on the table except for Shiloh and Atlanta. Shiloh is not listed in the question; therefore, Atlanta, Choice *A*, is the correct answer.

21. A: This question is asking you to compare the Union and Confederate casualties and find the one listed where the Union casualties most exceeded the Confederate ones. At Cold Harbor, there were approximately 8,142 more Union casualties than Confederate. At Chancellorsville, there were approximately 3,844 more Union casualties. At Atlanta the number of Confederate casualties exceeded the Union number, so it cannot be the correct answer. At Shiloh there were approximately 2,378 more Union casualties. Thus, the number of Union casualties most greatly exceeded the Confederate number at Cold Harbor, making Choice *A* the correct answer.

22. D: To calculate the total American casualties, we combine the Union and Confederate casualties since it was a civil war with Americans on both sides. There were approximately 51,112 (Union + Confederate losses) American casualties at Gettysburg; thus, the correct answer will be a battle with approximately 25,556 casualties, which is half of that number. Shiloh is the closest with a total of 23,716 casualties, making Choice *D* the correct answer.

23. B, D: Relevant information refers to information that is closely related to the subject being researched. Students might get overwhelmed by information when they first begin researching, so they should learn how to narrow down search terms for their field of study. Both Choices *A* and *E* are incorrect because they start with a range that is far too wide; the student will spend too much time sifting through unrelated information to gather only a few related facts. Choice *C* introduces a more limited range, but it is not closely related to the topic that is being researched. Choices *B* and *D* are correct because the student is choosing media and books that are closely related to the topic.

24. D: An actuary assesses risks and sets insurance premiums. While an actuary does work in insurance, the passage does not suggest that actuaries have any affiliation with hospitalists or working in a hospital, so all other choices are incorrect.

25. A: The purpose is to inform the reader about what assault is and how it is committed. Choice *B* is incorrect because the passage does not state that assault is a lesser form of lethal force, only that an assault can use lethal force, or alternatively, lethal force can be utilized to counter a dangerous assault. Choices *C* and *D* are incorrect because the passage is informative and does not have a set agenda.

26. C: The situation of the man who is attacked in an alley by another man with a knife would most merit the use of lethal force. If the man being attacked used lethal force in self-defense, it would not be considered illegal. The presence of a deadly weapon indicates malicious intent, and because the individual is isolated in an alley, lethal force in self-defense may be the only way to preserve his life. Choices *A* and *B* can be ruled out because in these situations no one is in danger of immediate death or bodily harm by someone else. Choice *D* is an assault that does exhibit intent to harm, but this situation isn't severe enough to merit lethal force; there is no intent to kill.

27. B: As discussed in the second passage, there are several forms of assault, like assault with a deadly weapon, verbal assault, or threatening posture or language. Choice *A* is incorrect because lethal force and assault are separate, as indicated by the passages. Choice *C* is incorrect because anyone is capable of assault; the author does not state that one group of people cannot commit assault. Choice *D* is incorrect because assault is never justified. Self-defense resulting in lethal force can be justified.

28. D: If true, the statement in Choice *D* would most undermine the last part of the passage because it directly contradicts how the law evaluates the use of lethal force. Choices *A* and *B* are stated in the paragraph, and therefore do not undermine the explanation from the author. Choice *C* does not necessarily undermine the passage, but it does not support the passage either. It is more of an opinion that does not strengthen or weaken the explanation.

29. C: Choice *C* clearly establishes what both assault and lethal force are and gives the specific way in which the two concepts meet. Choice *A* is incorrect because lethal force doesn't necessarily result in assault. This is also why Choice *B* is incorrect. Not all assaults would necessarily be life-threatening to the point where lethal force is needed for self-defense. Choice *D* is compelling but ultimately too vague; the statement touches on aspects of the two ideas but fails to present the concrete way in which the two are connected to each other.

30. D: This is the correct answer because the "gov" indicates that this is a government website. If you are traveling overseas, the U.S. government would be a reliable and up-to-date source of information, especially in regard to travel safety. While the other websites may contain some helpful information, blogs and wikis are often not as reliable as government websites.

31. A: In the first pie chart, the percentage of the European Union population that lived in Germany was 17%. In the second pie chart, we can see that this percentage drops to 16%. Therefore, there was a one percent decrease.

32. D: To find the correct answer, ask what yields the most information and is relevant to the task at hand: finding out about Harper Lee. A dictionary's main purpose is to define words, provide tenses, and establish pronunciation. A newspaper article might offer some information about Harper Lee, but it would be limited in scope to a specific topic or time period. A study guide would focus on literary elements of *To Kill a Mockingbird*, not Harper Lee's life. A biography would be the most comprehensive. It would cover the author, from birth to death, and touch on topics such as upbringing, significant achievements, and societal impacts.

33. D: Choice D is the best answer. It resolves the paradox by explaining that the two equally talented performers work in areas with different population densities. Choice A is irrelevant since the argument states that Gob and Bobo are equally talented; it does not matter if Bobo is an experienced clown. Choice B looks promising, but it only mentions preferences to children's birthday parties and not all possible shows. Choice C is a strong answer choice, but it is too general for our purposes.

34. B: Unlike all the other words on the list, the word *are* is a being verb. In addition, *are* is in the present tense. The words *mixed*, *thrown*, *grown*, *beaten*, and *jumped* are all action verbs, and they are all in the past tense. The past tense of *are*, of course, is *were*. Therefore, *are* does not fit for two reasons: verb type and tense.

35. A: The word *patronage* most nearly means auspices, which means protection or support. Choice *B*, *aberration*, means abnormality and does not make sense within the context of the sentence. Choice *C*, *acerbic*, means sour or sharply critical, and it also does not make sense in the sentence.

Choice *D*, *adulation*, is a positive word meaning *praise*, and thus does not fit with the word *condescending* in the sentence.

36. D: *Working man* is most closely aligned with Choice *D*, *bourgeois.* In the context of the speech, the word *bourgeois* means working or middle class. Choice A, athlete, does suggest someone who works hard, but it does not make sense in this context. Choice *B***,** *viscount*, is a European title used to describe a specific degree of nobility. Choice *C*, *entrepreneur*, is a person who operates their own business.

37. C: In the context of the speech, the term *working man* most closely correlates with Choice *C*, *working man is someone who works for wages among the middle class.* Choice *A* is not mentioned in the passage and is off-topic. Choice *B* may be true in some cases, but it does not reflect the sentiment described for the term *working man* in the passage. Choice *D* is not a definition, and the topics of the field, factory, and screen are not mentioned in the passage.

38. D: *Enterprise* most closely means cause. Choices *A, B,* and *C* are all related to the term *enterprise*. However, Dickens speaks of a *cause* here, not a *company*, *courage*, or a *game*. "He will stand by such an enterprise" is a call to stand by a cause to enable the working man to have a certain autonomy over his own economic standing. The very first paragraph ends with the statement that the working man "shall... have a share in the management of an institution which is designed for his benefit."

39. B: Recall from the first paragraph that the speaker is there to "accompany [the audience]... through one of my little Christmas books," making him an author there to entertain the crowd with his own writing. The speech preceding the reading is the passage itself, and, as the tone indicates, it is a serious speech addressing the working man. Although the passage speaks of employers and employees, the speaker himself is not an employer of the audience, so Choice *A* is incorrect. Choice *C* is also incorrect, as the salutation is not used ironically, but sincerely, as the speech addresses the wellbeing of the crowd. Choice *D* is incorrect because the speech is not given by a politician, but by a writer.

40. B: Choice A is incorrect because that is the speaker's first desire, not his second. Choices C and D are tricky because the language of both of these is mentioned after the word second. However, the speaker doesn't get to the second wish until the next sentence. Choices C and D are merely preliminary remarks before the statement of the main clause, Choice B.

41. 3: According to the table, there are three Heather Gray T-shirts ordered in a size small in the month of January.

42. 1: There were five shirts ordered in size medium and four shirts ordered in size small, so we can determine that there was one more medium size shirt ordered than small size.

43. C: Pathos refers to the author's appeal to the audience's or reader's emotions. Ethos refers to the level of credibility of a piece of writing. Logos refers to the author's appeal to the audience's or reader's logic. Kairos refers to the most opportune moment to do something. Therefore, the correct answer is pathos.

44. A: Firsthand accounts are given by primary sources—individuals who provide personal or expert accounts of an event, subject matter, time period, or individual. They are viewed more as objective accounts than subjective. Secondary sources are accounts given by an individual or group of individuals who were not physically present at the event or who did not have firsthand knowledge of an individual or time period. Secondary sources are sources that have used research in order to create a written work. *Direct sources* and *indirect sources* are not standard terms.

45. C: Choice *A* is incorrect. The Conservative Politician definitely believes that spending on social welfare programs increases the national debt. However, the Liberal Politician does not address the cost of those programs. Choice *B* is a strong answer choice. The Liberal politician explicitly agrees that certain classes of people rely on social welfare programs. The Conservative politician does agree that people rely on the programs but thinks this reliance is detrimental. This answer choice is slightly off base, so it can be eliminated. Choice *C* improves on Choice *B*. The Liberal Politician definitely believes that certain classes of people would be irreparably harmed. In contrast, the Conservative Politician asserts that the programs are actually harmful since people become dependent on the programs. The Conservative Politician concludes that people don't need the assistance and would be better off if left to fend for themselves. This is definitely the main point of disagreement. Choice *D* is not the main point of dispute. Neither of the politicians discusses whether *all* of the nation's leaders have bootstrapped their way to the top, so it can be eliminated.

Mathematics

1. B: The first step is to make all exponents positive by moving the terms with negative exponents to the opposite side of the fraction. This expression becomes:

$$\frac{4b^3b^2}{a^1a^4} \times \frac{3a}{b}$$

Then the rules for exponents can be used to simplify. Multiplying the same bases means the exponents can be added. Dividing the same bases means the exponents are subtracted. Thus, after multiplying the exponents in the first fraction the equation becomes:

$$\frac{4b^5}{a^5} \times \frac{3a}{b}$$

Then, the two fractions can be multiplied, and the variable terms must be divided to find $\frac{12b^4}{a^4}$.

2. C: The product of two irrational numbers can be rational or irrational. Sometimes the irrational parts of the two numbers cancel each other out, leaving a rational number. For example, $\sqrt{2} \times \sqrt{2} = 2$ because the roots cancel each other out. Technically, the product of two irrational numbers is a complex number, because real numbers are a type of complex number. However, Choice *D* is incorrect because the product of two irrational numbers is not an imaginary number.

3. B: The car is traveling at a speed of 5 meters per second. On the interval from 1 to 3 seconds, the position changes by 10 meters. This is 10 meters in 2 seconds, or 5 meters in each second.

4. C: The terms "whole numbers" and "natural numbers" include all the ordinary counting numbers (1, 2, 3, 4, 5, ...), and sometimes zero depending on the definition used, but no negative numbers. The term "integers" includes all those numbers, their negatives, and zero. So –4 is not a whole number or a natural number, but it is an integer. It is also rational because it can be written as a ratio of two integers ($-\frac{4}{1}$); all integers are rational. It is a real number because it does not have an imaginary component (symbolized by the letter i); all integers are real numbers.

5. C:

$$4\frac{5}{7}+6\frac{5}{8}$$

Start by adding the whole numbers.

$$10+\left(\frac{5}{7}+\frac{5}{8}\right)$$

Then, add the fractions by cross multiplying the numerators with the denominators and the denominators with each other:

$$10+\left(\frac{5\times 8}{7\times 8}=\frac{5\times 7}{8\times 7}\right)$$

$$10+\left(\frac{40}{56}+\frac{35}{56}\right)$$

Then add the numerators together:

$$10+\frac{75}{56}$$

Since the fraction is improper, convert it to a mixed number:

$$10+1\frac{19}{56}$$

Finally, add these together:

$$11\frac{19}{56}$$

6. 31.4: To calculate the circumference of a circle, use the formula $2\pi r$, where r equals the radius (or half of the diameter) of the circle and $\pi \approx 3.14$. Substitute the given information to get:

$$2\times 3.14\times 5=31.4$$

7. B: To convert miles to kilometers, we can multiply the number of miles by the miles-per-kilometer conversion factor:

$$4.67\text{ mi}\times\frac{1.609\text{ km}}{1\text{ mi}}=7.51403\text{ km}$$

Because the question asks for an answer with three significant digits, 7.51 kilometers is the correct answer.

8. B: $\frac{5}{2} \div \frac{1}{3} = \frac{5}{2} \times \frac{3}{1} = \frac{15}{2} = 7.5$.

9. A: The total fraction taken up by green and red shirts will be $\frac{1}{3} + \frac{2}{5} = \frac{5}{15} + \frac{6}{15} = \frac{11}{15}$. The remaining fraction is:

$$1 - \frac{11}{15} = \frac{15}{15} - \frac{11}{15} = \frac{4}{15}$$

10. A: The Pythagorean theorem tells us that $8^2 + b^2 = 10^2$, where b is the unknown leg. This simplifies to $64 + b^2 = 100$, so $b^2 = 100 - 64$. After subtracting, $b^2 = 36$. Therefore, $b = \sqrt{36}$, which is equal to 6 inches.

11. C: The average is calculated by adding up each month's sales and dividing the sum by the total number of months in the time period. Dealer 1 sold 2 cars in July, 12 in August, 8 in September, 6 in October, 10 in November, and 15 in December. The sum of these sales is:

$$2 + 12 + 8 + 6 + 10 + 15 = 53 \text{ cars}$$

To find the average, divide this sum by the total number of months, which is 6. 53 is divided by 6, it yields 8.8333... Since we are told to round to the nearest whole number, we round the answer to 9 cars.

12. D: A given number divides evenly by each of its factors to produce an integer (no decimals). To find the factors of 12, determine what whole numbers when multiplied equal 12. 1x12, 2x6, and 3x4 are all the ways to multiply to 12 using whole numbers, so the factors of 12 are: 1, 2, 3, 4, 6, 12.

13. 1: This problem can be solved using basic arithmetic. Xavier starts with 20 apples, then gives his sister half, which is 20 divided by 2.

$$20 - \frac{20}{2} = 20 - 10 = 10$$

He then gives his neighbor six apples, so 6 is subtracted from 10.

$$10 - 6 = 4$$

Finally, he uses $\frac{3}{4}$ of his remaining apples to make a pie. Since $\frac{3}{4}$ of 4 is 3, he uses 3 apples, so 3 is subtracted from 4.

$$4 - 3 = 1$$

14. A: The hundredths place value is located two digits to the right of the decimal point (the digit 9 in the original number). To decide whether to round up or keep the digit, examine the digit to the right, and if it is 5 or greater, round up. In this case, the digit to the right is 6, so the hundredths place is rounded up. When rounding up, if the digit to be increased is a 9, the digit to its left is increased by one, and the digit in the desired place value is made a zero. Therefore, the number is rounded to 847.90.

15. B: Fractions must have like denominators to be added. The common denominator is the least common multiple (LCM) of the two original denominators. In this case, the LCM is 15, so both fractions should be changed to equivalent fractions with a denominator of 15. Multiply the bottom of each fraction by whatever number is needed to produce 15 and multiply the top of each fraction by that same number:

$$\frac{1 \times 5}{3 \times 5} = \frac{5}{15} \text{ and } \frac{2 \times 3}{5 \times 3} = \frac{6}{15}$$

Now, add the numerators and keep the denominator the same:

$$\frac{5}{15}+\frac{6}{15}=\frac{11}{15}$$

16. D: Denote the width as w and the length as l. Then, $l = 3w + 5$. The perimeter is $2w + 2l = 90$. Substituting the first expression for l into the second equation yields:

$$2(3w+5)+2w=90$$

$$6w+10+2w=90$$

$$8w=80$$

$$w=10$$

Putting this into the first equation, it yields:

$$l=3(10)+5=35$$

17. A: Putting the scores in order from least to greatest, we have 60, 75, 80, and 85, as well as one unknown. The median is 80, so 80 must be the middle data point out of these five. Therefore, the unknown data point must be the fourth or fifth data point, meaning it must be greater than or equal to 80. The only answer that fails to meet this condition is 60.

18. A: Divide 54 by 15:

$$\begin{array}{r} 3 \\ 15\overline{)54} \\ -45 \\ \hline 9 \end{array}$$

The result is 3 with a remainder of 9, which is equivalent to $3\frac{9}{15}$. Reduce the fraction $\frac{9}{15}$ for the final answer, $3\frac{3}{5}$.

19. A: Using the order of operations, multiplication and division are computed first from left to right. Multiplication is on the left; therefore, multiplication should be performed first.

20. D: The original number was $8\frac{3}{7}$. Multiply the denominator by the whole number portion. Add the numerator, and put the total over the original denominator.

$$\frac{(8\times 7)+3}{7}=\frac{59}{7}$$

21. B: Audit Services makes up 40% of total income, and Taxation Services makes up 30%, so together they make up $40\% + 30\% = 70\%$ of total income. To find 70% of \$500,000, change the percentage to a decimal and multiply: $0.7 \times \$500{,}000 = \$350{,}000$.

22. A: Let the unknown score be x. The average will be:

$$\frac{5\times 50+4\times 70+x}{10}=\frac{530+x}{10}=55$$

Multiply both sides by 10 to get $530 + x = 550$, or $x = 20$.

23. A: We use the place value to the right of the thousandths place, which would be the ten-thousandths place. The value in the thousandths place is 7. The number in the place value to its right is greater than 4, so the 7 is bumped up to 8. Everything to its right is removed, which gives us 245.268.

24. C: It may help to look at this problem as a fraction:

$$\frac{1.2 \times 10^{12}}{3.0 \times 10^{8}}$$

We can calculate,

$$\frac{1.2}{3} = 0.4$$

Using the rules of exponents, we can see that,

$$\frac{10^{12}}{10^{8}} = 10^{12-8} = 10^{4}$$

This gives us an answer of 0.4×10^4, which is Choice *A*, but our answer is not yet in scientific notation because the first term, 0.4, is not between 1 and 10. We can rewrite 0.4×10^4, multiplying the first term by 10 and subtracting 1 from the exponent, which gives 4.0×10^3, Choice *C*.

25. A: The relative error can be found by finding the absolute error and making it a percent of the true value. The absolute error is $36 - 35.75 = 0.25$. This error is then divided by 35.75—the true value—to find 0.7%.

26. D: The slope from this equation is 50, and it is interpreted as the cost per gigabyte used. Since the g-value represents the number of gigabytes and the equation is set equal to the cost in dollars, the slope relates these two values. For every gigabyte used on the phone, the bill goes up 50 dollars.

27. D: This problem can be solved by using unit conversions. The initial units are miles per minute. The final units need to be feet per second. Converting miles to feet uses the equivalence statement $1 \text{ mile} = 5{,}280 \text{ feet}$. Converting minutes to seconds uses the equivalence statement 1 minute = 60 seconds. Setting up the ratios to convert the units is shown in the following equation:

$$\frac{72 \text{ miles}}{90 \text{ minutes}} \times \frac{1 \text{ minute}}{60 \text{ seconds}} \times \frac{5280 \text{ feet}}{1 \text{ mile}} = 70.4 \text{ feet per second}$$

The initial units cancel out, and the new, desired units are left.

28. B: The formula can be manipulated by dividing both sides by the length, l, and the width, w. The length and width will cancel on the right, leaving height, h, by itself.

29. 50: Setting up a proportion is the easiest way to represent this situation. The proportion is $\frac{20}{x} = \frac{40}{100}$, and cross-multiplication can be used to solve for x. Here, $40x = 2{,}000$, so $x = 50$.

30. B: The formula for the area of the circle is πr^2, and 13 squared is 169. Choice *A* is not the correct answer because that is 13×2. Choice *C* is not the correct answer because that is 13×10. Choice *D* is not the correct answer because that is $2 \times 13 \times 10$.

31. B: The domain is all possible input values, or x-values. For this equation, the domain is every number greater than or equal to zero. There are no negative numbers in the domain because taking the square root of a negative number results in an imaginary number.

32. C: The question states that red cans are \$1 each and blue cans are \$2 each. Since the total cost is \$16, we can say that $r \times 1 + b \times 2 = 16$, where r is the number of red cans and b is the number of blue cans. It can be written more simply as $r + 2b = 16$.

Because Jessica buys 10 cans total, $r + b = 10$, so $b = 10 - r$. Substituting in $10 - r$ for b in the original equation gives $r + 2(10 - r) = 16$. Simplifying and solving for r gives the answer:

$$r + 20 - 2r = 16$$

$$20 - r = 16$$

$$r = 4$$

33. B: The volume of a rectangular prism is $length \times width \times height$, and $3\text{cm} \times 5\text{cm} \times 11\text{cm}$ is $165\ \text{cm}^3$.

34. A: To find the fraction of the bill that the first three people pay, the fractions need to be added, which means finding the common denominator. The common denominator is 60.

$$\frac{1}{5} + \frac{1}{4} + \frac{1}{3} = \frac{12}{60} + \frac{15}{60} + \frac{20}{60} = \frac{47}{60}$$

The remainder of the bill is:

$$1 - \frac{47}{60} = \frac{60}{60} - \frac{47}{60} = \frac{13}{60}$$

35. B: Using the Pythagorean Theorem, we can determine the length of the hypotenuse by plugging in the lengths of the sides: $a^2 + b^2 = c^2$, or $3^2 + 4^2 = c^2$=25. The square root of 25 is 5. Choice *A* is not the correct answer because that is $3 + 4$. Choice *C* is not the correct answer because that is stopping at $3^2 + 4^2$ is $9 + 16$, which is 25. Choice *D* is not the correct answer because that is 3×4.

36. B: Multiplying by 10^{-3} means moving the decimal point three places to the left, putting in zeros as necessary.

37. A: If each man gains 10 pounds, every original data point will increase by 10 pounds. Therefore, the man with the original median will still have the median value, but that value will increase by 10. The smallest value and largest value will also increase by 10, so the difference between the two (the range) will remain the same.

38. D: When you simplify $\left(\frac{\pi}{5}\right) \times \left(\frac{180}{\pi}\right)$, you get 36°. Choice *A* is not the correct answer because 10° is $\frac{\pi}{18}$. Choice *B* is not the correct answer because 20° is $\frac{\pi}{9}$. Choice *C* is not the correct answer because 30° is $\frac{\pi}{6}$.

Science

1. C: A hypothesis is a statement that makes a prediction between two variables. The two variables here are the amount of poison and how quickly the rat dies. Choice *C* states that the more poison a rat is given, the more quickly it will die, which is a prediction. Choice *A* is incorrect because it's simply an observation. Choice *B* is incorrect because it's a question posed by the observation but makes no predictions. Choice *D* is incorrect because it's simply a fact.

2. B: The independent variable is the variable manipulated, and the dependent variable is the result of the changes in the independent variable. Choice *B* is correct because the amount of poison is the variable that is changed, and the speed of rat death is the result of the changes in the amount of poison administered. Choice *A* is incorrect because that answer states the opposite. Choice *C* is false because the scientist isn't attempting to determine whether the rat will die *if* it eats poison; the scientist is testing how quickly the rat will die depending on *how much* poison it eats. Choice *D* is incorrect because the cage isn't manipulated in any way and has nothing to do with the hypothesis.

3. B: Models are representations of concepts that are impossible to experience directly, such as the 3D representation of DNA, so Choice *B* is correct. Choice *A* is incorrect because theories simply explain why things happen. Choice *C* is incorrect because laws describe how things happen. Choice *D* is false because an observation analyzes situations using human senses.

4. A: A control is the component or group in an experimental design that isn't manipulated—it's the standard against which the resultant findings are compared, so Choice *A* is correct. A variable is an element of the experiment that is able to be manipulated, making Choice *B* false. A constant is a condition of the experiment outside of the hypothesis that remains unchanged in order to isolate the changes in the variables; therefore, Choice *C* is incorrect. Choice *D* is false because collected data are simply recordings of the observed phenomena that result from the experiment.

5. C: An inference is a logical prediction of a why an event occurred based on previous experiences or education. The person in this example knows that plants need water to survive; therefore, the prediction that someone forgot to water the plant is a reasonable inference, hence Choice *C* is correct. A classification is the grouping of events or objects into categories, so Choice *A* is incorrect. An observation analyzes situations using human senses, so Choice *B* is incorrect. Choice *D* is incorrect because collecting is the act of gathering data for analysis.

6. A: The decimal point for this value is located after the final zero. Because the decimal is moved 12 places to the left in order to get it between the *8* and the *6*, then the resulting exponent is positive, so Choice *A* is the correct answer. Choice *B* is false because the decimal has been moved in the wrong direction. Choice *C* is incorrect because the decimal has been moved an incorrect number of times. Choice *D* is false because this value is written to three significant figures, not two.

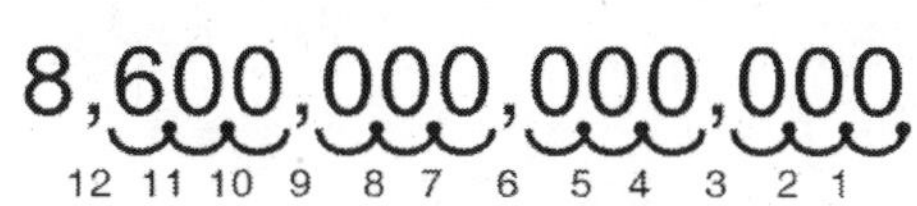

7. B: The set of results is close to the actual value of the acceleration due to gravity, making the results accurate. However, there is a different value recorded each time, so the results aren't precise, which makes Choice *B* the correct answer.

8. 0.57 M NaCl: To solve this, the number of moles of NaCl needs to be calculated:

First, to find the mass of NaCl, the mass of each of the molecule's atoms is added together as follows:

$$23.0 \text{ g Na} + 35.5 \text{ g Cl} = 58.5 \text{ g NaCl}$$

Next, the given mass of the substance is multiplied by one mole per total mass of the substance:

$$4.0 \text{ g NaCl} \times \frac{1 \text{ mol NaCl}}{58.5 \text{ g NaCl}} = 0.068 \text{ mol NaCl}$$

Finally, the moles are divided by the number of liters of the solution to find the molarity:

$$\frac{0.068 \text{ mol NaCl}}{0.120 \text{ L}} = 0.57 \text{ M NaCl}$$

9. C: According to the ideal gas law ($PV = nRT$), if volume is constant, the temperature is directly related to the pressure in a system. Therefore, if the pressure increases, the temperature will increase in direct proportion. Choice *A* would not be possible, since the system is closed and a change is occurring, so the temperature will change. Choice *B* incorrectly exhibits an inverse relationship between pressure and temperature, or $P = \frac{1}{T}$. Choice *D* is incorrect because even without actual values for the variables, the relationship and proportions can be determined.

10. D: An atom is structured with a nucleus in the center that contains neutral neutrons and positive protons. Surrounding the nucleus are orbiting electrons that are negatively charged. Choice *D* is the only correct answer.

11. C: Molecules that are soluble in lipids, like fats, sterols, and vitamins (A, D, E, and K), for example, are able to move in and out of a cell using passive transport. Water and oxygen are also able to move in and out of the cell without the use of cellular energy. Complex sugars and non-lipid-soluble molecules are too large to move through the cell membrane without relying on active transport mechanisms. Molecules naturally move from areas of high concentration to those of lower concentration. It requires active transport to move molecules in the opposite direction, as suggested by Choice *D*.

12. C: These are the coefficients that follow the law of conservation of matter.

13. C: A catalyst functions to increase reaction rates by decreasing the activation energy required for a reaction to take place. Inhibitors would increase the activation energy or otherwise stop the reactants from reacting. Although increasing the temperature usually increases a reaction's rate, this is not true in all cases, and most catalysts do not function in this manner.

14. D: Meiosis has the same phases as mitosis, except that they occur twice—once in meiosis I and once in meiosis II. During meiosis I, the cell splits into two. Each cell contains two sets of chromosomes. Next, during meiosis II, the two intermediate daughter cells divide again, producing four total haploid cells that each contain one set of chromosomes.

15. B: The secondary structure of a protein refers to the folds and coils that are formed by hydrogen bonding between the slightly charged atoms of the polypeptide backbone. The primary structure is the sequence of amino acids, similar to the letters in a long word. The tertiary structure is the overall shape of the molecule that results from the interactions between the side chains that are linked to the polypeptide backbone. The quaternary structure is the complete protein structure that occurs when a protein is made up of two or more polypeptide chains.

16. B: A solid produced during a reaction in solution is called a precipitate. In a neutralization reaction, the products (an acid and a base) react to form a salt and water. Choice *A*, an oxidation reaction, involves the transfer of an electron. Choice *C*, a synthesis reaction, involves the joining of two molecules to form a single molecule. Choice *D*, a decomposition reaction, involves the separation of a molecule into two other molecules.

17. C: Generally, all sensory pathways that extend from the sensory receptor to the brain are composed of three long neurons called the primary, secondary, and tertiary neurons. The primary one stretches from the sensory receptor to the dorsal root ganglion of the spinal nerve, and the secondary one stretches from the cell body of the primary neuron to the spinal cord or the brain stem. The tertiary one stretches from the cell body of the secondary one into the thalamus. Each type of sense, such as touch, hearing, and vision, has a different pathway designed specifically for that sensation.

18. C: Visual processing begins in the retina. When an individual sees an image, it is taken in through the cornea and lens and then transmitted upside down onto the retina. The cells in the retina process what is being seen and then send signals to the ganglion cells, whose axons make up the optic nerve. The optic nerve cells connect the retina to the brain, which is where the processing of the visual information is completed and the images are returned to their proper orientation.

19. A: Photosynthesis is the process of converting light energy into chemical energy, which is then stored in sugar and other organic molecules. The photosynthetic process takes place in the thylakoids inside chloroplasts in plants. Chlorophyll is a green pigment that in the thylakoid membranes and absorbs photons from light.

20. C: The somatic nervous system is the voluntary nervous system, which is responsible for voluntary movement. It includes nerves that transmit signals from the brain to the muscles of the body. Breathing is controlled by the autonomic nervous system. Thought and fear are complex processes that occur in the brain, which is part of the central nervous system.

21. D: Catabolism is the process of breaking down large molecules into smaller molecules to release energy for work. Carbohydrates and fats are catabolized to provide energy for exercise and daily activities. Anabolism synthesizes larger molecules from smaller constituent building blocks. Bioenergetics and metabolism are more general terms involving overall energy production and usage.

22. A: Platelets are the blood components responsible for clotting. There are between 150,000 and 450,000 platelets in healthy blood. When a clot forms, platelets adhere to the injured area of the vessel and promote a molecular cascade that results in adherence of more platelets. Ultimately, the platelet aggregation results in recruitment of a protein called fibrin, which adds structure to the clot. Too many platelets can cause clotting disorders. Too few platelets leads to bleeding disorders.

23. A: Choice *B* might be an attractive answer choice, but neutrophils are part of the innate immune system and are not considered part of the primary immune response. The first event that happens in a primary immune response is that macrophages ingest pathogens and display their antigens. Then, they secrete interleukin 1 to recruit helper T cells. Once helper T cells are activated, they secrete interleukin 2 to stimulate plasma B and killer T cell production. Only then can plasma B make the pathogen specific antibodies.

24. C: The epididymis stores sperm and is a coiled tube located near the testes. The immature sperm that enters the epididymis from the testes migrates through the 20-foot long epididymis tube in about two weeks, where viable sperm are concentrated at the end. The vas deferens is a tube that transports mature sperm from the epididymis to the urethra. Seminal vesicles are pouches attached that add fructose to the ejaculate to provide energy for sperm. The prostate gland excretes fluid that makes up about a third of semen released during ejaculation. The fluid reduces semen viscosity and contains enzymes that aid in sperm functioning; both effects increase sperm motility and ultimate success.

25. A: All three joint types given are synovial joints, allowing for a fair amount of movement (compared with fibrous and cartilaginous joints). Of the three given, hinge joints, such as the elbow, permit the least motion because they are uniaxial and permit movement in only one plane. Saddle joints and condyloid joints both have reciprocating surfaces that mate with one another and allow a variety of motions in numerous planes, but saddle joints, such as the thumb carpal-metacarpal joint, allow more motion than condyloid joints. In saddle joints, two concave surfaces articulate, and in a condyloid joint, such as the wrist, a concave surface articulates with a convex surface, allowing motion in mainly two planes.

26. C: The qualitative definition of ionization energy is the amount of energy needed to remove a the one most loosely bound valence electron from a gaseous atom or molecule to form a cation. Choice *A* refers to atomic radius, Choice *B* refers to electronegativity, and Choice *D* refers to electron affinity. All four of these properties follow trends on the periodic table.

27. C: Conversion within the metric system is as simple as the movement of decimal points. The prefix *kilo-* means "one thousand," or three zeros, so the procedure to convert kilometers to the primary unit (meters) is to move the decimal point three units to the right. To get to centimeters, the decimal point must be moved an additional two places to the right: 0.78 → 78,000. Choice *A* is false because the decimal point has only been moved one place to right. Choice *B* is incorrect because the decimal point is moved one unit in the wrong direction. Choice *D* is false because the decimal has only been moved three units to the right. The problem can also be solved by using the following conversion equation:

$$0.78 \text{ km} \times \frac{1{,}000 \text{ m}}{1 \text{ km}} \times \frac{100 \text{ cm}}{1 \text{ m}} = 78{,}000 \text{ cm}$$

The kilometer (km) units cancel each other out, as do the meter (m) units. The only units left are centimeters (cm).

28. D: The natural tendency in the universe is to increase entropy and disorder, so organisms undergo biochemical processes and use free energy and matter to stabilize their internal environment against this changing external environment in a process called homeostasis. Organisms strive to maintain physiologic factors such as body temperature, blood pH, and fluid balance in equilibrium or around a set point. Choice *A* is incorrect because homeostasis in organisms involves trying to maintain internal conditions around their set point, which doesn't always involve increasing body temperature, blood pH, and fluid balance; the organism may need to work to decrease these values. Choice *B* is incorrect because maintaining homeostasis expends energy; it does not absorb it. Choice *C* is incorrect because homeostasis involves maintaining order in the organism's internal, not external, environment.

29. A, B, C, D: All three types of muscle tissue (skeletal, cardiac, and smooth) share four important properties: they are contractile, meaning they can shorten and pull on connective tissue; excitable, meaning they respond to stimuli; elastic, meaning they rebound to their original length after a contraction; and extensible, meaning they can be stretched repeatedly but maintain the ability to contract. While skeletal muscle is under voluntary control, both cardiac and smooth muscle are involuntary.

30. C: The graph shows that as the value of x increases, the value of y decreases, which is the definition of a negative correlation, so Choice *C* is correct. A positive correlation is when the value of y increases as the value of x increases, so Choice *A* is incorrect. Choices *B* and *D* both show no determinable relationship between two variables.

31. C: When conducting scientific research, it is best to rely on sources that are known for honest, ethical, and unbiased research and experimentation. Most laboratories and universities must have their work validated through independent means in order to publish or claim results. Anyone can publish things on the Internet—it does not mean their work has been validated, and therefore, their work may not be correct.

32. A: The renal pelvis acts like a funnel by delivering the urine from the millions of collecting tubules to the ureters. It is the most central part of the kidney. The renal cortex is the outer layer of the kidney, while the renal medulla is the inner layer. The renal medulla contains the functional units of the kidneys—nephrons—which function to filter the blood. Choice *D,* Bowman's capsule, is the name for the structure that covers the glomeruli.

33. The lower margin of the liver can be found in the right upper quadrant of the abdomen. During palpation, the nurse should ask the patient to take a deep breath; this causes the liver to be displaced downward, and it can be further palpated in the right lower quadrant.

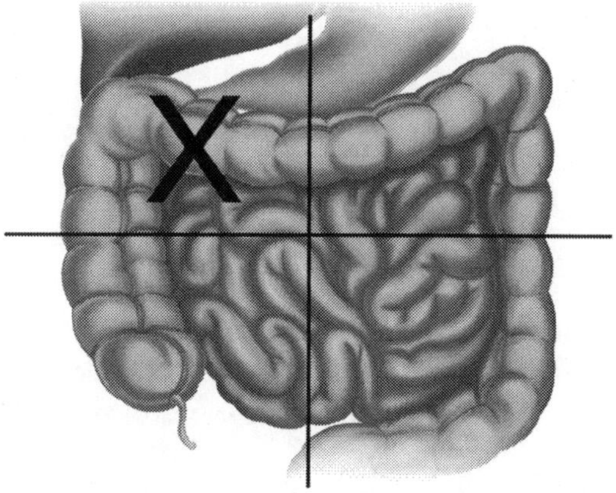

34. B: An amphoteric substance can act as an acid or a base depending on the properties of the solute. Water is a common example; because of its amphoteric property, it serves as a universal solvent. Choice *A* is incorrect because it describes electrolytes. Choices *C* and *D* are incorrect because they both describe an acid.

35. C: The body has a variety of touch receptors that detect tactile information, which gets carried via general somatic afferents and general visceral afferents to the CNS. Meissner's corpuscles respond to light touch and slower vibrations. Choice *A* is incorrect because Merkel's discs respond to sustained pressure. Choice *B* is incorrect because Pacinian corpuscles detect rapid vibration in the skin and fascia, and Choice *D* is incorrect because Ruffini endings detect deep touch and tension in the skin and fascia.

36. C: The uterus and ovaries aren't part of the birth canal, so Choices *A* and *D* are false. The cervix is the uppermost portion of the birth canal, so Choice B is incorrect, making Choice C the correct answer. The vagina is the muscular tube on the lowermost portion of the birth canal that connects the exterior environment to the cervix.

37. C: A cluster of capillaries that functions as the main filter of the blood entering the kidney is known as the glomerulus, so Choice *C* is correct. The Bowman's capsule surrounds the glomerulus and receives fluid and solutes from it; therefore, Choice *A* is incorrect. The loop of Henle is a part of the kidney tubule where water and nutrients are reabsorbed, so *B* is false. The nephron is the unit containing all of these anatomical features, making Choice *D* incorrect as well.

38. A: An alteration in the normal gene sequence is called a DNA point mutation. Mutations can be harmful, neutral, or even beneficial. Sometimes, as seen in natural selection, a genetic mutation can improve fitness, providing an adaptation that will aid in survival. DNA mutations can happen as a result of environmental damage, for example, from radiation or chemicals. Mutations can also happen during cell replication as a result of incorrect pairing of complementary nucleotides by DNA polymerase. There are also chromosomal mutations as well, where entire segments of chromosomes can be deleted, inverted, duplicated, or sent or received from a different chromosome.

39. B: According to the Punnett square, the child has a 2 out of 4 chance of having A-type blood, since the dominant allele I^A is present in two of the four possible offspring. The type O blood allele is masked by the type A blood allele since it is recessive.

I^A i	ii
I^A i	ii

40. D: Let's label *R* as the right-handed allele and *r* as the left-handed allele. Esther has to have the combination rr since she's left-handed. She had to get at least one recessive allele from each parent. So, her mom could either be Rr or rr (right-handed or left-handed), and her dad can also be Rr or rr. As long as each parent carries one recessive allele, it is possible that Esther is left-handed. Therefore, all answer choices are possible.

41. A: The process of cell division in somatic cells is called mitosis. In interphase, which precedes mitosis, cells prepare for division by copying their DNA. Once mitotic machinery has been assembled in interphase, mitosis occurs, which has five distinct phases: prophase, prometaphase, metaphase, anaphase, and telophase, followed by cytokinesis, which is the final splitting of the cytoplasm. The two diploid daughter cells are genetically identical to the parent cell.

42. D: Human gametes each contain 23 chromosomes. This is referred to as a haploid, which is a cell that has half the number of chromosomes as the original germ cell (46). Germ cells are diploid precursors of the haploid egg and sperm. Meiosis has two major phases, each of which is characterized by sub-phases similar to mitosis. In meiosis I, the DNA of the parent cell is duplicated in interphase, just like in mitosis. Starting with prophase I, things become a little different. Two homologous chromosomes form a tetrad, cross over, and exchange genetic content. Each shuffled chromosome of the tetrad migrates to the cell's poles, and two haploid daughter cells are formed. In meiosis II, each daughter undergoes another division more similar to mitosis (with the exception of the fact that there is no interphase), resulting in four genetically-different cells, each with only half of the chromosomal material of the original germ cell.

43. C: The alveoli are small sac-shaped structures at the end of the bronchioles where gas exchange takes place. The bronchioles are tubes through which air travels. The kidneys and medulla oblongata do not directly affect oxygen and carbon dioxide exchange.

44.

1. **Lungs**
2. **Left atrium**
3. **Mitral Valve**
4. **Left Ventricle**
5. **Aorta**
6. **Arteries and capillaries**
7. **Tissues**

The correct order is lungs to the left atrium, through the mitral valve into the left ventricle, pumped into the aorta upon contraction, then dispersed to tissues via a network of arteries and capillaries

45. A: This node is the primary stimulator of electrical activity in the heart. The other structures listed play a role in blood flow, but do not deal with electrical stimulation.

46. D: The primary function of the endocrine system is to maintain homeostasis, which means it makes constant adjustments to the body's systemic physiology to maintain a stable internal environment. Homeostasis requires an adequate heart rate, respirations, and water and electrolyte balance, as well as many other physiological processes; therefore, Choice *D* is the correct answer. The other answers are false because they represent only one aspect of homeostasis.

47. D: Thyroid hormone is responsible for regulating metabolism, so Choice *D* is the correct answer. Insulin is involved in glucose uptake into tissues, testosterone is for sperm production and secondary male sexual characteristics, and adrenaline is responsible for mechanisms in the flight-or-fight response, making Choices *A*, *B*, and *C* incorrect.

48. C: To make a solution from a pure solid, the total molecular weight of the substance must be calculated and then the proper mass of the substance in grams must be added to water to make a solution. To calculate the total molecular weight, the individual molecular weights must be added. Finally, the mass of substance needed to make the solution can be calculated.

$$\left(1 \times 40.07\frac{\text{g}}{\text{mol}}\text{Ca}\right) + \left(1 \times 12.01\frac{\text{g}}{\text{mol}}\text{C}\right) + \left(3 \times 15.99\frac{\text{g}}{\text{mol}}\text{O}\right) = 100.05\frac{\text{g}}{\text{mol}}\text{CaCO}_3$$

$$600\text{ mL CaCO}_3 \times \frac{1\text{ L CaCO}_3}{1{,}000\text{ mL CaCO}_3} \times \frac{0.350\text{ mol CaCO}_3}{\text{L CaCO}_3} \times \frac{100.05\text{ g CaCO}_3}{1\text{ mol CaCO}_3} = 21.0\text{ g CaCO}_3$$

The calculations reveal that Choice *C* is the correct answer. All other reported values are incorrect.

49. D: Preparing a solution from a stock is simply a process of dilution by adding a certain amount of the stock to water. The amount of stock to use can be calculated using a formula and algebra with the given values for the stock molarity (12.0 M), the diluted volume (250 ml), and diluted molarity (1.50 M):

$$V_S = \frac{M_D V_D}{M_S}$$

$$\text{V}_\text{S} = \frac{(1.50\text{ M})(250\text{ ml})}{12.0\text{ M}} = 31.3\text{ ml}$$

Because the given values are written to three significant figures, the answer should also be written in three significant figures, making Choice *D* the correct answer. The other answer choices are either incorrect values or reported to an incorrect number of significant figures.

50. C: Disruptive selection occurs when both extremes of a phenotype are selected. In Cameroon, the finches had both large and small beaks, but did not survive well with medium beaks. If medium beaks were selected, it would have been stabilizing selection, Choice *A*. If only one of the extremes had been favored, it would have been directional selection, Choice *B*.

English and Language Usage

1. C: A complex sentence joins an independent or main clause with a dependent or subordinate clause. In this case, the main clause is "The restaurant is unconventional." This is a clause with one subject-verb combination that can stand alone as a grammatically complete sentence. The dependent clause is "because it serves both Chicago style pizza and New York style pizza." This clause begins with the subordinating conjunction because and also consists of only one subject-verb combination. Choice A is incorrect because a simple sentence consists of only one verb-subject combination—one independent clause. Choice B is incorrect because a compound sentence contains two independent clauses connected by a conjunction. Choice D is incorrect because a compound-complex sentence consists of two or more independent clauses and one or more dependent clauses.

2. A: Parallelism refers to consistent use of sentence structure or word form. In this case, the list within the sentence does not utilize parallelism; three of the verbs appear in their base form—*travel*, *take*, and *eat*—but one appears as a gerund—*going*. A parallel version of this sentence would be "This summer, I'm planning to travel to Italy, take a Mediterranean cruise, go to Pompeii, and eat a lot of Italian food." *B* is incorrect because this description is a complete sentence. *C* is incorrect as a misplaced modifier is a modifier that is not located appropriately in relation to the word or words they modify. *D* is incorrect because subject-verb agreement refers to the appropriate conjugation of a verb in relation to its subject.

3. D: Swell. A tissue that is *engorged* is swollen with fluid. For example, a new mom will have breasts engorged with milk to nurture her baby.

4. C: The main idea of a piece is its central theme or subject and what the author wants readers to know or understand after they finish reading. Choice *A* is incorrect because the primary purpose is the reason that a piece was written, and while the main idea is an important part of the primary purpose, the above elements are not developed with that intent. Choice *B* is incorrect because while the plot refers to the events that occur in a narrative, organization, tone, and supporting details are not used only to develop plot. Choice *D* is incorrect because characterization is the description of a person.

5. D: The problem in the original passage is that the second sentence is a dependent clause that cannot stand alone as a sentence; it must be attached to the main clause found in the first sentence. Because the main clause comes first, it does not need to be separated by a comma. However, if the dependent clause came first, then a comma would be necessary, which is why Choice *C* is incorrect. Choices *A* and *B* also insert unnecessary commas into the sentence.

6. A: A noun refers to a person, place, thing, or idea. Although the word *approach* can also be used as a verb, in the sentence it functions as a noun within the noun phrase "a fresh approach," so *B* is incorrect. An adverb is a word or phrase that provides additional information about the verb, so Choice *C* is incorrect. An adjective is a word that describes a noun. Thus, Choice *D* is also incorrect.

7. A, B, D: Prewriting, Choice *A*, refers to brainstorming, researching, and organizing before the actual writing begins. Revising, Choice *B*, involves making changes to the text that improve content, clarity, and flow. Conferencing, Choice *D*, involves getting feedback from others. Sourcing, Choice *C*, is not a term used to describe a step in the writing process.

8. B: In this case, the phrase functions as an adverb modifying the verb report, so Choice *B* is the correct answer. *To the student center* does not consist of a subject-verb combination, so it is not a clause; thus, Choices *A* and *C* can be eliminated. This group of words is a phrase. Phrases are classified by either the controlling word in the phrase or its function in the sentence. Choice *D* is incorrect because a noun phrase is a series of words that describe or modify a noun.

9. D: A noun phrase consists of the noun and all of its modifiers. In this case, the subject of the sentence is the noun *puppy*, but it is preceded by several modifiers—adjectives that give more information about what kind of puppy, which are also part of the noun phrase. Thus, Choice *A* is incorrect. Charlotte refers to the owner and modifies the word *puppy*, so Choice *B* is false. Choice *C* is incorrect because it contains some, but not all, of the modifiers pertaining to the puppy.

10. C: Because Emma quoted excerpts from the play, she needs to insert citations that give proper credit to the original work being quoted. Failing to do so would constitute plagiarism. The remaining choices are incorrect because they are steps that Emma would have completed earlier in the writing process.

11. A: The affix circum– originates from Latin and means "around" or "surrounding. It is also related to other words that indicate something round, such as *circle* and *circus*.

12. D: Since the sentence contains two independent clauses and a dependent clause, the sentence is categorized as compound-complex:

Independent clause: *I accepted the change of seasons*

Independent clause: *I started to appreciate the fall*

Dependent clause: *Although I wished it were summer*

13. D: Students can use context clues to make a careful guess about the meaning of unfamiliar words. Although all of the words in a sentence can help contribute to the overall meaning, in this case, the adjective that pairs with ubiquitous gives the most important hint to the student: cars were first rare, but now they are ubiquitous. The inversion of rare is what gives meaning to the rest of the sentence; ubiquitous means "existing everywhere" or "not rare." *A* is incorrect because *ago* only indicates a time frame. *B* is incorrect because *cars* does not indicate a contrasting relationship to the word *ubiquitous* to provide a good context clue. *C* is incorrect because it also only indicates a time frame, but used together with *rare*, it provides the contrasting relationship needed to identify the meaning of the unknown word.

14. B: For this question, place the underlined sentence in each prospective choice's position. Leaving the sentence in place is incorrect because the father "going crazy" doesn't logically follow the fact that he was a "city slicker." Choice *C* is incorrect because the sentence in question is not a concluding sentence and does not transition smoothly into the second paragraph. Choice *D* is incorrect because the sentence doesn't necessarily need to be omitted since it logically follows the very first sentence in the passage.

15. D: Choice *D* is correct because "As it turns out" indicates a contrast from the previous sentiment, that the RV was a great purchase. Choice *A* is incorrect because the sentence needs an effective transition from the paragraph before. Choice *B* is incorrect because the text indicates it *is* surprising that the RV was a great purchase because the author was skeptical beforehand. Choice *C* is incorrect because the transition *furthermore* does not indicate a contrast.

16. B: This sentence calls for parallel structure. Choice *B* is correct because the verbs *wake*, *eat*, and *break* are consistent in tense and parts of speech. Choice *A* is incorrect because the words *wake* and *eat* are present tense while the word *broke* is in past tense. Choice *C* is incorrect because this turns the sentence into a question, which doesn't make sense within the context. Choice *D* is incorrect because it breaks tense with the rest of the passage. *Waking*, *eating*, and *breaking* are all present participles, and the context around the sentence is in past tense.

17. C: Choice *C* is correct because it is clear and fits within the context of the passage. Choice *A* is incorrect because, "We rejoiced as 'hackers,'" does not explain what was meant by "hackers" or why it was a cause for rejoicing. Choice *B* is incorrect because it does not mention a solution being found and is therefore not specific enough. Choice *D* is incorrect because the meaning is eschewed by the helping verb "had to rejoice," and the sentence suggests that rejoicing was necessary to "hack" a solution.

18. A: The original sentence is correct because the verb tense and the meaning both align with the rest of the passage. Choice *B* is incorrect because the order of the words makes the sentence more confusing than it otherwise would be. Choice *C* is incorrect because "We are even making" is in present tense. Choice *D* is incorrect because "We will make" is future tense. The surrounding text of the sentence is in past tense.

19. B: Choice *B* is correct because there is no punctuation needed if a dependent clause ("while traveling across America") is located behind the independent clause ("it allowed us to share adventures"). Choice *A* is incorrect because there are two dependent clauses connected and no independent clause, and a complete sentence requires at least one independent clause. Choice *C* is incorrect because of the same reason as Choice *A*. Semicolons have the same function as periods; therefore, there must be an independent clause on either side of the semicolon. Choice *D* is incorrect because the dash simply interrupts the complete sentence.

20. C: The rule for *me* and *I* is that one should use *I* when it is the subject pronoun of a sentence and *me* when it is the object pronoun of the sentence. Break the sentence up to see if *I* or *me* should be used. To say "Those are memories that I have now shared" is correct, rather than "Those are memories that me have now shared." Choice D is incorrect because *my siblings* should come before *I*.

21. B: The overall tone of this passage is Choice *B*, informal. The writer uses casual wording such as "city-slicker" to connect with the audience in an informal way.

22. D: Choice *D* is correct because Fred Hampton becoming an activist was a direct result of him wanting to see lasting social change for Black people. Choice *A* doesn't make sense because "In the meantime" denotes something happening at the same time as another thing. Choice *B* is incorrect because the text's tone does not indicate that becoming a civil rights activist is an unfortunate path. Choice *C* is incorrect because "Finally" indicates something that comes last in a series of events, and the word in question is at the beginning of the introductory paragraph.

23. C: Choice *C* is correct because there should be a comma between the city and state, as well as after the word "Illinois." Commas should be used to separate all geographical items within a sentence. Choice *A* is incorrect because it does not include the comma after "Illinois." Choice B is incorrect because the comma after "neighborhood" interrupts the phrase, "the Maywood neighborhood of Chicago." Finally, Choice *D* is incorrect because the order of the sentence designates that Chicago, Illinois is in Maywood, which is incorrect.

24. C: The paragraph is incorrect as-is because it is too long and thus loses the reader as it changes focus halfway through. Choice *C* is correct because if the new paragraph began with "While studying at Triton," we would see a smooth transition from one paragraph to the next. We can also see how the two paragraphs are logically split in two. The first half of the paragraph talks about where he studied. The second half of the paragraph talks about the NAACP and the result of his leadership in the association. If we look at the passage as a whole, we can see that there are two main topics that should be broken in two.

25. B: We can determine this answer by using context clues. We know that the BPP was "similar in function" to the NAACP. To find out what the NAACP's function is, we must look at the previous sentences. We know from above that the NAACP is an activist group, so we can assume that the BPP was also an activist group.

26. A: Choice C is incorrect because it misplaces the apostrophe. While Choice D contains proper construction of a possessive, it changes the name of the organization from the Black Panther Party to the Black Panther Parties. Choice B also changes the name of the organization, and it doesn't use a possessive form. Choice D is incorrect because, again, the word "parties" should not be plural; instead, it is one unified party.

27. C: Choice *C* is correct because the passage is in the past tense and "enabled" is a past tense verb. Choice *A*, "enable," is present tense. Choice *B*, "are enabling," is a present participle, which suggests a continuing action. Choice *D*, "will enable," is future tense.

28. D: Choice *D* is correct because the conjunction "and" is the best way to combine the two independent clauses. Choice *A* is incorrect because the word "he" becomes repetitive since the two clauses can be joined together. Choice *B* is incorrect because the conjunction "but" indicates a contrast, and there is no contrast between the two clauses. Choice *C* is incorrect because the introduction of the comma after "project" with no conjunction creates a comma splice.

29. A, C: "Seperate" is a common misspelling of the word "separate". The word "acheivement" is misspelled. Remember the rules for "*i* before *e* except after *c*." Choices *B* and *D*, "greatest" and "leader," are both spelled correctly.

30. A: The tone of this passage is more formal because it is using more elevated language, as opposed to an informal tone which would read more conversationally.

31. B: This sentence, while short like the others, gives us the most detail ("red" sign) and is therefore the most specific answer option.

32. C: While this statement acknowledges the individual's shortcomings, it does so in a way that makes them feel included rather than singled out. Additionally, it does not put the student on the defensive during conversation.

33. A: The answer is punctual, which specifically means "on time." All of the other answer choices mean to arrive either early or late.

34. D: Writers must use citations when including content that is not their own original work. This includes paraphrasing, summarizing, and directly quoting the ideas of another author. Citations are not necessary when stating an original conclusion about another author's work (unless, of course, the conclusion involves a direct referral to the other author's content). They are also not necessary in original short stories because no outside information is borrowed. Finally, citations are not required when stating facts that are considered common knowledge, such as *George Washington was the first president of the United States* or *The Earth revolves around the Sun*.

35. B: Editing refers to checking a piece of writing for grammatical changes such as spelling, incomplete sentences, punctuation, etc. Revising refers to making changes to the content and clarity of a text. Writers should both revise and edit the entirety of their work before submitting a final draft.

36. A: Blog posts are not appropriate sources for a research paper because they have no accountability measures for truth or validity. Anyone can have a blog and post anything on it without being peer-reviewed or fact checked. When writing a research paper, one should only use the most reputable sources that have been professionally vetted for accuracy, including government websites, peer-reviewed journal articles, and documentaries.

37. D: Prewriting is the first step of the writing process. It involves preparing to write by determining the purpose and topic of writing, brainstorming ideas, researching, and organizing thoughts with an outline or similar organizational tool. Revising and conferencing come at the end of the writing process and involve making content changes and getting feedback from readers. Writing involves fleshing out the ideas that were researched and outlined, providing evidence to support main points, and making sure that each paragraph of text flows seamlessly into the next.

Practice Tests #3–#11

To keep the size of this book manageable, save paper, and provide a digital test-taking experience, practice tests #3–#11 can be found online. Scan the QR code or go to this link to access it:

testprepbooks.com/online387/teas

SCAN ME

The first time you access the test, you will need to register as a "new user" and verify your email address.

If you have any issues, please email support@testprepbooks.com.

Index

Abdominal, 96, 98
Abdominal Cavity, 96
Absolute Value, 39, 58
Accuracy/Reliability, 28
Acromial, 98
Action, 60, 111, 196, 197, 200, 201, 204, 205, 216, 273, 342
Active Immunization, 126
Adhesiveness, 170, 177
Adjective, 24, 39, 195, 200, 201, 253, 254, 281, 282, 316, 340, 343
Adrenal Gland, 119
Adverbs, 202
Algebraic Equations, 61
Amphoteric, 177, 312, 337
Anatomy, 96
Anecdotes, 15
Anion, 169
Antecedent, 199, 200
Anterior, 96, 97, 118
Antonyms, 23
Arc of a Circle, 86
Area, 83, 84, 85, 88, 101, 102, 131, 132, 164, 181, 191, 246, 273, 298, 317, 335
Articles, 27, 34, 35, 199, 205, 282
Artificial, 126
Atomic Radius, 164, 166
Author, 15, 24, 26, 27, 28, 29, 30, 31, 32, 222, 223, 225, 226, 227, 228, 261, 262, 263, 288, 325, 326, 341
Bar Graph, 19, 73, 74, 75
Base, 44, 54, 55, 84, 85, 87, 90, 91, 149, 150, 156, 171, 182, 202, 264, 275, 312, 327, 337, 340
Behaves, 178
Bias, 22, 26, 28, 32, 34, 185, 260
Bile, 106, 107
Bimodal, 80
Bling-Bling, 24
Blood, 128
Bolus, 105
Brachial, 98
Brainstorming, 213, 214
Building Blocks, 150, 211, 335
Cardiac Muscle, 115, 314
Carpal, 98
Cartesian Plane, 74
Catalysts, 176, 248, 275, 334
Cation, 169
Caudal, 97
Cell Walls, 131, 134, 154
Cells, 99, 100, 102, 103, 105, 106, 107, 112, 115, 116, 118, 119, 123, 125, 126, 127, 130, 131, 132, 133, 134, 149, 150, 152, 154, 155, 163, 244, 247, 253, 273, 274, 276, 279, 308, 309, 313, 334, 335, 338
Cellulose, 153, 154
Cephalic, 97
Cerebrum, 109
Cervical, 96, 222
Chart, 20, 35, 74, 75, 76, 90, 152, 156, 162, 183, 237, 290, 294
Cheap, 24
Chitin, 154
Chloroplasts, 134
Chromatin, 131
Chromosomes, 115, 131, 149, 273, 313, 334, 337, 338
Chyme, 105, 106, 107
Cilia and Flagella, 133
Clavicular, 98
Coenzymes, 176
Cofactors, 176, 248, 275
Cohesiveness, 170, 177
Colloquial, 210, 258, 283
Colors, 103
Comma, 193, 194, 195, 203, 254, 279, 280, 282, 340, 342
Common Denominator, 43, 56, 57, 332
Common Noun, 199
Complete Subjects, 203
Complex Sentence, 193, 198
Compound, 204
Compound Sentence, 198, 253, 257, 280, 282
Compound Subjects, 204
Compound-Complex Sentence, 198
Conclusions, 17, 28, 29, 32, 78, 182, 221, 226, 262, 324
Condensation, 166, 167, 168, 277
Conjunctions, 198, 203
Connective, 103, 112, 116, 118, 128, 130, 274, 336
Connotation, 24
Consistent Flow, 211
Context Clues, 23, 24, 342
Contractions, 105, 191, 196, 205, 210
Contrast, 30, 83, 131, 207, 210, 227, 261, 262, 264, 283, 327, 341, 342

Conversion Factor, 68, 91, 92
Coordinating Conjunctions, 203
Costs, 62, 63, 65, 261
Counter-Argument, 32
Covalent Bond, 152, 169, 170, 248, 275
Covariance, 83
Coverage, 28, 279
Cranial, 96, 97, 111
Cubital, 98
Decimal Number, 40, 44, 49, 54
Decimal Place, 44, 51, 52, 54, 85, 301
Decimal Point, 40, 44, 45, 54, 55, 60, 183, 184, 265, 267, 332, 333
Decimal System, 44
Decimals, 39, 40, 43, 44, 45, 46, 49, 51, 52, 54, 59, 67
Decimals and Percentages, 45
Declarative, 197
Deduction, 323
Deep, 98, 337
Definitions, 23, 39
Degrees, 22, 67, 86, 206, 284
Demonstrative Pronouns, 199
Denotation, 24
Dense, 112, 130, 177, 178, 274
Depend, 73, 177, 295
Dependent, 73, 74, 77, 81, 113, 182, 185, 187, 193, 198, 203, 207, 248, 273, 307, 316, 327, 340, 341
Dependent Clause, 207
Dependent Variable, 73, 74, 77, 81, 307
Dependent Variables, 73
Deposition, 168
Dipoles, 170, 248, 275
Direct Objects, 204
Direct Subjects, 203
Discombobulated, 23
Distal, 97, 105, 123
Distance, 58, 78, 83, 85, 86, 164, 206, 281
Distinct Section, 211
Dorsal, 97
Drafting, 213, 214, 215, 225
Duodenum, 106, 107
EBSCO, 34
Electron Affinity, 164, 166, 169
Electronegative, 177
Electronegativity, 164, 166
Electrons, 162, 163, 164, 166, 169, 170, 177, 178, 248, 250, 275, 277
Ellipsis, 193
Empirical, 26, 185
Emulsify, 106
Enzymes, 106, 115, 127, 133, 154, 176, 224, 248, 273, 275, 277, 279, 335
Epigastric, 98, 99
Epithelial, 103, 116, 249
Estimation, 64, 65, 66
Ethnocentric, 31
Even Numbers, 39
Exclamations Point (!), 210
Exclamatory, 197
Expiration, 102
Explanations, 23, 182, 185, 261
Expository Writing, 26, 261
Extensive, 23, 78, 177, 178, 260
Fact, 285, 323
Fact and Opinion, 22, 32
Facts, 15, 16, 17, 22, 24, 32, 213, 234, 263, 264, 265, 325
Femoral, 98
First, 249, 250, 260, 262, 263, 265, 266, 270, 271, 286, 290, 295, 303, 306, 309, 325, 326, 330, 332, 335, 340, 341, 342
First Person, 199, 210, 306
First-Person Point of View, 31, 210
Format, 17, 59, 214
Four-Year College, 20
Fractions and Decimals, 46
Fractions and Percentages, 45
Frankenstein, 31
Freezing, 168
Frugal, 24
GCF, 41, 42
Geniculate, 98
Ginormous, 24
Glycogen, 154
Golgi Apparatus, 133, 245, 273
Hamlet, 30, 31
Harry Potter, 31
Headings, 18
Helping (Auxiliary), 201
Herd, 190
Heterozygous, 151, 152, 276
High Heat of Vaporization, 177
High Specific Heat, 177
High Surface Tension, 177
Homophones, 191
Homozygous, 151, 249
Horizontal Axis, 73, 74, 81
Hundredths, 40, 44, 183, 265, 266
Hyphen, 195, 255, 281
Hypogastric, 98, 99

Hypothalamus, 109, 110, 116, 118
Ileum, 107
Imperative, 197, 199, 210
Imperative Sentences, 204
Implied, 24, 29, 197
Improper Fraction, 41, 43
In Medias Res, 26
In the First Place, 26
Indefinite Pronouns, 199, 206
Independent, 73, 74, 77, 81, 152, 187, 193, 194, 198, 203, 207, 280, 282, 307, 341, 342
Independent Assortment, 152
Independent Clause, 207
Indirect Objects, 204
Indirect Subjects, 203, 204
Inexpensive, 24
Inferior, 97, 101, 105, 222, 274
Integers, 39, 40, 41, 43, 48
Intensive, 177, 178
Interjection, 203, 210
Interjections, 194, 203
Interrogation, 197
Interrogative, 197, 199
Interrogative Pronouns, 199
Intrinsic Factor, 107
Ion, 123, 164, 169, 170, 181, 182, 272, 277
Ionic Bond, 169, 170, 248, 275
Ionization Energy, 164, 166, 169
Irregular Plurals, 191
Jargon, 26, 258
Jejunum, 107
Lastly, 34, 40, 60, 150, 166, 183, 265, 276
Lateral, 96, 97, 246, 274
Layout, 18
LCM, 41
Left Hypochondriac, 98, 99
Left Inguinal, 98, 99
Left Lower Quadrant (LLQ), 99
Left Lumbar, 98, 99
Left Upper Quadrant (LUQ), 99
Line Graph, 19, 73, 74, 77, 78
Line Plot, 75
Lumen, 106, 132
Lymph, 127, 128
Lymph Nodes, 127
Lymphatic System, 127
Lysosomes, 131, 133, 273
Main, 15, 16, 31, 32, 90, 119, 123, 131, 133, 193, 196, 200, 201, 203, 210, 212, 213, 227, 233, 264, 295, 299, 312, 323, 327, 337, 340, 342
Main Idea, 15, 16, 31, 32, 213
Mathematically, 65
Mean, 23, 74, 78, 79, 80, 81, 210, 241, 262, 267, 271, 295
Medial, 97, 246, 274
Median, 78, 79, 80, 81, 239, 241, 271
Melting, 168, 169, 170, 178
Merriam-Webster's, 24
Message, 30, 31, 102
Metathesis Reaction, 170
Misspelled, 191, 192, 282, 321, 343
Mitochondria, 100, 131, 133, 150, 245, 273
Mixed Number, 41, 43, 56
Mode, 78, 79, 80, 241, 271, 274
Muscle, 102, 105, 112, 113, 115, 116, 133, 154, 163, 246, 273, 274, 276, 310, 314, 336
Muscular System, 112, 130
Narrative, 26, 30, 31, 72, 223, 261
National Geographic, 28, 287, 324
Natural, 125, 126, 127, 151, 182, 186, 213, 226, 232, 262, 264, 300, 307, 319, 336, 337
Nervous, 102, 107, 109, 111, 113, 117, 118, 130, 133, 186, 200, 251, 253, 255, 278, 279, 281, 309
Neutrons, 162, 163, 166, 277
No, 285
Nucleolus, 132, 133
Nucleosome, 132
Nucleus, 113, 115, 131, 132, 133, 149, 150, 162, 164, 166, 250, 277
Ocular, 98
Odd Numbers, 39
Ones, 24, 44, 47, 49, 50, 117, 183, 184, 222, 227, 292, 323, 324
Opinion, 22, 24, 32, 223, 227, 284, 325
Organ Systems, 99
Organs, 96, 99, 103, 105, 111, 115, 123, 126, 127, 130, 131, 200, 279
Origin, 74, 200
Oropharynx, 127
Osmotic Potential, 147
Outliers, 78, 79, 80, 81, 241, 271
Outline, 15, 213, 214, 286
Palmar, 98
Pancreas, 105, 106, 107, 119
Paragraph, 15, 72, 211, 212, 262, 297, 325, 326, 341, 342
Parathyroid Glands, 119
Parentheses, 46, 49, 57, 195, 196
Participles, 202
Particles, 117, 126, 132, 166, 167, 168, 185, 201

Passive Immunity, 126
Past, 19, 166, 168, 182, 202, 216, 217, 235, 295
Past Participle, 202
Pedal, 98
Pelvic, 96, 98
Pelvic Cavity, 96
Perimeter, 83, 84, 85, 87, 239, 243, 244
Peristalsis, 105
Personal Pronouns, 199, 210
Persuasive, 16, 26, 223, 261
PH, 102, 106, 123, 163, 176, 177, 181, 182, 246, 248, 272, 274, 275, 310, 336
Phrase, 204
Physiology, 96, 339
Picture Graph, 75
Pie, 294
Pie Chart, 294
Pie Charts, 294
Pineal Gland, 119
Pituitary Gland, 96, 118
Places, 18, 30, 45, 48, 49, 51, 52, 54, 60, 199, 281, 332, 333
Plantar, 98
Points, 15, 16, 18, 71, 73, 74, 76, 78, 79, 80, 81, 86, 169, 170, 178, 212, 213, 235, 261, 323
Polar, 132, 154, 177
Possessive Nouns, 201
Possessive Pronouns, 199, 200, 201
Posterior, 96, 97, 118, 119, 246, 274
Predicate Adjective, 204
Predicate Nominative, 204
Predicates, 204
Prefix, 90, 91, 191, 201, 215, 216, 255, 281, 317
Prepositional Phrases, 202, 204
Prepositions, 202, 282
Pronoun, 199, 200, 201, 202, 211, 257, 280, 281, 282
Pronoun Reference, 200, 211
Pronoun-Antecedent Agreement, 200
Proper Fraction, 41, 43
Proper Name, 199
Proper Noun, 192, 199
Proteins, 103, 105, 106, 107, 123, 125, 126, 131, 132, 133, 149, 150, 152, 154, 170, 176, 181, 248, 249, 250, 273, 275, 276, 277
Protons, 162, 163, 164, 166, 169, 177, 250, 277
Proximal, 97, 123
Pubic, 98
Publisher, 28, 214
Pyloric Sphincter, 106
Quotation Marks, 18
Rate of Change, 70, 78
Rational Numbers, 40, 59, 60
Ratios, 20, 41, 42, 66, 68, 331
Real Numbers, 40, 305
Reciprocal Pronouns, 199
References, 28, 164, 211, 274, 291
Reflex Arc, 111, 245, 273
Relationship, 62, 66, 68, 77, 81, 191, 211, 222, 242, 246, 250, 255, 293, 334, 341
Relative Pronouns, 199
Repeating, 40, 153, 154, 163, 190
Revenue, 63
Ribosomes, 132, 133, 149, 150
Right Hypochondriac, 98
Right Inguinal, 98
Right Lower Quadrant (RLQ), 98
Right Lumbar, 98
Right Upper Quadrant (RUQ), 98
Rough Endoplasmic Reticulum, 133
Rounding, 65, 66, 85, 183, 301, 304
Scale Factor, 62, 66, 68
Scientific Notation, 55, 183, 307
Second, 24, 26, 50, 52, 55, 56, 57, 58, 64, 66, 68, 71, 78, 150, 152, 183, 185, 190, 194, 195, 196, 198, 199, 210, 225, 250, 255, 281, 284, 292, 295, 300, 305, 306, 325, 331, 340, 342
Second Person, 26, 199, 210, 255, 281, 306
Second-Person Point of View, 210
Secretory Vesicles, 133
See Above, 195
Segregation, 152
Self-Ionizable, 177
Semicolon, 194, 203, 342
Semi-Engineer, 195
Sentence, 15, 23, 192, 193, 194, 195, 196, 197, 198, 200, 201, 202, 203, 204, 205, 207, 211, 212, 213, 215, 220, 221, 253, 256, 257, 258, 279, 280, 281, 282, 315, 316, 317, 340, 341, 342
Sequence, 21, 26, 104, 131, 149, 150, 207, 235, 246, 312, 334, 337
Significant, 31, 125, 167, 183, 184, 287, 307, 315, 333
Simple Sentence, 198, 213
Simple Subjects, 203
Simplified, 42, 43, 85, 86, 270
Single Theme, 211
SIRS, 34
Skeletal Muscles, 111, 112, 113
Slang, 210, 258
Slice, 76
Smooth Endoplasmic Reticulum, 133

Smooth Muscles, 113, 116
Solute Potential, 147
Sounds, 102, 197, 258
Spinal Cavity, 96
Spread, 65, 79, 81, 226, 260, 279
Square Root Symbol, 56
Starch, 154
State of Being, 196, 201
Stomach, 127
Subject, 15, 24, 31, 32, 196, 197, 198, 200, 203, 204, 205, 206, 207, 210, 221, 261, 280, 282, 291, 315, 325, 340
Subjects, 203, 207
Sublimation, 168
Subordinate, 193, 203, 284
Subordinating Conjunctions, 203
Substitution Reaction, 170
Superficial, 97, 98, 246, 274
Superior, 31, 97, 101, 105, 210, 274
Supporting Details, 15, 16, 28, 31
Surface Area, 83, 101, 246, 273
Synapses, 108
Synonyms, 23, 211
Tally Chart, 75
Technical, 17, 26, 197, 220, 223, 261
Tenths, 40, 44, 265, 266
Terminating, 100
Testes and Ovaries, 119
Textual Evidence, 32
The National Enquirer, 28
the Scarlet Letter, 30
Theme, 29, 30, 31, 211, 233
Third, 24, 31, 44, 52, 55, 57, 58, 64, 155, 199, 210, 211, 297, 306, 335
Third Person, 31, 199, 210, 306
Third-Person Limited, 31, 210
Third-Person Objective, 211
Third-Person Omniscient, 211
Third-Person Point of View, 210
Thoracic, 96, 98
Thousandths, 40, 44, 265
Thymus Gland, 118
Thyroid Gland, 119
Tissues, 99, 103, 105, 117, 125, 130, 339
Title, 18, 19, 72, 73, 192, 214, 326
To Kill a Mockingbird, 192
Topic, 15, 16, 18, 26, 27, 28, 34, 195, 211, 212, 213, 214, 230, 232, 290, 325, 326
Topic Sentence, 211, 212
Transcription, 149, 150, 157
Translation, 149, 150, 157, 255, 281
Two-Year College, 20
Type, 23, 26, 33, 35, 39, 56, 63, 64, 68, 77, 103, 115, 126, 130, 134, 151, 155, 170, 171, 182, 186, 197, 210, 248, 251, 253, 258, 274, 276, 279, 293, 317, 334, 338
Types, 15, 23, 26, 30, 35, 59, 63, 64, 72, 73, 103, 105, 107, 111, 112, 115, 118, 125, 127, 130, 149, 154, 155, 166, 169, 170, 177, 181, 194, 197, 199, 203, 212, 222, 308, 310, 335, 336
Umbilical, 98, 99
Unemployed, 20
Unified, 211, 342
Unimodal, 80
Unit Rates, 68
Universal Lesson, 30
Vacuoles, 134
Vaporization, 166, 168, 177, 277
Ventral, 97
Verb, 24, 196, 198, 199, 200, 201, 202, 203, 204, 205, 206, 207, 211, 216, 217, 254, 258, 279, 280, 282, 315, 316, 340
Vertical Axis, 73, 74, 81
Vocational School, 20
Waste, 100, 102, 107, 116, 117, 123, 125, 133, 134, 272, 276
Whole, 285
Whole Numbers, 39, 41, 51, 52, 56, 59
Wikipedia, 34
Workforce, 20
X-Axis, 73, 74, 77, 81
X-Y Diagram, 81
Y-Axis, 73, 74, 77, 81

Dear ATI TEAS Test Taker,

Thank you for purchasing this practice test book for your ATI TEAS exam. We hope that we exceeded your expectations.

We strive to make our practice questions as similar as possible to what you will encounter on test day. With that being said, if you found something that you feel was not up to your standards, please send us an email and let us know.

We would also like to let you know about other books in our catalog that may interest you.

TEAS 7 Flashcards

This can be found on Amazon: amazon.com/dp/1628453109

HESI

This can be found on Amazon: amazon.com/dp/1637751931

We have study guides in a wide variety of fields. If the one you are looking for isn't listed above, then try searching for it on Amazon or send us an email.

Thanks Again and Happy Testing!
Product Development Team
support@testprepbooks.com

Online Resources & Audiobook

Included with your purchase are multiple online resources. This includes the practice tests in an interactive format and this book in audiobook format. There is also a convenient study timer to help you manage your time.

Scan the QR code or go to this link to access this content:

testprepbooks.com/online387/teas

SCAN ME

The first time you access the page, you will need to register as a "new user" and verify your email address.

If you have any issues, please email support@testprepbooks.com.

Thank you for letting us be a part of your studying journey!

Made in the USA
Monee, IL
16 September 2026

63182435R10207